Ultimate
Nutrition
for Health

*Your complete guide to health,
diet, nutrition & natural foods*

MANFRED URS KOCH

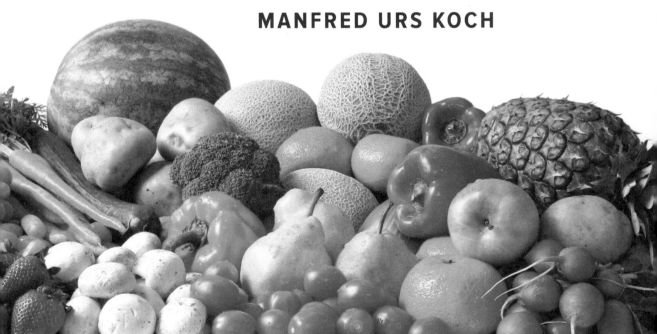

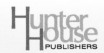

PUBLISHERS

Hunter House Inc., Publishers
PO Box 2914
Alameda CA 94501-0914

Library of Congress Cataloging-in-Publication Data

Koch, Manfred Urs.
[Laugh with health]
Ultimate nutrition for health : your complete guide to health, diet,
nutrition, and natural foods / Manfred Urs Koch.
          pages cm
Previously published as: Laugh with health, 1984.
Includes bibliographical references and index.
    ISBN 978-0-89793-681-1 (pbk.) —
    ISBN 978-0-89793-690-3 (ebook)
    1. Nutrition. 2. Natural foods. I. Title.
TX353.K7 2013
641.3'02 — dc23   2013012240

Project Credits
Designed by Tracey Gibbs
Illustrations by Manfred Urs Koch
Photographs courtesy of Shutterstock
2014 Edition Editor: Kelley Blewster

Printed and bound by Bang Printing, Brainerd, Minnesota
Manufactured in the United States of America

9 8 7 6 5 4 3 2 1   First Edition   14 15 16 17 18

PREFACE

Manfred Urs Koch first published this book in Australia in 1981, under the title *Laugh with Health*.

Initially, he devoted four years of intense research into nutrition to understand the subject and to develop the basic outline of the book. During the winter months, he traveled north to the warmer parts of Australia and spent many days at a time in remote areas, using his fully restored Holden car as a mobile office.

The first edition was hand-folded by volunteers from Metung, a yachting village in Victoria. Local people came to the "wood cottage" for two weeks, and finally the 234,000 folded sheets were taken to Melbourne for binding. From the first edition of 1,000 books, 500 were given away to friends, shops, and the numerous helpers. One year later, bookshops asked for more copies and the second printing took place. In 1983 the book was published in the USA and the UK. It has been self-published fourteen printings by the author and for six printings by other Australian publishers.

Manfred has also self-published two other books: *The Health Index,* in 1983, and *Natural to Juice,* in 2000.

This book is a bestseller throughout health shops in Australia and is used as a reference book for school students and for naturopaths. It is endorsed by many in the medical profession as well as by naturopaths.

A total of 140,000 copies of this book have been sold worldwide. It has progressed into a complete guide to health, diet, nutrition, and natural foods.

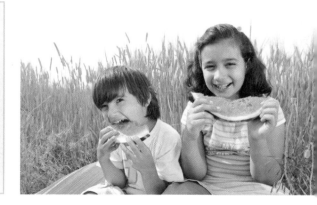

TABLE OF CONTENTS

NUTRITION INTRODUCTION

WHAT IS HEALTH?

Health is defined as soundness of body and mind.

WHAT MAIN FACTORS PROMOTE GOOD HEALTH?

1. regular physical activity
2. a regular and balanced diet of nutritious foods
3. regular intake of water
4. a variety of foods from the five main food groups

HOW DO I OBTAIN A BALANCED DIET?

Enjoy a variety of foods from the five main food groups.

WHAT ARE THE FIVE MAIN FOOD GROUPS?

1. grains group
2. vegetable group
3. fruit group
4. milk, yogurt, and cheese group
5. meat, poultry, fish, dry beans, eggs, and nuts group

WHAT IS NUTRITION?

Nutrition is the supply of the essential nutrients from foods.

WHAT FOODS SUPPLY THE ESSENTIAL NUTRIENTS?

A variety of foods from the five main food groups will supply all the essential nutrients.

WHAT ARE THE ESSENTIAL NUTRIENT GROUPS?

1. carbohydrates
2. proteins
3. fats and oils
4. minerals
5. vitamins
6. water

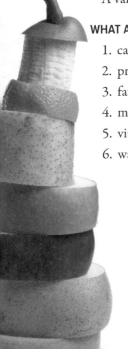

HOW DO I OBTAIN A NUTRITIOUS DIET?

1. Eat plenty of vegetables, legumes, and fruits.
2. Eat plenty of grains including breads, rice, pasta, and noodles, preferably whole grain.
3. Include lean meats, fish, poultry, and/or alternatives.
4. Include milk, yogurt, cheeses, and/or alternatives.
5. Drink plenty of water.

WHAT OTHER FACTORS ARE IMPORTANT?

1. Limit intake of saturated fat and moderate total fat intake.
2. Choose foods low in salt.
3. Consume only moderate amounts of sugars and foods containing added sugar.
4. Prevent weight gain: be physically active and eat according to your energy needs.
5. Prepare and store food safely.

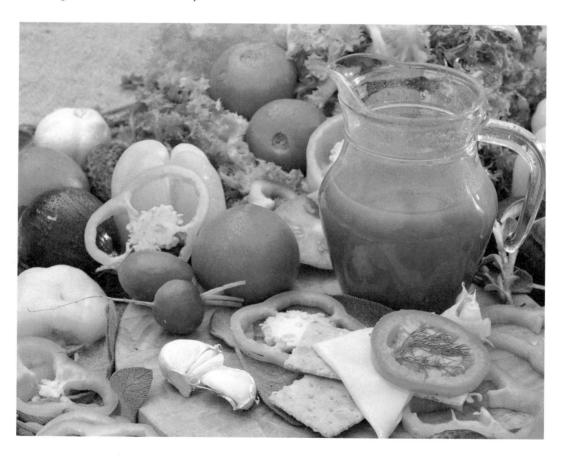

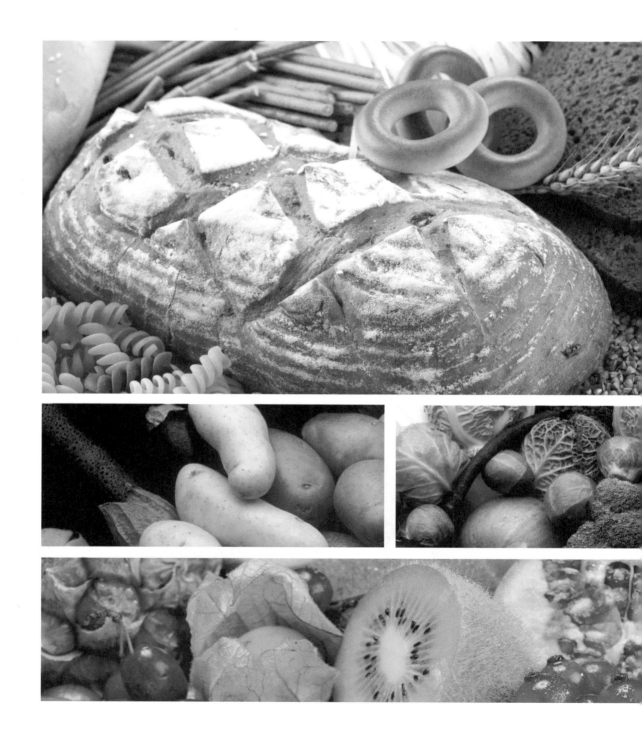

WHAT FOODS ARE IN THE MAIN FOOD GROUPS?

GROUP 1 – GRAINS
Whole grains:

   Barley: barley bread, barley soup.

   Corn: cornmeal, sweet corn, whole-grain corn bread.

   Millet: whole millet bread, millet cookies.

   Oats: rolled oats, oat bread, oatmeal cookies, muesli.

   Rice: brown rice, wild rice.

   Rye: rye bread, pumpernickel.

   Wheat: whole-wheat flour, whole-grain bread, bulgur, whole-wheat pasta, whole-grain bakery products, whole-grain cereals.

Refined grains:

   Corn tortillas, corn flakes, white rice, rice crackers, white bread, rolls, pizza crust, pasta, biscuits, crackers, pretzels, pita bread, couscous, breakfast cereals.

GROUP 2 – VEGETABLES

   Artichoke, asparagus, beets, bok choy, broccoli, Brussels sprouts, cabbage, carrots, cauliflower, celery, cucumbers, eggplant, leeks, lettuce, mushrooms, onions, parsnips, peppers, potatoes, pumpkin, radishes, spinach and other leafy greens, sweet potatoes, taro, turnips, zucchini.

GROUP 3 – FRUITS

   Apples, apricots, avocadoes, bananas, blueberries, cantaloupe, cherries, currants, dates, figs, grapefruit, grapes, guava, kiwi, lemons, limes, mango, melons, olives, oranges, papaya, peaches, pears, pineapple, plums, strawberries, tangerines, tomatoes, watermelon.

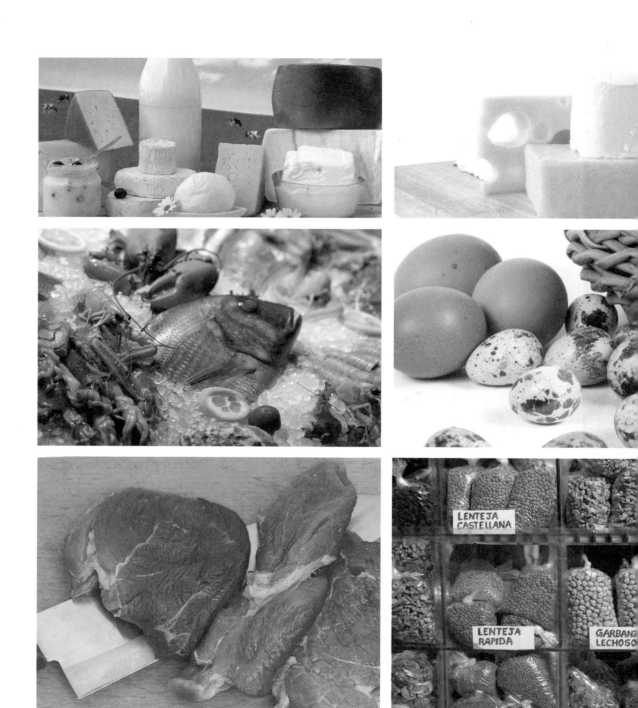

WHAT OTHER FOODS ARE IN THE MAIN FOOD GROUPS?

GROUP 4 – MILK, YOGURT, AND CHEESE

Milk: whole milk, reduced-fat milk, fat-free milk, low-fat milk, lactose-free milk, lactose-reduced milk, soy milk.

Yogurt: whole-milk yogurt, fat-free, low-fat, reduced-fat yogurt.

Cheese: American, cheddar, cottage, cream, edam, emmenthal, feta, gruyère, mozzarella, parmesan, ricotta, Swiss, jarlsburg.

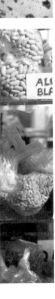

GROUP 5 – MEAT, POULTRY, FISH, SEAFOOD, EGGS

Meats: <u>Beef</u>: fillet, roasts, steak, ground, sausages, ribs, stew meat. <u>Veal</u>: cutlets, shank, chops. <u>Pork</u>: sausage, ham, leg roast, loin, spare ribs. <u>Lamb</u>: chops, sausages, cutlets, fillets, rack, roast.

Game: bison, pheasant, quail, rabbit, venison, elk.

Poultry: chicken, duck, goose, turkey.

Fish: bass, catfish, cod, flounder, haddock, halibut, herring, mackerel, perch, pollock, salmon, sardines, sea bass, snapper, swordfish, trout, tuna.

Shellfish and Seafood: clams, crab, crayfish, lobster, mussels, octopus. prawns, squid.

Eggs: free-range, factory-cage, home-raised.

GROUP 5 – NON-ANIMAL-BASED PROTEIN ALTERNATIVES

Dried Beans and Peas: black beans, black-eyed peas, chickpeas, falafel, kidney beans, lentils, lima beans, navy beans, pinto beans, soybeans, split peas, tofu, white beans, tempeh.

Nuts: almonds, Brazil, cashew, chestnuts, hazelnuts, hickory, macadamia, pecan, pine, pistachio, walnuts.

Seeds: pumpkin (pepitas), sesame, sunflower.

MYPLATE GUIDELINES

MyPlate is the U.S. government's initiative to remind Americans to eat healthfully. You may remember the food guide pyramid. It was replaced with MyPlate in 2011 (see the illustration on the opposite page).

Here are the main points of the MyPlate program. These come from the website ChooseMyPlate.gov, where you can find a complete discussion of the recommendations. I've added some comments of my own, which appear in parentheses and which are meant to highlight the primary message of this book: Rely on natural foods in their most simple and nutritious forms by utilizing delicious recipes and proper food combinations that are well balanced throughout a day, a week, and a lifetime.

BALANCING CALORIES

- Enjoy your food, but eat less. (Enjoy natural foods, and be naturally satisfied.)
- Avoid oversized portions. (Eat naturally, and fill your plate and appetite properly.)

FOODS TO INCREASE

- Make half your plate fruits and vegetables. (Consume fruits for fitness, vegetables for strength.)
- Make at least half your grains whole grains. (Enjoy whole grains for clever brains.)
- Switch to fat-free or low-fat (1%) milk. (But children should drink whole milk.)

FOODS TO REDUCE

- Compare sodium in foods like soup, bread, and frozen meals—and choose foods with lower numbers.
- Eat fewer foods that are high in solid fats. (Eat more nuts and seeds.)
- Drink water instead of sugary drinks. (If you want a sweet taste, remember that freshly squeezed juices are the sweetest.)

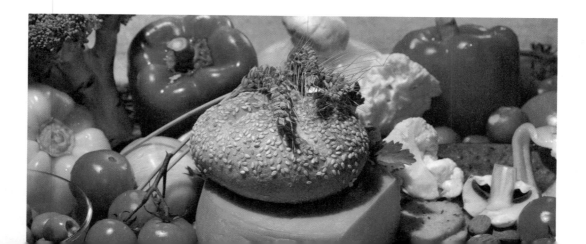

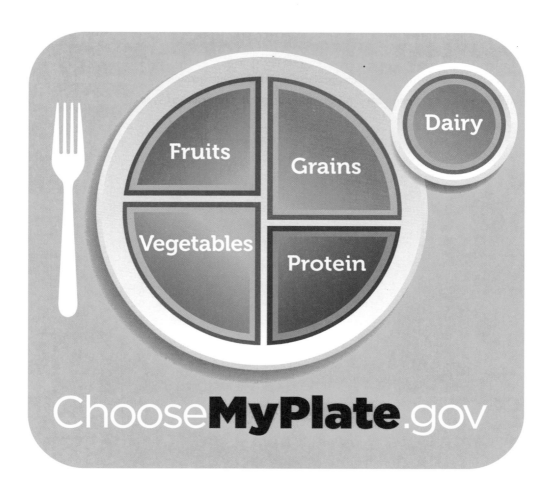

This illustration appears on and the information on the previous page is adapted from the USDA Center for Nutrition Policy and Promotion's ChooseMyPlate.gov website.

RECOMMENDED NUMBER OF SERVINGS

The U.S. government recommendations (MyPlate) don't list specific numbers of servings you should eat each day from the different food groups. You may find this information helpful, so I've included some guidelines from other experts. The chart below shows the recommended number of servings per day from each of the five main food groups. A variation in the number of servings allows for different daily levels of physical activity and differences in body mass. Serving sizes are described on page 13. In addition, the group of extras includes a large number of foods that are usually cooked or processed, or that include added fats, oils, or sugar. These foods are not recommended for daily intake and are best consumed only occasionally.

Food Groups	Children			Women				Men	
	Ages 4–8	Ages 8–11	Ages 12–18	Ages 19–60	Age 60+	Pregnant	Lactating	Ages 19–60	Age 60+
Servings									
Cereals, bread, rice, pasta, noodles	5–7	6–9	5–11	4–9	4–7	4–6	5–7	6–12	4–9
Vegetables, legumes	2	3	4	5	5	5–6	7	5	5
Fruit	1	1	3	2	2	4	5	2	2
Milk, yogurt, cheese	2	2	3	2	2	2	2	2	2
Lean meat, fish, poultry, eggs, nuts, legumes	½	1	1	1	1	1½	2	1	1
Extra foods: processed or with added fats or sugar (have no more than)	1–2	1–2	1–3	0–2½	0–2	0–2½	0–2½	0–3	0–2½

RECOMMENDED SERVING SIZES

Specific serving sizes aren't included in the MyPlate guidelines, but I've included that information here, based on the recommendations of many governmental and nongovernmental expert sources.

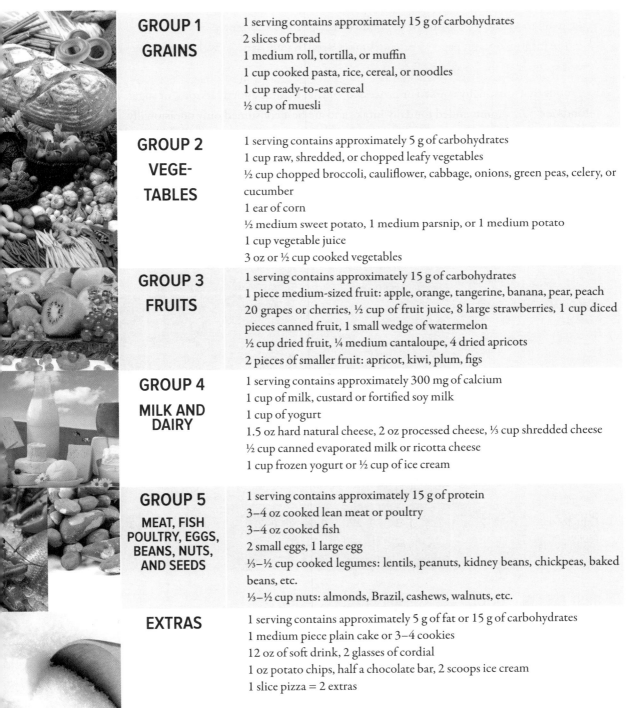

GROUP 1
GRAINS

1 serving contains approximately 15 g of carbohydrates
2 slices of bread
1 medium roll, tortilla, or muffin
1 cup cooked pasta, rice, cereal, or noodles
1 cup ready-to-eat cereal
½ cup of muesli

GROUP 2
VEGE-TABLES

1 serving contains approximately 5 g of carbohydrates
1 cup raw, shredded, or chopped leafy vegetables
½ cup chopped broccoli, cauliflower, cabbage, onions, green peas, celery, or cucumber
1 ear of corn
½ medium sweet potato, 1 medium parsnip, or 1 medium potato
1 cup vegetable juice
3 oz or ½ cup cooked vegetables

GROUP 3
FRUITS

1 serving contains approximately 15 g of carbohydrates
1 piece medium-sized fruit: apple, orange, tangerine, banana, pear, peach
20 grapes or cherries, ½ cup of fruit juice, 8 large strawberries, 1 cup diced pieces canned fruit, 1 small wedge of watermelon
½ cup dried fruit, ¼ medium cantaloupe, 4 dried apricots
2 pieces of smaller fruit: apricot, kiwi, plum, figs

GROUP 4
MILK AND DAIRY

1 serving contains approximately 300 mg of calcium
1 cup of milk, custard or fortified soy milk
1 cup of yogurt
1.5 oz hard natural cheese, 2 oz processed cheese, ⅓ cup shredded cheese
½ cup canned evaporated milk or ricotta cheese
1 cup frozen yogurt or ½ cup of ice cream

GROUP 5
MEAT, FISH POULTRY, EGGS, BEANS, NUTS, AND SEEDS

1 serving contains approximately 15 g of protein
3–4 oz cooked lean meat or poultry
3–4 oz cooked fish
2 small eggs, 1 large egg
⅓–½ cup cooked legumes: lentils, peanuts, kidney beans, chickpeas, baked beans, etc.
⅓–½ cup nuts: almonds, Brazil, cashews, walnuts, etc.

EXTRAS

1 serving contains approximately 5 g of fat or 15 g of carbohydrates
1 medium piece plain cake or 3–4 cookies
12 oz of soft drink, 2 glasses of cordial
1 oz potato chips, half a chocolate bar, 2 scoops ice cream
1 slice pizza = 2 extras

WHAT NUTRIENTS DO THE MAIN FOOD GROUPS SUPPLY?

The table on this page shows the main food groups together with a color-coded guide to their supply of the primary nutrient groups. It is obvious from the table that a variety of foods from the main food groups is required to obtain all the primary nutrients.

The information on page 15 provides more detail on nutrients as well as references to relevant sections of the book.

Main Food Groups	Carbo-hydrates	Protein	Fats & Oils	Minerals	Vitamins	Water
Group 1 Breads & Cereals	Whole grains	Whole grains	Whole grains	Whole grains	Whole grains	POOR except sweet corn
Group 2 Vegetables	Potato, pumpkin, winter squash, most vegetables	FAIR especially potato	POOR	All vegetables	All vegetables	All vegetables especially celery, lettuce, carrots
Group 3 Fruits	Dates, bananas, figs, apples, avocado	POOR except dates	POOR except avocado, olives	All fruits	All fruits	All fruits especially melons
Group 4 Milk & Milk Products	POOR	Cheese, milk, yogurt	Cheese, butter	Cheese, yogurt; milk is a FAIR source	Cheese, yogurt	Milk
Group 5 Meats	POOR	Fish, beef, chicken	Fish	Fish, beef, chicken	Fish, beef, chicken	POOR
Group 5 Protein Alternatives	Legumes	Seeds, nuts, legumes, eggs	Seeds, nuts	Seeds, nuts, eggs, legumes	Seeds, nuts, eggs, legumes	Fresh beans, peas, sprouts

BEST GOOD FAIR POOR

WHAT OTHER NUTRIENTS DO THE MAIN FOOD GROUPS SUPPLY?

All whole grains are very good suppliers of carbohydrates: Wheat is approximately 70% carbohydrate content, oats are approximately 66%. Whole grains supply a good amount of protein, approximately 12% for wheat. Whole grains supply good amounts of minerals and are a fair source of vitamins. Refined grains and cereals are a poor source of the essential nutrients, except for carbohydrates.

Starchy vegetables supply approximately 14% carbohydrate content. Leafy and salad vegetables supply approximately 3%, and brassica vegetables supply approximately 5% carbohydrate content. Most vegetables are a very good source of minerals and vitamins. (Refer to pages 156–160 and 175–176.) The potato supplies approximately 17% carbohydrate content and 3% protein content.

Fresh fruits supply approximately 12% carbohydrate content. Dried fruits supply approximately 65% carbohydrate content. Dates supply a small amount of complete protein. Olive oil and avocado are a very good source of fats and oils. All fruits are very good suppliers of numerous minerals and vitamins. (Refer to pages 156–160 and 175–176.) Most fruits, especially melons, are an excellent source of water.

Milk and dairy products are a poor source of carbohydrates. Cheese, milk, and yogurt are good suppliers of protein: Cheddar cheese is 25% protein. Butter and cheese are rich sources of saturated fats. Cheese and yogurt are excellent sources of the mineral calcium. (Refer to pages 114–120 for more details on the nutrient content of milk and dairy foods.)

Meat, chicken, eggs, and fish contain no carbohydrate content. They are all very good sources of protein: Chicken is approximately 21% protein, beef 24%, and fish 22%, with tuna at 28%. (Refer to pages 122–130.) Fish, especially oily fish, are an excellent source of the essential oil omega-3 (refer to page 124). Meat, chicken, and fish supply only a few of the essential minerals and vitamins (refer to pages 156–160 and 175–176). Cooked meats may supply excess saturated fats.

Legumes are very good suppliers of carbohydrates—approximately 12–20%—and fiber. Seeds, nuts, and eggs are a very good source of protein (refer to pages 92–94). Legumes supply approximately 20–26% protein (refer to pages 92–94). Seeds and nuts are very good source of the essential oils omega-3 and omega-6 (refer to pages 134–135). Seeds, nuts, and legumes are very good sources of most minerals and some vitamins. (Refer to pages 156–160 and 175–176.)

WHAT IS A CARBOHYDRATE?

An energy-producing organic compound of carbon, oxygen, and hydrogen.

HOW ARE CARBOHYDRATES MADE?

Carbohydrates are mainly produced by plants.

WHAT ARE THE MAIN TYPES OF CARBOHYDRATES?

Sugars and starches.

HOW DOES THE BODY USE CARBOHYDRATES?

Carbohydrates are converted into glucose, which is used by the brain and muscles for energy. Take a look at the figure below:

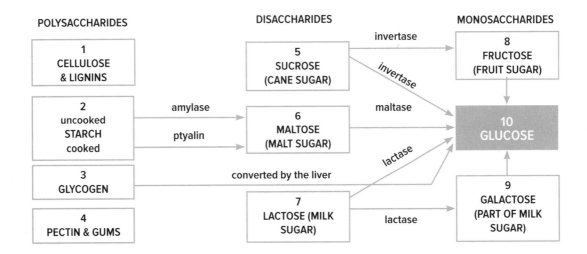

1. Cellulose and lignins are both insoluble fibers. They protect against digestive problems.
2. There are two types of starch:
   Amylose: takes longer to convert to glucose; it has a lower GI.
   Amylopectin: converts quickly into glucose; it has a high GI.
3. Glycogen is stored in the liver and muscles and converted into glucose when the body requires extra energy.
4. Pectin and gums are water-soluble fibers. They bind cholesterol and prevent its absorption.
5. Sucrose: from sugar cane.
6. Maltose: malt from grains.
7. Lactose: milk sugar; it is hard to convert for many people, due to a lack of the enzyme lactase.
8. Fructose: a simple sugar from fruits; it is easy to convert.
9. Galactose: part of milk sugar.
10. Glucose: the primary energy fuel for the brain and muscles.

Grains have been used for thousands of years as a main provider of food, energy, and nourishment. The discovery of grains as a source of food by primitive people enabled them to settle in one place and rely on a food supply from the "crop that did not wander." People shared the task of crop cultivation until such time when machinery took over.

Nowadays, some people rarely eat whole grains. Processed and refined foods have flooded the food aisles, and as they are great profit-making foods, advertising of them is both competitive and compelling. Breakfast cereals can make giants out of dwarfs, cookies can become mother's best helper, and white bread can be so spongy that the more you eat, the more flexible and active you become—well, that's advertising!

Grains are a compact carbohydrate food, an energy source. For many people, their regular diet will include only one main grain, usually wheat, often in the form of sandwiches. Rice is also a common addition to the diet; however, the other grains rarely get a chance to contribute their nutritional benefits and unique taste.

The routine of modern-day living can have a detrimental effect on health. Time goes so quickly in the morning before work or school that some people compensate by relying on the quickest and most convenient packaged breakfast foods.

Be prepared for breakfast and give whole grains a chance to start your day well. You need energy to get through a busy day, and breakfast is the ideal time to obtain the stamina of whole grains. Grains supply long-lasting energy, and apart from being an excellent source of carbohydrates, they also supply a fair percentage of primary protein.

At least two meals a day should be based around whole grains. There are many forms of whole grain, some of which are seldom included or even thought of as a substitute for commercially prepared and refined breakfast cereals. A rolled grain is a whole grain, with all the essential nutrients in proper balance.

The following pages provide a detailed nutritional survey of the main whole grains: barley, corn, millet, oats, rice, rye, and wheat, listing the best attributes of each whole grain and its products, with negative factors also mentioned. The glycemic index (GI) of each grain is also listed. GI refers to how quickly a carbohydrate affects your blood sugar. Some nutrition experts recommend avoiding foods with a high GI. Foods ranked by the GI are given scores:

High: 70+

Medium: 56-69

Low: 55 and under

Generally speaking, whole grains are absorbed more slowly by the body; hence, they usually have a lower GI.

The boxes labeled "C.P.L." indicate the percentages of calories that come from carbohydrate, protein, and lipids.

The balanced diet requires approximately 50% carbohydrates. Whole grains provide approximately 70–80% carbohydrate content, 10% protein, and a low fat content of 5%. Therefore, such foods as milk, cheese, butter, cream, and oil can be added to grains, moderately, without problems.

Most grains need added fats to make them appetizing, such as the basic bread and cheese combination. In addition, fats lower the glycemic index, providing a slower conversion of the starch content into glucose.

Refined grains lack valuable fiber and nutrients; plus they increase blood sugar levels quickly, as they are mainly starch. Refer to the figure on page 16.

Whole grains are the ideal energy food, providing stamina and a great supply of life-supporting nutrients. Page 30 provides a guide to the daily intake of grains as part of a balanced diet.

Serve up the full benefits and flavor of whole grains today!

NOTE: Nutrient amounts are listed as milligrams (mg) per 100 grams (g), unless otherwise stated.

BARLEY – *Hordeum vulgare*

Barley made its name in history long before wheat and rye, as it was used by the Egyptians over 8,000 years ago. Barley grain was used for the daily bread of Greek, Roman, Chinese, and Hebrew civilizations from 4,000 BC onward, and it was also traded as payment for a day's work.

Today, barley is mainly used for the brewing of beer, vinegar, and whiskey. The true value of barley's unique nutritional qualities and flavor is untapped.

The best way to obtain barley in the diet is from barley grass juice. This is very similar to wheatgrass juice in its healing power (see page 112).

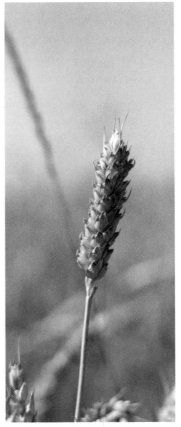

Barley sprouts have helped in the discovery of nations: Captain Cook recognized that sprouted grains protected his hard-working men from illness, especially scurvy. Barley sprouts make an excellent addition to bread, casseroles, and soups.

Barley flakes, or rolled barley, are ideal for hot cereal and, when blended, for vegetarian pâté. Barley provides a unique body-warming effect; it was "fast food" for athletes and gladiators during the Roman empire.

Barley has the ability to decrease the risk of colon cancer, as the barley fiber promotes the growth of "friendly" bacteria in the colon. Beneficial fatty acids, termed butyric acids, are formed, which promote colon health by stimulating cells. These beneficial bacteria also retard the action of harmful bacteria. In addition, barley offers a good supply of the mineral selenium, known to protect against colon cancer.

Barley fiber is a good source of beta glucan, which helps eliminate bile acids, chemicals produced by the liver and stored in the gallbladder to process fats. The removal of bile actually lowers blood cholesterol, as the liver will utilize stored cholesterol in the manufacture of more bile acids. Barley provides approximately 60% of recommended daily dietary fiber intake from 1 cup of cooked rolled barley, and nearly 20% of daily protein when combined with milk. Rolled barley is best presoaked in water overnight and cooked for breakfast with milk added. If you have to add a dash of sugar, don't worry, as the barley fiber slows the rise in blood sugar levels. However, barley is rich in maltose, or malt sugar, providing good natural sweetness.

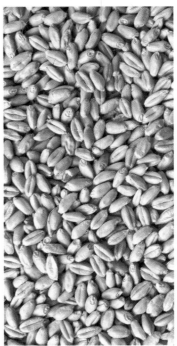

The supply of organic copper from barley is ideal for the health of the joint system, the blood vessels, and the skeletal system. A 1-cup serving of barley provides over 25% of one's daily copper requirements.

A rolled-barley breakfast will protect against rheumatoid arthritis, due to its good supply of copper, while the phosphorus content (296 mg) is abundant and beneficial for the brain and nervous system. It also contains magnesium (37 mg).

Barley water has proved beneficial for asthmatics as it contains the substance hordenine, an antispasmodic. It can be made by boiling barley grains for 1 hour, then allowing to cool before drinking the water.

Be brave: Try barley for breakfast, and in winter, place a pot of barley grains on the stove and get the true old-fashioned slow-cooked flavor: Simmer for two hours for soups, add your veggies, spices, and herbs in the last 20 minutes.

Barley brings a bounty of beautiful body benefits!

BARLEY

NOTE: DV amounts listed refer to the daily value for women 25–50 years; refer to DRI tables on pages 95–96 for adult male and child values.

GLYCEMIC INDEX: 56	TOTAL CALORIES PER 100 G: 365	CALORIES FROM		
		CARB: 300 82%	PROTEIN: 26 7%	FAT: 39 11%

CORN/MAIZE

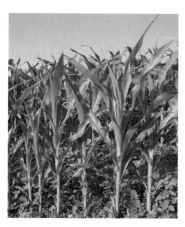

Corn is the "daughter of life" according to the American Indians, and for 10,000 years it was their staple grain. In Mexico it is consumed in the form of tortillas and in North America as hominy. Corn was exported to China, Africa, Japan, and India during the sixteenth century, but it was scorned when compared to wheat and rye for breadmaking.

Corn flour contains no gluten and is low in two essential amino acids: tryptophan and lysine. In addition, the niacin in corn flour is poorly absorbed.

There are five main types of corn: *Dent corn* is used for breadmaking; *flint corn* for animal fodder; *flour corn* is the best quality for breadmaking; *popcorn* is the most popular and least nutritious; and the wonderful *sweet corn* is by far the most nutritious and delicious. Sweet corn, also known as corn on the cob, is full of benefits: The folate content (19 mcg) is a great bonus for children or people who don't like to eat their greens. Folate is vital for healthy growth in children, and it is essential during pregnancy and also for the brain and nervous system.

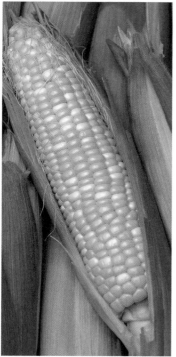

Sweet corn is the best grain source of vitamin A (400 IU), and this combined with its high sulfur content (368 mg) will protect the body against infections, especially when eaten raw or steamed lightly.

The vitamin A in corn is mainly in the form of beta-cryptoxanthin, a carotenoid. One report showed a 37% reduction in the risk of lung cancer in smokers who regularly consumed beta-cryptoxanthin–rich foods.

Sweet corn is a good source of potassium (280 mg). For children with a sweet tooth, a cob of corn for an after-school snack might hit the spot. The magnesium it contains (48 mg) might be just enough to help them concentrate and be creative with their homework, too! Sweet corn is a natural treat with few calories (96) and a low fat content (1 g), so add a dab of butter and get eating. It is available nearly all year round, but it's best and sweetest in summer.

The vitamin C (12 mg) plus the good supply of fiber (0.07 g) both add to the benefits of sweet corn. Unlike flour corn, sweet corn also contains a good supply of vitamin B3 (1.7 mg) and this, combined with its phosphorus and magnesium content, means sweet corn is food for the brain. Vitamin B3 is required for the synthesis of the nerve transmitter acetylcholine, which is required for memory and protection from Alzheimer's disease, senility, and age-related mental deterioration. It's great for the elderly! Fortunately, vitamin B3 is stable to heat, so you can cook up a storm. Even canned corn provides a portion of the benefits.

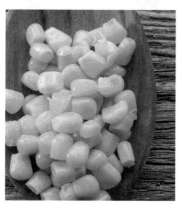

Corn chips and tacos have become popular, and even though they provide mostly a tasty crunch on their own, added ingredients can make them a complete healthy meal. I have noticed children eating lettuce, grated carrot, peppers, kidney beans, and cheese on their tacos, so they're a great way to help children obtain proper nutrition. Fast and simple nachos are also a delight. Crispy tortilla chips can be full of flavor and natural ingredients. Corn bread is also a great option.

Try corn pancakes combined with steamed apples, a sprinkle of chopped almonds, and a spoonful of cream.

NOTE: Nutrient amounts are listed as milligrams (mg) per 100 grams (g), unless otherwise stated.

MILLET – *Pennisetum glaucum*

Millet is, botanically speaking, a mixed bag of grains: finger millet, bullrush millet, common millet, and foxtail millet. The common characteristics are the very small grains on a drought-resistant plant that can be grown in poor soils.

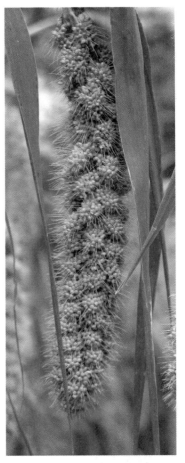

Because half the world's soils are now depleted, millet may become more of a necessity in the future rather than simply enjoying its current status in the developed world as bird food or cattle feed. Millet is cultivated on a large scale in the arid areas of India, Sri Lanka, Zimbabwe, and other parts of Africa. Finger millet in particular can be stored for up to five years, which makes it a great famine reserve food in the dry tropics.

Millet has four times the amount of the essential mineral silicon (160 mg) as wheat. Silicon is required for hair growth, blood circulation, protection from mental fatigue, arthritis, and infection.

Millet provides over twice the iron content (3–6.8 mg) of whole wheat and four times that of rice. Millet contains the same magnesium content (162 mg) as whole wheat, twice that of rice, and seven times that of white bread. Magnesium is known to reduce migraine attacks and the severity of asthma, plus it reduces high blood pressure and is vital for the nervous system, memory, and strong bone development.

Millet will continue to have an expanding role in our future diet due to its being gluten free. For people with wheat allergies, celiac disease, and yeast intolerances, the millet grain can provide a breakfast meal that is low in fat (4.2 g), is high in fiber (8.5 g, or 34% DV), and affords complete protein (11 g), with a great carbohydrate supply (72 g).

The question is, how does it taste? Like any food, if it's prepared properly and you're hungry, it tastes magnificent. Rinse half a cup of millet in a sieve, place half a cup of millet, 1 cup of water, and 1 cup of milk in a saucepan; simmer for 10–15 minutes while stirring. Add extra milk or water when required, as millet requires nearly 5 cups liquid per a 1-cup serving. Add a dash of cinnamon and nutmeg, and serve in a bowl with stewed apples, slivered almonds, and a dribble of sweetened cream—a breakfast that will beat any processed cereal nutritionally. Millet can take the place of rice with vegetable dishes, or add it to muffins. Refer to page 218 for a few simple millet recipes. In India, millet is made into a bread called *roti* and in Africa into *injera*. For a French-style recipe try Normandy millet, or grind millet and add it to a bread mixture.

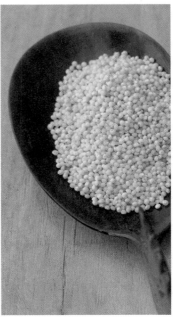

Millet is also a good source of folate (85 mcg—more than cooked broccoli). During pregnancy, the combination of millet's great iron and folate content makes it a sensible food to use regularly, instead of toast. Millet also provides the mineral zinc (1.7 mg), which is required for improved function of the immune system, reproductive system, good skin condition, and general body healing. Millet provides copper (0.7 mg, or 37% DV). That's more than meat, oysters, or bread.

Millet provides an abundance of phosphorus (285 mg, or 47% DV), which is essential for the nervous system, memory, and energy distribution. Millet is the ideal gluten-free grain and therefore a good substitute for wheat and bran. It is also a nonallergenic food. So don't get stuck in a rut with wheat for breakfast, lunch, or evening—the tiny millet grain is ready in a jiffy!

NOTE: DV amounts listed refer to the daily value for women 25–50 years; refer to DRI tables on pages 95–96 for adult male and child values.

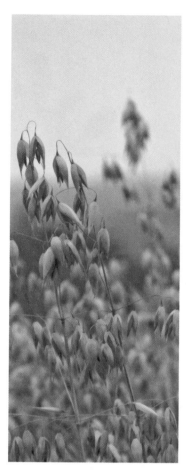

OATS – *Avena sativa*

Oats have a short history compared to other grains. They were first cultivated about 3,000 years ago in Europe. Oats must be prepared quickly after harvesting due to a fat-dissolving enzyme within the grain that causes spoilage. Only 5% of the oats produced are used for human consumption. Thoroughbred horses get the balance, so no wonder they are winners!

Oats are now recognized as a great nutritional food. Scottish people have kept fit and strong for centuries with oats as a staple. Oats are prepared into various forms such as oat groats, which provide the whole-grain benefit. Quick-cooking oats are precooked and finely cut. Oat bran provides numerous health benefits. The old-fashioned rolled oats are basically the whole grain that has been steamed and flattened by rolling. Ideally, use the best quality rolled oats.

Oats for breakfast can balance your daily energy levels. Oats contain a special ingredient in the fiber, known as beta glucan. It helps to slow the rise in blood sugar levels, which is ideal for diabetics. These days, with so many foods loaded with sugar, the use of oats is more a necessity than a choice. For children, giving in to cravings for sugar and soft drinks can eventually trigger the onset of diabetic symptoms: hyperactivity, inability to concentrate, and a miserable attitude, to mention a few.

A bowl of well-prepared porridge for breakfast can really balance the body for an active day. Place 1 cup of quality whole rolled oats in a saucepan with 1 cup of water and 1 cup of milk. Slowly bring to a low simmer, while stirring regularly. Add extra milk to ensure a smooth consistency. Add a splash of cinnamon, a dash of salt, and serve with stewed apples and sweetened cream. For adults, try raw rolled oats, soaked overnight or for at least 10 minutes in goat's milk or "pure milk." Where do you get "pure milk"? You make it. Find a top-quality plain acidophilus yogurt made from raw milk—check the labels, as only a few are made from raw milk. Mix 3 tablespoons of the yogurt in a jar with 1 cup of pure water, stir very well, shake, and pour over the raw rolled oats. Add sliced peaches or canned apricots on top, and serve with a dribble of sweetened cream. Now that's the best balanced breakfast.

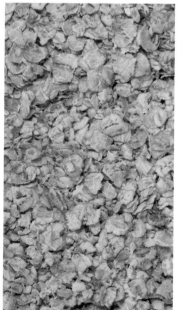

Apart from stabilizing blood sugar levels, the beta glucan in rolled oats can reduce blood cholesterol by 8–23%, according to one study. Oats are the best grain source of complete protein (17 g, or 34% DV), and that's from a small 100-gram serving, not even counting the extra protein value when the milk is added. Just imagine if you added a few ground almonds or sunflower seeds—you'd be obtaining over half your daily protein requirements at breakfast.

Oats are also an excellent source of fiber (10.5 g, or 42% DV). For those concerned about colon cancer, fiber is vital. The rich supply of selenium from oats (35% DV) and oat bran (45 mcg, or 55% DV) has an important role, along with glutathione peroxidase, in promoting antioxidant power and a decreased risk of bowel cancer. (White bread, meat, and chicken are all common foods with one common negative factor: They provide no fiber.)

There's an old Scottish proverb: "The whiter the bread, the sooner you're dead." Don't delay, get your oats today!

OATS

NOTE: Nutrient amounts are listed as milligrams (mg) per 100 grams (g), unless otherwise stated.

GLYCEMIC INDEX: 56	TOTAL CALORIES PER 100 G: 340	CALORIES FROM		
		CARB: 257 76%	PROTEIN: 39 11%	FAT: 44 13%

OATS (MUESLI)

Oats are the main ingredient in muesli, a recipe invented by Dr. Bircher-Benner of Switzerland in the late 1900s. The name "muesli" translates to mean "mixture." Dr. Bircher-Benner developed a sanatorium for healing, and the muesli recipe was designed specifically as a complete health-restoring meal.

The original recipe was prepared on a daily basis and was given to the patients throughout the day or night. Initially, the method included rolled oats being soaked in pure milk overnight. Later, the recipe changed, and freshly extracted fruit juice replaced the milk. In the morning, raw hazelnut or almond pieces were added, plus an abundance of grated apple, a few grapes, and berries.

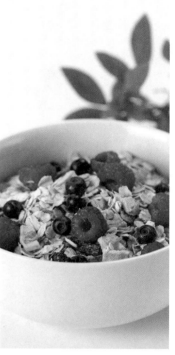

The original muesli recipe can be refrigerated for up to two days and contains no sugar. Processed muesli formulas are often toasted and have too many ingredients in poor combinations, causing poor digestion.

Oats are the greatest "brain grain," the abundance of inositol (12 mg), a B-complex vitamin, is vital for nourishment of brain cells as it assists in the transfer of neurotransmitters between brain cells. Inositol can be manufactured by the body from glucose, and with oats, the great supply of carbohydrates (66 g, or 22% DV) is converted into glucose. This provides a stable supply of brain energy; in fact, the brain utilizes up to 90% of all glucose; the remainder is used by muscles during activity. Oats' excellent supply of magnesium (177 mg, or 44% DV) adds weight to the "brain grain" title. This mineral is not only required for conversion of carbohydrates into glucose but is also vital for a good memory, as it activates brain activity and nourishes the white nerve fibers of the brain.

Oats are an excellent source of phosphorus (523 mg, or 52% DV). A lack of phosphorus can lead to poor memory and poor concentration. Processed breakfast cereals are low in phosphorus, and added sugar causes a depletion of this vital mineral.

Oats are an excellent source of manganese (4.9 mg, or 100% DV), the "memory mineral." Manganese also helps stabilize glucose levels; it is very important for people with diabetes. Manganese is essential for brain function as it coordinates nerve impulses, plus it is a natural antioxidant and essential for the reproductive system. The ample supply of copper in oats (0.6 mg, or 31% DV) assists the nervous system. Copper is likely to be the missing mineral causing postpartum depression. Serum copper levels rise considerably during pregnancy due to elevated estrogen levels, which can take months to stabilize. The bonus with oats is that the copper is balanced with the mineral zinc (4 mg, or 26% DV), as they both compete for absorption within the digestive tract.

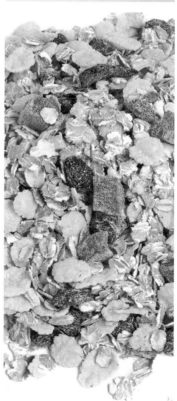

Oats' good iron content (4.7 mg, or 26% DV) is vital, especially during menstruation, pregnancy, and after childbirth. For maximum benefits, add strawberries to the muesli breakfast, as the added vitamin C and the good protein from oats (17 g) will greatly assist absorption of the iron. The vitamin B1 (0.8 mg, or 51% DV) supply is very good and promotes mental efficiency and nerve cell function. Oats also provide B5 (1.3 mg), folate (56 mcg), and B6 (0.1 mg). The potassium content (429 mg) assists muscle and nerve function. The fat content of oats (7 g) provides the wonderful creamy texture.

Muesli is ready to start your day right!

NOTE: DV amounts listed refer to the daily value for women 25–50 years; refer to DRI tables on pages 95–96 for adult male and child values.

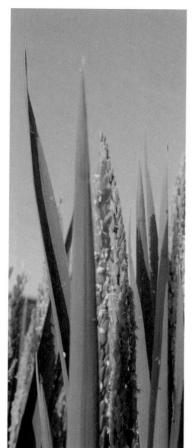

RICE (WHITE) – *Oryza sativa*

Rice feeds half the world's population. It was first cultivated in China over 6,000 years ago. Rice is the only grain grown underwater. Initially, planting and harvesting were done by hand and with water buffalo. This method is still in use in some cultures.

Whole rice can be stored for up to six months, unless it is processed into white rice, which can be stored even longer. The outer layers of whole rice contain the rice bran and the oil-rich germ layer, which are susceptible to oxidation and rancidity. There are three main types of rice: long grain, medium, and short grain. They can all be eaten as either whole brown rice or refined white rice.

Nutritionally speaking, there is a vast difference between brown and white rice with approximately 60% loss of nearly all nutrients in white rice. White rice needs added vitamins to be approved for sale. Enriched rice has added B vitamins and iron; however, over ten other nutrients that are milled out are not replaced.

White, polished rice is basically pure granules of starch. During the Spanish colonial wars, the British soldiers were fed white rice, while their servants lived off the rice water from cooking. The soldiers developed beriberi, a vitamin B1 deficiency. The servants worked harder but did not develop beriberi.

Fortunately, white rice is usually served as a base ingredient for numerous dishes in which a variety of other ingredients can supply nutrients, thereby reducing the risk of problems. However, in some places, where rice makes up nearly 90% of the daily diet, white rice is barely enough to maintain life. The added nutritional benefits of whole-grain brown rice can really be a deciding factor for health.

Rice was behind the initial discovery of B vitamins. In 1897 Dr. Eijkman proved that men who ate whole-grain rice did not contract beriberi. The Japanese navy lost thousands of sailors following the regular daily use of polished or white rice. Dr. R.R. Williams first extracted vitamin B1 from the rice bran. After receiving an award he commented, "Man commits a crime against nature when he eats the starch and throws away the mechanism necessary for the metabolism of that starch."

Apart from the B1 deficiency in white rice, the loss of major minerals and other vitamins is obvious (refer to the table to the left). White rice cannot be considered a nutritious food. But if that's the only way *children* will eat rice, be sure to use enriched rice, pile on the carrots, peas, corn, beans, or cheese, or make a peanut sauce. Or add a dash of nutritional yeast or rice bran, because B1 is vital for children's growth, memory, concentration, and appetite. A prolonged deficiency of B1 can also lead to irritability and depression.

Basically, white rice and white bread are the classic "empty calorie" foods. They do not even provide the essential nutrients to support the proper digestion and absorption of their own starch content. For example, B1 is essential for proper digestion/absorption of starch, B2 essential for secretion of gastric juices and absorption of carbohydrates, B3 assists the function of many digestive enzymes, B5 is required for enzyme development for carbohydrate utilization, manganese for digestive and enzyme reactions, phosphorus for energy distribution, and iron for protein metabolism. All the essential fatty acids (or vitamin F) plus fiber are lacking from white rice. White rice is nice and filling but nasty in its lack of ability to provide nutrition.

Except for calories and protein, all amounts are measured in mg per 100 grams, dry weight approx. *added nutrients	BROWN RICE	WHITE RICE	WHITE ENRICHED	RICE BRAN	BROWN RICE FLOUR	WILD RICE
Calories	359	357	363	276	292	353
Protein	7.5	6.5	6.7	13	5.6	14
Calcium	32	17	8.7	76	8.6	19
Phosphorus	256	111	108	1,386	271	432
Potassium	259	110	86	1,495	233	426
Iron	1.6	0.7	4.3*	19	1.5	1.9
Vitamin B1	0.34	0.08	0.5*	2.3	0.35	0.11
Vitamin B2	0.05	0.03	0.04*	0.25	0.06	0.02
Vitamin B3	4.6	1.6	5*	30	5.1	6.1

NOTE: Nutrient amounts are listed as milligrams (mg) per 100 grams (g), unless otherwise stated.

RICE (BROWN) – *Oryza sativa*

Whole-grain brown rice is full of remarkable benefits, and the alkaline balance it provides after digestion is a real bonus for health. Nearly all foods, except almonds, fruits, vegetables, soy, and millet, are classed as acid-forming foods. The ideal diet needs 75% alkaline-forming foods. Brown rice is a miracle worker in health-restoring benefits due to this one factor alone. Use a rice cooker or steamer to gain a soft texture—it only takes 15 minutes longer to cook than most white rice.

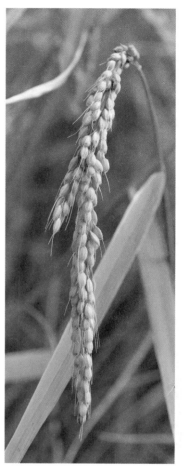

Brown rice provides complete protein (8 g), and compared to all grains, it has the best percentage of available protein (70% npu; npu stands for net protein utilization [as explained on page 91]). When such foods as cheese or milk are added, the protein value increases another 30%, and with legumes the increase is 40%. One 7-ounce serving of cooked brown rice topped with kidney beans and cheese will provide over half the adult daily protein requirement at one quarter the price of beef. Brown rice provides 140% more fiber than white rice and nearly three times the iron content (1.5 mg). The manganese content (3.7 mg) of brown rice will provide over 50% of the daily requirement (2–5 mg) Manganese is essential for the nerves, hormone production, and as a component of an antioxidant enzyme termed superoxide dismutase, which is required to protect against free radicals that result during the production of energy from cells. Brown rice is also a good source of selenium (23 mcg), which has an RDI of 70–85 mcg and is required for protection from heart disease and free radicals.

The phosphorus content (333 mg, or 33% DV) of brown rice is beneficial for blood circulation, the nervous system, the brain, and the skin. But processing destroys over half the value of this vital mineral. The magnesium content (143 mg, or 36% DV) is over four times that of white rice; no wonder stress is booming, as magnesium is essential for relaxed nerves. (As an aside, alcohol depletes magnesium.)

Brown rice is one of the easiest foods to digest (in two hours). It actually takes less time to digest than white rice (which takes two and a half hours). If you are looking for a power-packed powder, try a sprinkle of rice bran on your white rice dish, or in a sauce or gravy, and retrieve the abundance of missing nutrients. Rice bran provides nearly eight times the B-vitamin content of brown rice and 40 times that of white rice. Rice bran is potent in phosphorus (1,386 mg), iron (19 mg), silicon (885 mg) and potassium (1,495 mg)—now that's nutrition. Rice bran needs to be kept in the fridge to maintain its benefits. Try a sprinkle in sauces, breads, cookies, pancakes, or on breakfast cereal. Whenever you have white rice, a dash of rice bran can provide a great balance to all that soft white starch.

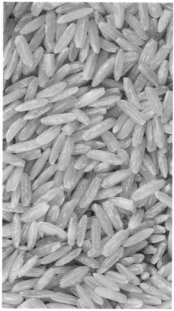

Another rice, called wild rice (*Zizania aquatica*), is more expensive but prized in the best restaurants and the home kitchen. Technically, wild rice isn't rice at all but is, in fact, the grain from a type of grass. The protein (14 g) is double that of brown rice, but it has a similar carbohydrate value (75 g). Most nutrients are present in an approximately 20% greater value except for calcium (19 mg). Wild rice is a good source of iron (4.2 mg), and it has a similar caloric value (353).

It's good to note that all rices are gluten free, making them ideal for those with celiac disease, yeast infections, and wheat intolerances. Ideally, let brown rice replace numerous other wheat or meat meals to gain alkaline balance. If you have to get takeout, it's better to have rice than a hamburger. The price of brown rice is another major benefit. Yes, brown rice is all right tonight!

NOTE: DV amounts listed refer to the daily value for women 25–50 years; refer to DRI tables on pages 95–96 for adult male and child values.

RYE – *Secale cereale*

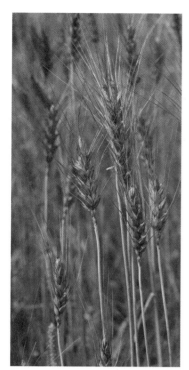

Rye is a grain that can withstand cold, acid soil, and low rainfall. Rye has been a staple grain in Europe, Scandinavia, and Russia for centuries. It was first cultivated by the Romans around 400 BC. Rye also has a dark history due to a fungus, *ergot,* that attacked the grains, producing a virus in humans and animals. During the Middle Ages, and even until 1953 in France, the virus caused severe problems with the central nervous system. Modern science has eliminated this disease in the rye plant. Remember, the potato also caused problems at one time, so don't be put off by this natural whole grain.

Today, rye is gaining popularity as a replacement for wheat bread. It is also used to make whiskey. Whole-grain rye is referred to as rye groats; they are best presoaked prior to cooking or steaming, like rice, and then added to soups, bread, or stews. The protein content (14.8 g, or 30% DV) of whole rye is a great benefit; it provides complete protein with a low fat content (2.5 g, or 4% DV). A vegetable soup with rye groats may sound unappetizing, but once the rye has been soaked overnight and simmered in vegetable stock for one hour and then cooked with winter vegetables and spices for 30 minutes, then served with a splash of cream, rye soup is on its way to being a delicious provider of flavor and nourishment.

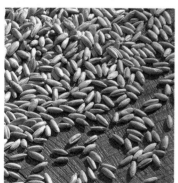

Rye bread is available in numerous varieties. They all have a low gluten content compared to wheat. However, some rye breads also include either wheat flour or added gluten, to give the bread a soft and lighter texture. The best rye bread is made with organic rye flour, sour rye dough, water, and no yeast. Another benefit of rye bread is its excellent fiber content (14 g, or 55% DV). The bran and germ are difficult to separate from the grain during milling compared to wheat. The fiber content will help protect against colon cancer, as fiber binds with toxins in the colon to regularly eliminate possible cancer-causing substances. Rye is the second-best grain source of the mineral phosphorus (374 mg, or 37% DV). When you add a slice of cheese to rye bread, the benefits for the bones, skeletal system, and nervous system are excellent.

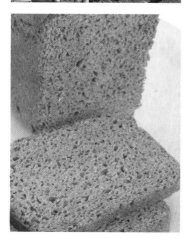

Rye is also a source of lignan, a natural estrogen that can be very beneficial during menopause to stabilize the body's estrogen levels. During menopause, normal estrogen levels can diminish, causing discomfort and hot flushes. Lignan can also inhibit excess estrogen production, a possible cause of breast cancer, as it blocks the estrogen receptors. In addition, the supply of manganese found in rye (2.7 mg, or 50% DV) is vital for regulation of menstrual cycles and normal blood sugar levels. The good supply of magnesium (121 mg, or 30% DV) plus the valuable supply of zinc (3.7 mg, or 25% DV) and phosphorus all add up to make the rye grain ideal for strong bone development. Rye bread is full of selenium (35 mcg, or 30% DV), which promotes the function of the thyroid gland in regulating metabolism. White bread contains none of the above benefits nor any of the following nutrients found in rye bread: vitamin E (1.3 mg), folate (60 mcg), potassium (264 mg). As an added bonus, rye bread has a wonderful rich flavor. So shop around for the best rye bread and enjoy the benefits.

NOTE: Nutrient amounts are listed as milligrams (mg) per 100 grams (g), unless otherwise stated.

WHEAT – *Triticum* spp.

Wheat cultivation has spread around the world, with varieties that are grown in nearly all climates, from Arctic to subtropical. There are two main types of whole wheat: hard wheat and soft wheat. However, there are thousands of varieties of wheat, of which about three hundred are used commercially. Among the most common varieties is the *hard red winter wheat,* which originated in Canada and is now used worldwide. It is ideal for breadmaking, grows quickly, and may be harvested three months after sowing. The next common variety is *white wheat*. It is ideal for pastry making and for breakfast cereals, as it is starchy and contains less gluten protein. *Durum wheat* produces the world's best pasta; it is a very hard grain with an amber color, and grows mainly in warm, dry climates.

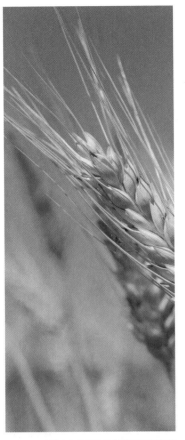

The whole-wheat grain can be prepared in an incredible variety of recipes, products, and forms. To gain the ultimate benefit from the wheat grain, there is nothing better than *wheatgrass juice* (refer to page 112). The second-best form of the wheat grain is the *sprouted wheat*. Used fresh on salads or mixed into mayonnaise, they are delightful and highly nutritious. They can also be added to breads and soups, but fresh is best.

Apart from these methods, wheat is also prepared into various forms such as *cracked wheat*, used in the famous and healthful *tabouli* recipe and in numerous soups. It is made from whole-wheat grain, cracked under pressure, and it provides the full grain benefits. *Kibbled wheat* is similar: It is produced from the whole-wheat grain, then placed through a machine that cracks the grain into tiny pieces. These are used in bread and in some breakfast cereals.

The most common use of wheat is as *flour*. The best quality flour is made from organic whole-grain wheat that is *stone-ground* into a flour containing the full value of the wheat grain, including the germ and bran. Stone-ground mills do not produce excess heat and therefore the flour is of better quality. Common milling uses steel rollers that move quickly, causing the whole-grain flour to heat, and the wheat germ content may turn rancid if not used promptly. *Whole-grain flour* does retain the entire wheat germ and bran layer, plus the starchy endosperm (the inner portion of the wheat grain). It needs to be used soon after milling.

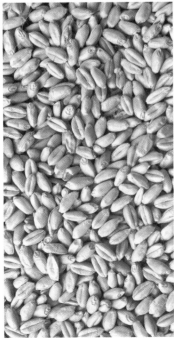

Varieties of *whole-meal bread* can vary considerably in their content, plus they may contain all the additives that are used in the production of white bread. Check the labels carefully until you find a loaf with life. Commercial bread, even top-quality stone-ground, whole-wheat bread, may contain a few additives to improve shelf life, but the fewer added, the better.

Due to the fact that the oil content in the *wheat germ* clogs up the steel mills, it is removed for better productivity. Wheat germ is then sold separately. It is the most nutritious part of the grain but must be kept fresh in a cool and airtight container and used within a few weeks. The *wheat bran* is also removed from the whole-wheat grain in the production of *white flour*, as it makes bread bulky. White flour is the biggest business, used in bread that comes in hundreds of different shapes and sizes as well as in other recipes.

NOTE: DV amounts listed refer to the daily value for women 25–50 years; refer to DRI tables on pages 95–96 for adult male and child values.

WHEAT (BREAD)

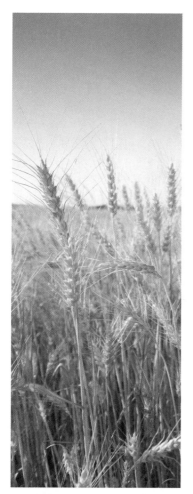

For 10,000 years the wheat grain has provided the "staff of life," the "daily bread," and it was usually obtained in the whole-grain form. The current milling of wheat produces incredibly fine white flour and wheat products. The common milling process removes all the wheat germ and bran plus at least 40% (and up to 60%) of all nutrients, depending on the refinement grade of the wheat flour. Government health authorities now require "enrichment" of flour for mass-produced bread; however, enriching returns only a small portion of a few B vitamins. When comparing the nutritional value of the whole-wheat grain to refined flour and white bread, it is obvious that "humans cannot live by bread alone" (refer to the table on page 29).

The nutritional value of whole-grain wheat flour may be lowered by the presence of *phytic acid* in the bran. An excess intake of bran or whole-grain products may cause problems, as phytic acid combines with minerals—especially calcium, iron, and zinc—forming insoluble compounds that are not easily absorbed. The supply of calcium (32–100 mg) in whole wheat may therefore be of no value, but the body can adapt to the phytic acid. For people who eat whole-grain breads as a staple food, it is more than likely that their digestive system has overcome this problem. For people who are used to eating white bread, however, it may take their bodies a few weeks to adjust to whole-grain bread and to properly absorb the calcium, iron, and zinc.

In any event, whole-wheat and especially white bread are poor sources of calcium (3–8% DV). A cheddar cheese sandwich is full of calcium (728 mg), and 100 g of pasta with cheese (728 mg) or tahini on bread (420 mg) both also provide great portions of the daily calcium requirement of 500–1,300 mg per day.

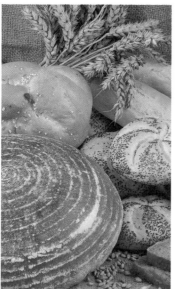

Wheat bread has a fair iron content (2.5 mg in both white and whole-meal bread; 3–4.6 mg, or 10–25% DV in whole-grain wheat), but iron may bind with the phytic acid in whole-grain bread, which can reduce iron absorption if your digestive system is not used to whole-grain bread. Foods such as parsley (6 mg of iron), pumpkin seeds (11 mg), tahini (9 mg), almonds (4.7 mg), cashews (3.7 mg), sunflower seeds (7 mg), and dried apricots (4.4 mg), when eaten regularly, will help provide iron, as the daily iron requirement is 8–18 mg (during pregnancy 27 mg). Foods such as beef (1.7 mg) and eggs (2 mg) only add a little to the daily iron requirement. Five slices of white bread will provide approximately 3 mg of iron. With five slices of whole-meal bread approximately 4.5 mg of iron is provided, but it may not be absorbed unless it is regularly part of the diet. In regards to zinc, white bread provides 0.68 mg and whole-grain bread 1.8 mg; the daily adult zinc requirement is 10–15 mg.

The carbohydrate content of white bread (72.5 g) and whole-grain bread (72.6 g) is nearly identical. The same applies to protein: white has 12 g and whole-grain 13.7 g. The main difference is the fiber content: White bread has 2.4 g and whole-grain has 12.2 g, or 50% DV. Whole-grain bread has nearly five times the fiber content!

A white-bread diet in combination with a regular meat diet (meat has no fiber) is a risky long-term diet, especially for colon health. One study showed that the "protective quantity" of fiber, for adults, needs to be more than 28 g a day. That's 48 slices of white bread.

NOTE: Nutrient amounts are listed as milligrams (mg) per 100 grams (g), unless otherwise stated.

GLYCEMIC INDEX: 41	TOTAL CALORIES PER 100 G: 339	CALORIES FROM		
		CARB: 269 80%	PROTEIN: 49 14%	FAT: 21 6%

WHEAT (PASTA)

Wheat is the main ingredient in pasta, and a special type of wheat—durum wheat—is used almost exclusively. The name "pasta" implies a "paste" of water and flour.

The main styles (shapes) of pasta are: cannelloni, lasagna, macaroni, rigatoni, spaghetti, tagliatelle, and vermicelli. Within these styles are numerous variations in size, shape, thickness, added ingredients, plus plain and whole-wheat versions. Some pasta has egg added to the mix (*al uovo*), but generally it is made from plain durum wheat.

Pasta and pizza are among the most common meals in the family home, not just in Italy but throughout the world. They are easy to make and numerous different ingredients can be added to make each dish different. Pasta or pizza, on its own, has about the same protein (12.8 g, or 26% DV), same carbohydrate (74 g), and same fiber content as white bread (2.4 g). As it has a very low fat content (1.6 g, or 2% DV), a serving of grated cheese will balance the meal plus add a good dose of calcium, especially if its parmesan (1,380 mg). But cheese supplies no fiber so, once again, the addition of fiber-rich foods is really beneficial. One serving of cheddar cheese (28 g) will add 9.4 g of fat—mainly saturated (6 g) and monounsaturated (2.6 g). And as the approximate daily requirement is 60–80 g, the added cheese is good value for the active person.

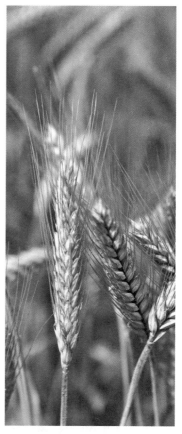

For children, a meal of pasta and cheese is great, but they also need vegetables and fruit, plus oats or other whole-grain cereals. Add some baby spinach or a dash of bran to the tomato sauce, or serve it with yummy whole-grain bread and butter. The protein content of pasta (12.8 g, or 26% DV) is good, and with added cheese (25 g) the protein increases to 38 g, nearly 60% DV for adults and approximately 80% DV for children. Now that's big value for a growing family!

The main benefit of pasta and pizza is the excellent carbohydrate content (approximately 72 g, or 25% DV). Both pasta and bread are energy-packed foods; however, as the body requires numerous nutrients to help utilize and produce the energy, plain white pasta, pizza, or bread on its own is fairly inadequate, due to a poor supply of essential nutrients. To overcome this problem, add ingredients that are full of nutrients. Pasta with mixed vegetables, parmesan, and a rich tomato sauce provides basic but good nutrition.

For a top-quality pasta meal, add some ground pumpkin seeds on top of the cheese. Delicious! The same applies to noodles: Add some stir-fried vegetables, blanched almonds, or cracked or finely ground pumpkin seeds, and you can be sure of gaining great nutrition and additional flavor.

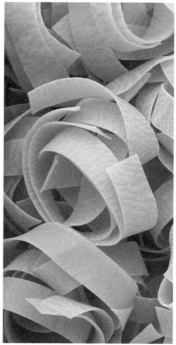

Foods such as pasta, pizza, noodles, and bread can comfortably provide one-third of our daily energy values. We can get another third from fruits and vegetables and the balance from fats, oils, and proteins. Pasta, bread, and noodles provide approximately 72 g of carbohydrates per 100 g. The daily average requirement for children and teenagers is about 300–350 g, for adults 300 g. Our calorie requirements per day are children 2,000, women 2,200, teenagers and men 3,000, an average person 2,400 calories. Pasta or bread provides approximately 340 calories per 100 g serving. So always remember that it's the topping that makes the bread, pasta, pizza, or noodles healthful.

NOTE: DV amounts listed refer to the daily value for women 25–50 years; refer to DRI tables on pages 95–96 for adult male and child values.

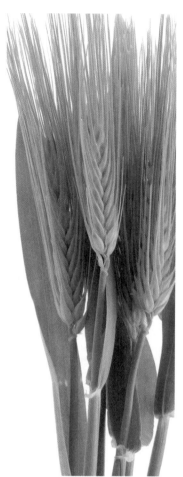

WHEAT (FLOUR NUTRIENTS)

Wheat in the whole form and as whole-grain flour is a power-packed food. The protein and carbohydrate value are well balanced, and the supply of minerals (except calcium) and fiber is beneficial. The main problems with white flour, bread, pastries, pizza, and pasta products are: the low fiber content, as mentioned; the low calcium and phosphorus content, as these minerals are essential for nerves, brain, bones, and digestion; the low magnesium content, as magnesium is vital for the nerves, digestion, bones, and brain; and the low potassium supply, as potassium is essential for the heart muscles, circulation, and nerves. The iron content is fair, but the manganese content, vital for blood development, memory, glands, and nerves, is deficient. The zinc content is low; zinc is vital for bone strength and growth, digestion, glands, and hormones. B vitamins are added to enrich white flour, but the vitamin E content is very low, and this vitamin is vital for the heart, healing, long life, antioxidation, and fertility. The number of common ailments associated with the above nutrient deficiencies is enormous, and white-flour products can be a major contributor to poor health if they are the staple food in the diet. Furthermore, refined white bread includes additives.

Products made from refined white flour cannot stand alone nutritionally; they need added ingredients to ensure proper health. In addition, the high glycemic index of pretzels (80), white bread (70), and muffins (70) adds further weight to the suggestion that beneficial foods need to be included with the white flour products. Ideally, whole grains such as oats can take the place of breakfast toast, or yeast extract can be added to the bread or toast, to give it a small boost for your nerves. Toast with tahini is great as it supplies a good dose of vitamin E and minerals, plus protein.

Let your bread be delightful, but healthful. Add natural ingredients to make the soft, spongy, white bread beneficial. May your daily bread be loaded with benefits and flavor.

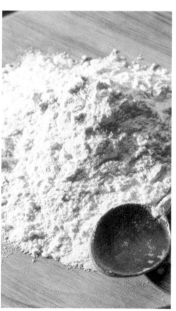

Nutrients per 100 g dry weight	Whole Grain Wheat White	Whole Grain Wheat Red	Whole Grain Wheat Flour	White Wheat Flour	Wheat Bran	Wheat Germ	Wheat Gluten	Pasta	Whole Grain Rye
Carbohydrate	75.9	68	72.6	72.5	64.5	51.8	13.8	74.7	69.8
Protein	11.3	15.4	13.7	12	15.5	23.1	75.2	12.8	14.8
Lipids (Fat)	1.7	1.9	1.9	1.7	4.3	9.7	1.9	1.6	2.5
Calories	342	329	339	361	216	360	370	371	335
Fiber	12.2	12.2	12.2	2.4	42.8	13.2	0.6	2.4	14.6
Calcium	32	25	34	15	73	39	142	18	33
Phosphorus	355	332	346	97	1013	842	260	150	374
Magnesium	93	124	138	25	611	239	25	48	121
Potassium	432	340	405	100	1182	892	100	162	264
Sodium	2	2	5	2	2	12	29	7	6
Manganese	3.8	4.1	3.8	0.8	11.5	13.3	—	0.7	2.7
Iron	4.6	3.6	3.9	4.4*	10.6	6.3	5.2	1.3	2.7
Selenium	—	—	70	39	77	79	39	62	35
Zinc	3.3	2.8	2.9	0.9	7.3	12.3	0.9	1.2	3.7
Vitamin B1	0.4	0.5	0.4	0.8*	0.5	1.9	0	0.1	0.3
Vitamin B2	0.1	0.1	0.2	0.5*	0.6	0.5	0	0.1	0.3
Vitamin B3	4.4	5.7	6.4	7.6*	13.6	6.8	0	1.7	4.3
Vitamin E	1	1	0.8	0.4	1.5	15.8	0	0	1.3

NOTE: Nutrient amounts are listed as milligrams (mg) per 100 grams (g), unless otherwise stated.

The tables below (and the tables on pages 42, 60, 77, and 104) are provided as a guide to the daily amounts of the individual food groups that are suggested by three different dietary guidelines: 1. Ultimate Nutrition for Health (UNH) Diet, 2. U.S. MyPlate and DRIs, 3. Australian Guide to Healthy Eating. These tables are provided as a guide only and are not to be considered for an exact daily intake. The primary aim of these tables is to show that all the main food groups are required for a balanced diet. All three dietary guidelines suggest that a variety of foods be obtained on a daily basis, and over a period of one week a complete range of natural food groups can be obtained. Balance your life naturally!

Whole Grains	Main Health Benefits Plus Main Nutrients, Antioxidants, and Phytonutrients	Aids Which Body Systems
Barley	protects against colon cancer, arthritis, asthma, diabetes, high cholesterol	digestive, elimination
Corn—sweet	protects against infections, lung cancer, brain disorders, irritability	respiratory, brain
Millet	silicon, iron, gluten free, yeast free, alkaline, folate, phosphorus, zinc, copper	digestive, repair
Oats	fiber, lowers blood sugar levels and cholesterol, ideal for diabetics, magnesium, antioxidants, protein	digestive, blood, brain, nervous
Rice—brown	alkaline, manganese, selenium, phosphorus, gluten free, yeast free	digestive, blood
Rye	fiber, low gluten, natural estrogens, manganese, selenium, zinc	digestive, glandular
Wheat—whole	carbohydrates, fiber, potassium, manganese, selenium, vitamin E	muscular

RECOMMENDATIONS FOR DAILY CARBOHYDRATE INTAKE FROM GRAINS		Adult Male	Adult Female	Teenager	Child
Total Daily Carbohydrate Intake (based on typical guidelines)		340 g	280 g	400 g	270 g
1. *UNH* recommendation: 20% of carbohydrate intake from whole grains		68 g	56 g	80 g	54 g
Note the carb content of several common grain foods	100 g (3–4 oz) whole-wheat bread	approx. 39 g of carbohydrate			
	100 g white bread	approx. 51 g of carbohydrate			
	100 g pasta	approx. 75 g of carbohydrate			
	100 g rice	approx. 80 g of carbohydrate			
	100 g oats	approx. 68 g of carbohydrate			
2. U.S. MyPlate and DRIs		Whole grains at most meals. White rice, white bread, potatoes, pasta eaten sparingly.			
3. Australian Guide to Healthy Eating*		6–12 servings	4–9 servings	5–11 servings	5–9 servings

* 1 serving is equivalent to: 2 slices bread (60 g), 1 cup of rice, pasta, noodles (180 g), ⅓ cup of cereal (40 g), ½ cup of untoasted muesli, ¼ cup flour (40 g), 1 cup of oatmeal (230 g).

UNH RECOMMENDATION FOR DAILY PROTEIN INTAKE FROM GRAINS		Adult Male	Adult Female	Teenager	Child
Total Daily Protein Intake (based on typical guidelines)		60 g	47 g	65 g	45 g
1. *UNH* recommendation: 5% of protein intake from whole grains		3 g	2 g	3 g	2 g
Note the protein content of several common grain foods	100 g (3–4 oz) whole-wheat or white bread	approx. 9 g of protein			
	100 g pasta	approx. 12 g of protein			
	100 g rice	approx. 7 g of protein			
	100 g oats	approx. 16 g of protein			

UNH = Ultimate Nutrition for Health
DRIs = Dietary Reference Intakes

Legumes is another name for beans and peas. The following pages will provide you with information about the various types of legumes, and their nutritional value, historical information, and their methods of preparation. The main legumes discussed are: carob bean, chickpea, green bean, kidney bean, and its relatives, lentil, lima bean, mung bean, peanut, pea, and soybean. Dried legumes are one of nature's best stores of nutrition. They are basically a seed, and when water is added, new life will develop with every day of growth.

Presoaking legumes has many advantages. For some legumes it is essential in order to convert the concentrated starches, especially stachyose and raffinose, to promote better digestion. Otherwise these undigested starches get attacked by intestinal bacteria, forming carbon dioxide and hydrogen gas, and causing flatulence and a great loss of nutritional benefits.

Raw-dried legumes also contain such substances as alkaloids, glycosides, and saponin, which are detrimental to digestion but are eliminated with long soaking and proper cooking. Presoaking for a few days will greatly enhance the digestion and nutrient quality of the legume. If you are short on time to prepare legumes, use fresh beans or peas, or choose from a large variety of canned beans. They are very economical and can be stored in the pantry for those times when stocks are low or you need a big boost of energy and fiber.

Make sure that your kitchen is always well stocked with at least the basic legumes: chickpeas, kidney beans, lentils, lima beans, mung beans, and soybeans. The variety of legume products is abundant and their popularity is increasing due to the resurgence of many traditional recipes.

Legumes supply all the essential daily protein requirements, and their ability to reduce blood cholesterol is a major benefit.

Generally speaking, legumes are classed as a carbohydrate food. However, millions of people throughout the world rely on legumes for their daily protein requirements. An excess intake of animal proteins and insufficient legume consumption are possibly the main contributing factors toward the multitude of heart and arterial diseases that are prevalent today.

This chapter provides valuable information on the numerous benefits of legumes as well as ideas for methods of preparation. Once you have tried a few simple recipes, you will realize how so many people throughout the world enjoy their legume meals.

Legume meals could easily replace at least two animal protein meals per week. Ideally, a balanced diet requires 20% of carbohydrates to be obtained from legumes. The legume kingdom affords complete protein, numerous minerals, vitamins, abundant fiber, and a beneficial slow-releasing energy. If you have the chance to enjoy legumes, at home or when dining out, treat yourself.

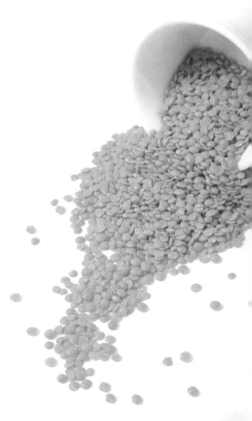

CAROB BEANS – *Ceratonia siliqua*

Carob beans have a remarkable history. The carob tree is said to be the oldest known fruit-bearing tree in the areas of Syria, Palestine, Spain, Egypt, and Sicily. Carob has provided generations of people with food, and it has been called "bread that grows on trees," "staff of life," and "St. John's bread." It is mentioned in the Bible as providing energy, nourishment, and food for thought during times in the wilderness.

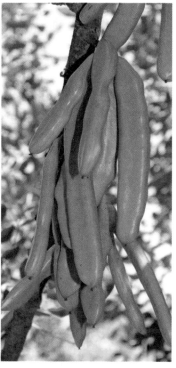

Carob is a hardy food source. It can be stored for long periods, and the large carob pods can be eaten as a sweet food, directly from the tree, when ripened to a very dark brown color. One of the greatest benefits of carob is the alkaline balance it provides to the digestive system. There's no need for antacids; carob actually reduces stomach acidity. Carob is an excellent source of natural pectin, vital for the treatment of stomach upsets and diarrhea and the reduction of cholesterol. Pectin removes toxins from the digestive system and promotes protein digestion by preventing digested protein from spoiling in the lower digestive system.

Carob is a compact carbohydrate food (89 g, or 30% DV) and it is full of fiber (40 g, or 159% DV), which is bulky and noticeable when making carob drinks. Ideally, for a smooth drink, allow the carob sediment to settle and then pour the liquid content into another cup. In contrast to chocolate, carob contains no caffeine and no oxalic acid; these two factors alone give carob the power to be an excellent replacement for chocolate or caffeine. For growing children especially, oxalic acid in chocolate binds with calcium, retarding the absorption of this mighty mineral.

Carob is a very good source of calcium (348 mg, or 35% DV, nearly three times that of cow's milk) and when combined with a milk shake, it provides a sweet flavor and does not require the loads of sugar normally associated with chocolate drinks. Carob provides excellent natural sweetness (49 g) with the bonus of vitamins B1, B2, B3, B5, and folate (30 mcg) and a very good supply of the alkaline mineral potassium (827 mg, or 24% DV), ideal for active muscles and improved blood circulation. Because potassium is heat sensitive, a carob drink will provide potent potassium, over twice that of bananas. The supply of the mineral copper (0.6–1 mg) is only a quarter that of chocolate (3.8 g), but the recommended daily intake of copper for adults is 1.5–3 mg, so don't overdose.

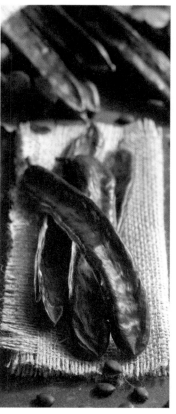

Carob and chocolate both provide approximately 1 g of zinc. The fat content of carob (1 g) is mainly polyunsaturated and low compared to chocolate (8.4 g) which is 60% saturated fat. When baking cookies, carob powder with complete protein (5 g) adds a sweet flavor and dark color to cookies. Make some carob crackles and you can be sure you're giving the children a great party food. Add a small amount of honey and ice cream to any carob milk shake, drink, or recipe; doing so promotes a smooth consistency. Carob also provides magnesium (54 mg), compared to chocolate with 13 mg; phosphorus (79 mg), compared to chocolate with 100 mg; and twelve times the iron content of milk chocolate (3 mg as opposed to 0.24 mg). For adults, try carob with goat's milk, soy milk, or acidophilus milk. Carob snack bars are the ideal replacement for chocolate bars as they are a great calcium food plus they will promote digestion.

Carob was once used to measure precious stones and gold—it's where the term "carat" comes from. Now it is an easy to obtain, healthy, and inexpensive sweet or snack.

NOTE: DV amounts listed refer to the daily value for women 25–50 years; refer to DRI tables on pages 95–96 for adult male and child values.

CHICKPEAS – *Cicer arietinum*

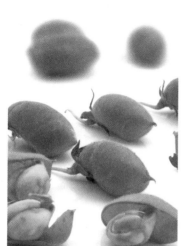

Chickpeas are famous for their inclusion as the main ingredient in hummus, now a common dip or spread, and one that has supported people from the Middle East for thousands of years. Another common name for chickpeas is garbanzos. They are available in various colors, such as the common light yellow, red, brown, and black, but all have a distinct pointed pod housing two or three peas, also with a pointed tip.

A famous recipe using chickpeas is the falafel. Here chickpeas are combined with sesame seeds, potato, onions, parsley, garlic, and various spices such as cayenne pepper and paprika. Next time you see falafel for sale, indulge in a truly amazing meal. Add some tahini sauce—it is full of health benefits. If you are making hummus at home, presoak the beans for two to four days, rinsing twice a day. You will increase the protein value and reduce the compounds that cause flatulence.

Chickpeas provide protein (19 g, or 40% DV), and with a dab of tahini on the falafel, the protein increases greatly, due to the balance of the amino acid methionine. For a fiber-rich food (17 g, or 70% DV), chickpeas are ideal. If you need to be on a cholesterol-free diet, you can gain extra benefits from chickpea fiber, as it binds with cholesterol-laden bile and eliminates it from the body. If you need a low-fat diet, chickpeas supply 6 g of fat (mainly unsaturated—5 g), or only 51 calories from its fat content.

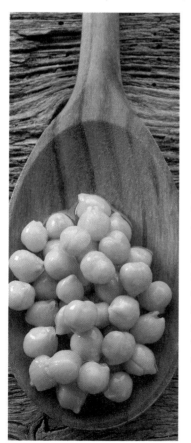

Chickpeas combine well with winter vegetables. For a tasty yet simple way to serve them, cook in water for one hour then place in an oven or skillet and lightly dry roast them. Sprinkle with pure olive oil and enjoy with a fresh salad or broccoli and cheese. The calcium content (105 mg) is fair and the phosphorus content (366 mg, or 37% DV) is ample to assist proper digestion of the compact nutrients. The iron content (6 mg, or 35% DV) is of great benefit during pregnancy, lactation, or any time you feel weary.

Chickpeas supply over three times the iron content of beef (1.9 mg). In addition, the manganese content (2 mg) and the very good copper content (1 mg, or 42% DV) are both vital for the production of new blood. Try some hummus as a dip and offset those feelings of fatigue.

As with all legumes, the potassium content (875 mg) is very good, but once again, it is a heat-sensitive nutrient, so sprout them first to reduce cooking time and increase nutrient values. The magnesium content (115 mg, or 29% DV) is another activating nutrient for the nervous system and brain; plus it is required to assist enzymes for digestion and hormone production.

Chickpeas supply five times the magnesium content of beef and milk. The supply of folate (557 mcg, or 139% DV) is excellent and vital for protection from heart attacks and for the proper functioning of the brain and nervous system. Folic acid is water soluble and required daily from the diet: for adults 200 mcg, during pregnancy 400 mcg, and during lactation 350 mcg. Spinach supplies only 95 mcg of folate, so chickpeas are the folate king. The supply of the trace mineral molybdenum is excellent—over 75% daily value from a 1-cup serving. Very few foods supply molybdenum, which is required for the nerves and brain and for fat metabolism.

Chickpeas are ready to please your nutritional appetite.

NOTE: Nutrient amounts are listed as milligrams (mg) per 100 grams (g), unless otherwise stated.

GREEN BEANS – *Phaseolus vulgaris*

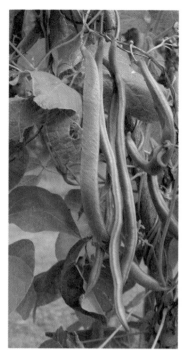

Green beans, commonly termed the French bean or string bean, belong to the same botanical species as the kidney bean. During the sixteenth century, the green bean was considered a luxury food for royalty. It is reported as one of the oldest known foods, dating back 7,000 years in Mexico and known to the American Indians. The green bean supported the survival of early settlers in America prior to the cultivation of corn and other crops.

Green beans are a good carbohydrate food (8 g), plus a fair source of dietary fiber (3.5 g), important for elimination of waste as it binds with cancer-causing toxins, usually as a byproduct of meat digestion, and cleanses the colon. Because meat, chicken, and fish provide no fiber, the addition of green beans to the menu is really a life saver in the long term.

The good supply of folate (40 mcg) is worth snapping into, especially for the expectant mother, as folate is vital for infant development and for the reproduction of body cells. Folate also promotes brain function and is essential for the nervous system and to prevent nervous exhaustion. Folate is water soluble and required regularly from the diet. The iron (1.1 mg) and vitamin K (22 mcg) supplied by the green bean is also important for an expectant mother, in addition to being vital for the circulatory system. If you freeze green beans, the vitamin K may disappear. Furthermore, antibiotics, aspirin, mineral oils, and X rays can all deplete the body's store of this fat-soluble vitamin. Green beans provide complete protein (2 g) with a very low fat content (0.013 g), so you can add butter or oil to the lightly steamed green beans and still have a well-balanced food.

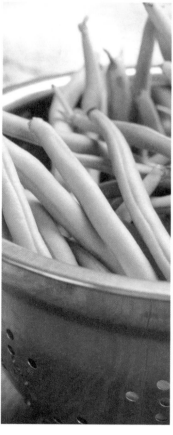

The supply of potassium (230 mg) means it is worth picking beans fresh from the vine as potassium is heat sensitive. In combination with the phosphorus content (42 mg), potassium provides benefits of increased oxygen to the brain for efficient mental function. Beans' magnesium content of 25 mg promotes nourishment to the white nerve fibers of the brain. The vitamin A content (700 IU) is fair. The supply of vitamin C (16 mg) makes the fresh French bean an antioxidant food, able to retard the oxidation of cholesterol, thereby warding off arterial plaque.

The green bean is a safe food for diabetics (50 GI), plus it is said to promote the production of natural insulin due to the supply of plant hormones in combination with the small amount of the mineral zinc (0.26 mg).

The green bean is very low in calories (34), and this combined with its supply of fiber means you can eat them all day and still feel satisfied that your waistline is on the decline! A short cooking time is ample to soften the texture. Immerse them in simmering water for two minutes. Add your favorite cream sauce, and serve with grilled ocean fish and roasted pumpkin for a colorful, healthful meal. Green beans supply a small amount of calcium (41 mg), so add a sprinkle of cheese for a satisfying and bone-building entrée. When in season, the green bean is a very economical food and children seem to like the taste. That's certainly a bonus for their health as green beans are the best legume source of vitamins A, K, and folate.

If a green bean snaps when you bend it, try it raw; if it's a few days old, lightly steam it for an excellent addition to any protein meal, such as with rice, chicken, meat, or fish. The green French bean will help you stay lean.

GREEN BEANS

NOTE: DV amounts listed refer to the daily value for women 25–50 years; refer to DRI tables on pages 95–96 for adult male and child values.

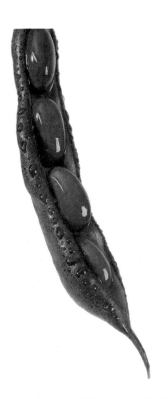

KIDNEY BEANS – *Phaseolus vulgaris*

Kidney beans have numerous cousins: the navy bean, pinto bean, Mexican black bean, cannellini bean, flageolet bean, and haricot bean, plus the fresh green bean and the snap bean. Originating in Peru, the *Phaseolus vulgaris* species spread around the world.

The red kidney bean is the most famous canned bean or baked bean, and today it lines the supermarket shelves from Ulmarra to Uganda, providing one of the cheapest and easiest to prepare meals: the British and Aussie favorite, baked beans on toast. The kidney bean is the main ingredient in numerous Mexican dishes; the bean taco with lettuce and cheese is a great meal that children like, and they gain great benefits from the excellent protein value it provides. On their own, kidney beans supply protein (24 g, or 47% DV), and with added cheese, two tacos will provide children aged 8 to 14 with all their daily protein requirements. In addition, kidney beans provide calcium (143 mg); with a good sprinkle of cheese, the taco can also provide all the daily calcium for growing children. The corn part of the taco shell is fairly low in nutrients but it provides the "crunch factor" that stimulates the appetite.

The carbohydrate content (60 g) of kidney beans is as good as it gets, due to the excellent supply of fiber (25 g, or 100% DV), which helps to gradually stabilize the supply of blood sugar, in contrast to the very common high glycemic index of white bread (70) and potato chips (52). Boiled kidney beans have a low glycemic index of 29; canned beans have a GI of 52. Corn taco shells have a high glycemic index of 72. Adding cheese to a taco will greatly reduce the GI of the corn shell and make it a safe food for children. For a very low-GI kidney bean meal, ideal for diabetics, use boiled kidney beans (29) with added cheese (0), onion (9), lettuce (5), tomato (35), and peppers (8). Kidney beans are very low in fat (1 g), with only 7 calories per 100 g serving, so you can add the cheese and still be confident of a very lean meal, plus an excellent supply of nutrients. The potassium content is 1,406 mg, or 40% DV, but it's a heat-sensitive nutrient, so sprout your legumes first to reduce cooking time by 70% and increase their nutrient balance and promote digestion. If kidney beans are not sprouted and/or cooked properly, that is, until soft, a toxic factor called *haemagglutinin* will remain in the bean, possibly leading to gastroenteritis. Sprouting alone reduces the haemagglutinin in kidney beans to a level equal to that of other legumes.

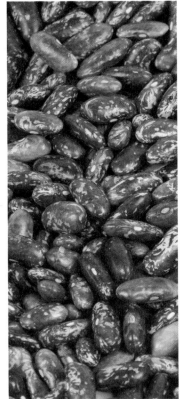

For people too busy to sprout and cook kidney beans, or other legumes, a wide range of well-cooked, canned legumes is available at a very low price. They should be a regular part of the shopping list, as they are quick to prepare into nourishing meals. A bean salad in summer, for example, will provide excellent folate (394 mcg, or 98% DV)—by contrast, lettuce only supplies 41 mcg of folate.

For an excellent supply of organic iron (8 mg, or 46% DV), kidney beans are really essential, supplying four times the iron content of beef and over ten times that of cheese (0.67 mg) or chicken. The supply of molybdenum is excellent (80% DV); plus there's phosphorus (407 mg, or 41% DV), magnesium (140 mg, or 35% DV), and copper (48% DV). Including kidney beans in your diet can help you reach the full benefit of true health.

Kidney beans will support your nutritional needs!

NOTE: Nutrient amounts are listed as milligrams (mg) per 100 grams (g), unless otherwise stated.

LENTILS – *Lens culinaris*

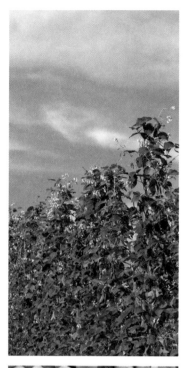

Lentils have been around for ages; they were one of the first cultivated foods over 8,000 years ago. Lentils helped to build the mighty pyramids; they were used by the Egyptians as a main food for the laborers. Further proof of the power of lentils comes from the Russian soldiers during both world wars: Lentils provided the major part of their battlefield diet.

Two basic types of lentils are available. There's the common reddish-brown lentil from India, and the pale green lentil from China. And while they might be tiny, they're power packed with nutritional benefits.

The protein value (28 g, or 56% DV) is complete in all the essential amino acids; however, lentils have a low net protein utilization of 30%. From the total protein in lentils, only one-third is usable unless other foods are combined to assist in the balance of the limiting amino acids (those that are in short supply). Such foods as rice or cheese or egg are most commonly used and can improve the lentil protein balance by 50%. The main limiting amino acids in lentils are methionine and tryptophan.

Lentils are compact and provide a great supply of calories (338, or 17% DV) with a very low fat content of 1 g. If you are a regular meat eater, you run a greater risk of cardiovascular and heart problems due to the saturated fat and cholesterol content of meat. Lentils provide none of those nasties, and in fact, the excellent fiber content helps to lower cholesterol, as fiber binds with the fat-dissolving enzyme bile and helps to rid the body of the cholesterol within the bile.

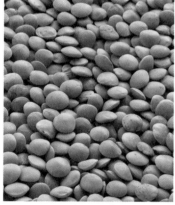

Lentils are also a good food for diabetics; the glycemic index is a low 27 for red lentils and 30 for brown or green lentils . Lentil vegetable soup or the famous Indian dish *dahl,* made from red lentils, onions, garlic, curry, tomatoes and a bay leaf, are really low on the GI scale. A small dab of sour cream or plain yogurt in the soup makes a simple and tasty snack or meal. Lentil burgers are another favorite.

Let lentils loose in your kitchen and be amazed! One advantage of lentils, compared to other legumes, is that they require far less cooking. Place the dried lentils on a large plate and check for any cracked or damaged seeds, then rinse them and place in boiling water. Allow the water to reboil, and then simmer, brown or green lentils for 50 minutes, red lentils for 30 minutes. Sprouting the lentils for two days is a good idea, but not essential. Sprouting and cooking converts the starches *stachyose* and *raffinose* into a simpler starch that can be absorbed into the bloodstream. Otherwise flatulence can occur as the intestinal bacteria will convert those starches into carbon dioxide and hydrogen—especially if lentils are not part of your regular diet.

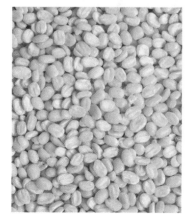

Lentils provide an excellent supply of organic iron (9 g, or 50% DV) and that's from a small 100-g serving. Beef only supplies 2 g iron! The secret behind the power of lentils is the potent iron content plus the supply of numerous minerals. From 1 cup of cooked lentils you obtain an excellent supply of phosphorus (50% DV), copper (25% DV), molybdenum (90% DV), manganese (30% DV), magnesium (25% DV), and zinc (20% DV). Try getting that value from takeout foods.

Lentils were once termed "poor man's meat"; they are now formally classified as the "rich, red, iron food"!

NOTE: DV amounts listed refer to the daily value for women 25–50 years; refer to DRI tables on pages 95–96 for adult male and child values.

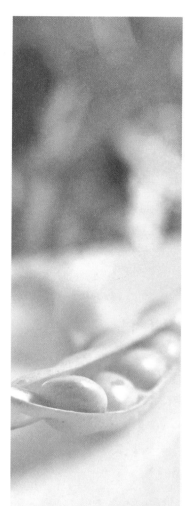

LIMA BEANS – *Phaseolus lunatus*

Lima beans gain their botanical name from the Greek word *phases*, for "aspect" or "appearance," and *lunatus,* derived from the Latin *luna*, meaning "moon." So lima beans "appear like the moon." They are available in white, red, brown, black, and purple varieties.

Lima beans are best soaked overnight, to reduce the *raffinose* starch, or oligosaccharides. Buy a few cans of cooked lima beans for a quick, easy added ingredient to many recipes.

Also known as butter beans, curry beans, pole beans, and sieva beans, lima beans originated from Lima, in Peru, over 7,000 years ago. They were discovered by Christopher Columbus and introduced to Europe and Asia. The protein content (21 g, or 43% DV) is complete in all essential amino acids, while the very low fat content (1 g, or 1% DV) means you can add butter to the beans, just before serving, and relax about the added calories. Lima beans provide only 6 calories from unsaturated fats; butter supplies 700 calories per 100 grams, or 100 calories per teaspoon. Because the recommended daily adult calorie intake is 2,500–3,000 kcal, a dab of butter with lima beans will easily fit into a balanced diet.

Lima beans are one of the foods richest in potassium (1,700 mg), containing an amount equal to soybeans and greater than any other legume or natural food. Potassium is heat sensitive and lima beans need to be cooked, but if they're presoaked and slow cooked, an abundance of potassium will still be supplied. The magnesium content (224 mg, or 56% DV) is not heat sensitive; neither is the phosphorus content (385 mg, or 38% DV). Both these major minerals are essential for the brain, nervous system, and heart muscles.

The manganese content (2 mg) is similar to that of sunflower seeds. After wheat germ, wheat bran, nuts, and seeds, lima beans are a very good source of this mineral. Manganese works with enzymes for energy production and as an antioxidant; the enzyme *superoxide dismutase* needs manganese to destroy free radicals within cells.

Even though they are white, lima beans are a rich source of organic iron (8 mg, or 42% DV). In addition, 1 cup of cooked lima beans provides the following nutrients: molybdenum (85% DV), folate (40%), phosphorus (30%), and copper (20%). Now that's a bean that's full of beans!

Lima beans do contain purines, naturally occurring substances that are broken down by the digestive system into uric acid. For people suffering from gout or kidney stones, it is best to avoid lima beans due to the purine content, but a healthy body can eliminate uric acid, which is also a by-product of meat consumption. In addition, lima beans provide no saturated fat or cholesterol.

The rich fiber content of lima beans actually lowers cholesterol and also promotes a steady supply of valuable starch energy—and all for a low price. Try a lima bean salad or the traditional native American dish succotash. Buy lima beans dried, canned, or frozen, and gain power from the protein, strength from the iron, and antioxidants from the manganese and molybdenum.

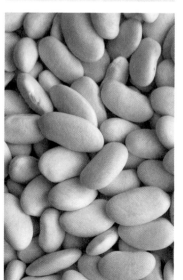

NOTE: Nutrient amounts are listed as milligrams (mg) per 100 grams (g), unless otherwise stated.

GLYCEMIC INDEX: 31	TOTAL CALORIES PER 100 G: 347	CALORIES FROM		
		CARB: 255 73%	PROTEIN: 83 24%	FAT: 10 3%

MUNG BEAN – *Vigna radiata*

Mung beans have been around since before recorded history. In India the mung bean was made into a flour or porridge, and in China mung bean sprouts were discovered thousands of years ago. Other names for the mung bean include golden gram, black gram, green gram, and Oregon pea. If you need protein, mung beans supply 24 g of complete protein, or 48% DV; mung bean sprouts supply 37 g of protein. Mung beans are full of dietary fiber (16 g, or 65% DV), making them beneficial for the elimination of toxic waste in the bowel. The iron content (7 mg, or 47% DV) is a bonus for the blood system, as are the manganese content (1 mg) and the supply of copper (1 mg, or 47% DV).

Mung beans are a very good source of magnesium (189 mg, or 47% DV), phosphorus (367 mg, or 37% DV), and folate (625 mcg, or 156% DV). In fact, they are one of the best sources of folate, which is essential for prevention of nervous fatigue, anemia, and blood disorders. It is also an essential nutrient for expectant mothers. Even a few cooked mung beans mixed into a soup or salad can make the world of difference to your well-being. The very good supply of potassium (1,246 mg, or 36% DV) and of zinc (3 mg) will help protect against infections and will improve blood circulation and nerve transmission. The fair amount of calcium (132 mg, or 13% DV) will assist digestion. Because mung beans provide a very low fat content of 1% by weight, you can easily add a cream sauce, mayonnaise, or salad dressing to boost the taste of the magnificent mung bean. Refer to page 111 for mung sprouts.

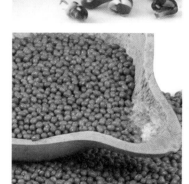

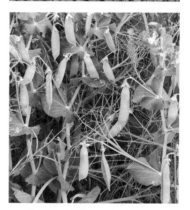

GLYCEMIC INDEX: 48	TOTAL CALORIES PER 100 G: 341	CALORIES FROM		
		CARB: 246 82%	PROTEIN: 85 25%	FAT: 10 3%

PEAS – *Pisum sativum/arvense*

Peas are possibly the most popular legume. Often considered a vegetable, botanically they belong to the pea and pod family (*Leguminosae*). Peas are a great companion to numerous foods—a steak meal would be very limited in numerous nutrients without peas, and the peas actually supply more iron (4 mg) than the steak (1.8 mg)! Peas are an excellent source of fiber (26 g, or 102% DV), magnesium (115 mg, or 30% DV), and potassium (981 mg, or 28% DV), whereas meat supplies no fiber, very little magnesium (20 mg), and only 318 mg of potassium. Peas are also a very good source of folate (274 mcg), another nutrient missing from meat. Folate stimulates the production of hydrochloric acid in the stomach, so a deficiency of this vitamin can reduce iron absorption and retard protein digestion. Eat your peas before the meat for better digestion.

Spring is pea season, so that's the time to stock up on the benefits of fresh snow peas and green peas and obtain a fair supply of vitamin K (19 mg), which is destroyed by freezing. The older we are, the more vitamin K we require. Meat and chicken supply no vitamin K, and digesting them can actually upset the intestinal bacteria that help manufacture vitamin K. The supply of copper from peas is good (1 mg, or 43% DV), whereas meat supplies only .007 mg of copper. Peas supply more protein (25 g, or 49% DV) than chicken (21 g) or beef (24 g), so pile on the peas. Fresh peas also deliver a sweet flavor due to their excellent carbohydrate (60 g) and sugar content (8 g). Oh, sweet pea!

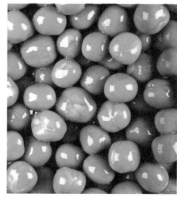

NOTE: DV amounts listed refer to the daily value for women 25–50 years; refer to DRI charts on pages 95–96 for adult male and child values.

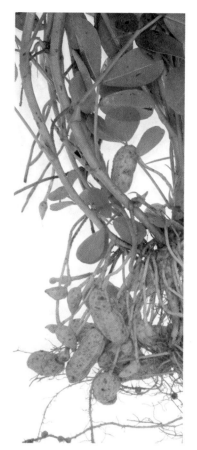

PEANUTS – *Arachis hypogaea*

Peanuts are often referred to as nuts; however, they are a member of the legume family (*Leguminosae*). Peanuts are unique among legumes because the seed or pea grows underground.

Peanuts provide more calories than any other legume, over 70% of which come from their fat content (49 g, or 76% DV). Peanuts provide a saturated fat content of 7 g, polyunsaturated 16 g, and monunsaturated 24 g. Most of the monunsaturated oils are in the form of oleic acid (70%), which is also contained in olive oil, and linoleic acid or omega-6 (20%), with only a trace of the essential and hard-to-get omega-3.

The most common use of peanuts is in the manufacture of peanut butter, whose rich supply of fats makes it a tempting food. Ideally, freshly made peanut butter—crunchy or smooth—can be enjoyed without any additives if you obtain it from a natural-foods store. The supermarket brands contain a lot of added salt (630 mg) and sugar (8.2 g), plus antioxidants (320) to retard spoilage. Furthermore, only 85% of conventional peanut butter is actually peanuts; the balance consists of added oils that have been hydrogenated to provide an even consistency. For the very best peanut butter, obtain it freshly ground, add a tablespoon of flaxseed oil, and mix well for a delicious spread on bread or toast. Note that peanuts provide protein (26 g, or 52% DV), but they are low in two essential amino acids: methionine and tryptophan. Peanuts have a net protein utilization of 43%.

Peanuts are a very good source of B vitamins, especially biotin, which is essential for fat metabolism and sugar metabolism, and which may prevent muscle cramps following excessive physical exertion. A quarter-cup serving supplies 26 mcg, or 87% DV, of this important nutrient. For active children, the biotin in peanut butter boosts power and coordination of muscles and also muscle tone. Vitamin B3 is very well supplied in peanuts (22 mg, or 120% DV), and because it is not heat sensitive the total value of this vitamin is available to assist in the production of energy from carbohydrates, protein, and fats. Pantothenic acid or vitamin B5 is also well supplied (2 mg, or 35% DV). It is required for energy production from foods but can be depleted during food processing.

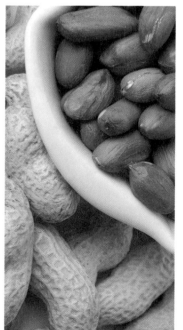

As a breakfast spread, peanut butter is great, but limit the spreading to less than twice a week, unless you add flaxseed oil for the omega-3 benefits. The supply of the trace mineral copper is very good from both peanuts (1.1 mcg, or 57% DV) and peanut butter (0.5 g). Copper is essential for the metabolism of fats. Isn't it remarkable how natural foods are balanced to "self-manage" their own digestion! Copper is also vital for the heart muscles and the nervous system. Peanuts' supply of folate (240 mcg, or 60% DV) is also very good. But how much peanut butter can you realistically eat? Ideally for children, about enough for two slices of toast, which provides approximately 20% of folate value. The rest of your folate is best supplied from broccoli, legumes, or cashews.

Peanuts also supply good amounts of magnesium (168 mg, or 42% DV), phosphorus (376 mg, or 38% DV), potassium (705 mg, or 20% DV), and zinc (3 mg, or 22% DV). Other benefits of peanuts are the supply of fiber (8 g, or 35% DV), vitamin E (8 mg, or 28% DV), and manganese (2 mg, or 70% DV).

Peanuts can cause severe allergic reactions in some people, and the oxalates they contain may cause problems with kidney stones and gallbladder conditions. Peanuts are an acidic food and thus are best eaten in moderation.

Peanuts provide protein and pure potential to promote power.

NOTE: Nutrient amounts are listed as milligrams (mg) per 100 grams (g), unless otherwise stated.

SOYBEANS – *Glycine max*

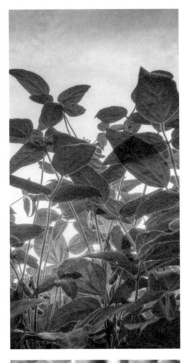

Soybeans are native to China, and for 4,000 years the Chinese have produced numerous foods and products from the cultivated soybean. Today, soybeans are available worldwide and are recognized as an excellent alkaline protein food; they provide 36 g, or 73% DV, from a small 100-g (3.5-oz) serving. Now that's protein power! In fact, soybeans are the fourth-best protein food, after tuna, other fish, and eggs (refer to pages 88–96).

Soybeans require a lot of cooking time and preparation. Fortunately, precooked, canned soybeans are very cheap. Soy products such as tofu—soybean curd—are an excellent protein food, easy to add to any stir-fry. Quickly fried, tofu acquires flavor and tastes great with green Asian vegetables and a splash of soy sauce.

Soybeans provide the essential fatty acids linoleic acid (omega-6) and linolenic acid (omega-3). That's a real bonus and a compelling reason to include more soy in the diet. Soy's excellent supply of lecithin is vital for protection from the excess cholesterol gained by consuming animal-product foods; soybeans supply no cholesterol, and soy oil provides a fair amount of omega-3 fatty acids (7 g). Ideally, add a tablespoon of flaxseed oil whenever you use soy oil.

Lecithin is a brain nutrient. If you are feeling fatigued, it may be due to a lack of iron, but also try adding a little lecithin to your breakfast cereal, omelet, or pancake mix to wake up your brain and nervous system. Most lecithin supplements are extracted from the mighty soybean.

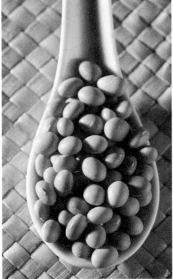

Soybeans are an excellent food for diabetics, especially those who are not insulin dependent, as the protein and fiber (9 g, or 37% DV) may help stabilize blood sugar levels. In some cases, regular use of soybeans has lowered diabetic patients' insulin medication requirements. In addition, soybeans can help to lower harmful high triglyceride levels in the blood, an important bonus for diabetics. For people with irritable bowel syndrome, soybean fiber may reduce symptoms such as diarrhea and constipation. Soybeans provide a nearly unique source of genistein, an isoflavone that may provide protection against prostate cancer by blocking cancer cells from reproducing.

Soy milk is a common alternative to dairy milk. For those with lactose intolerance or other dairy allergies, several varieties of soy milk are now available. Check the label to see if the soybeans used are genetically modified, and if so, avoid such products as they haven't been fully tested for safety.

Soybeans are an excellent source of the hard-to-find trace mineral molybdenum, which is vital for the brain and nervous system: 1 cup of soybeans provides nearly 80% DV Soybeans are a very good source of iron (8 mg), magnesium (280 mg, or 70% DV), and phosphorus (704 mg, or 70% DV). And as for folate, soybeans (375 mg) and soy flour (410 mg) are top providers. Soybeans also supply abundant vitamin K (190 mcg).

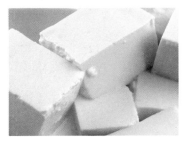

It takes time to get used to soy protein power, so start off with small servings of beans or tofu. In whatever form you choose, consume a soy-based meal at least weekly for a protein boost that surpasses any from beef. (Cows are often fed soy to promote growth.) For a dessert or sweet snack, try tofu ice cream, or make a milkshake from soy milk with a dash of added ice cream.

Soy can provide a range of benefits in most of its many edible forms (see opposite page). Soybeans are small in size but superior in sustenance.

SOYBEANS

NOTE: DV amounts listed refer to the daily value for women 25–50 years; refer to DRI charts on pages 95–96 for adult male and child values.

SOYBEANS | TRADITIONAL PRODUCTS

There are two types of soybeans: the edible bean and the commercial field variety. The majority of soy products are produced from the commercial field variety. Some of these products have been used for thousands of years and others have been developed only recently. Both the Chinese and the Japanese were using soy products long before the Western world even heard the word "soy."

TOFU: Developed by the Chinese, tofu is prepared from ground soybeans to which powdered gypsum is added to promote a curdled effect. It can be eaten at this stage or fermented to produce a high-protein tofu cheese.

MISO: Used by the Japanese for over 2,000 years, miso is prepared from fermented soybeans, cooked rice, and sea salt. Miso preparation is a very lengthy process: the mixture is placed in large wooden vats and slowly fermented with the organism *Aspergillus oryzae*. Miso is available at most natural-food stores. It supplies excellent amounts of protein and can be suitably combined with other ingredients to enhance soups, spreads, and gravies, or diluted and mixed with a salad dressing.

HAMANATTO: Also known as "miso beans," hamanatto was developed in Korea. It is made from steamed soy beans and roasted wheat which are combined and fermented. The mixture is poured into large wooden buckets and placed in the sun; salt and ginger are added. Fermenting takes about one year, and then the mixture is placed on wooden trays and allowed to dry. Hamanatto supplies excellent amounts of protein and combines well with most cooked meals.

NATTO: Developed by Buddhist monks over 2,000 years ago. The process uses cooked soybeans inoculated with *Bacillus subtilis*. The mixture is wrapped in thin sheets of pinewood and allowed to ferment for a few days.

SOY SAUCE: The most widely used soy product, soy sauce is prepared from cooked soybeans mixed with roasted wheat and then impregnated with the organism *Aspergillus oryzae*. The mixture is placed in wooden vats. Salt is added, and the brew is allowed to ferment for a minimum of six months, and sometimes up to five years. The finished product is strained and stored in glass containers. Soy sauce combines very well with savory rice dishes, salad dressings, gravies, and many meals. It is full of salt, however, so take it easy!

TAMARI: A similar product to soy sauce, but fermented for at least three years, tamari enhances the taste of rice dishes, fresh garden salads, and many other meals, cooked or raw. Tamari is available at most natural-food stores. Try the taste sometime; it's an excellent substitute for table salt. Fermented foods promote digestion and health.

SOY MILK: An excellent substitute for either powdered or pasteurized cow's milk, soy milk is prepared from presoaked, ground soybeans. The mixture is then boiled, strained, and reboiled. Commercial soy milk is available in either a dry powdered form or a liquid form. Compared to cow's milk, soy milk is not mucus forming, far richer in the mineral iron (containing over eight times more), and more compatible with human digestion. The taste is different from cow's milk: try a 50–50 combination to start, and slowly wean yourself off the cow's milk. You will obtain the best of both taste and nutrients. Avoid those winter coughs: Avoid cow's milk.

SOY GRITS: An essential food for every kitchen, soy grits are prepared from cracked soybeans. The main advantage over whole beans is that they require far less cooking time—less than half an hour at moderate heat. Soy grits will enhance the protein value of all meals. Serve them as a side dish mixed with steamed vegetables, combined with any soup or casserole, or alongside cooked mung beans.

SOY FLOUR: An excellent source of complete protein, soy flour comes in three varieties: full-fat (20% fat content); medium-fat (5%); or the popular fat-free variety. Soy flour contains no gluten, so it produces a very compact homemade bread. In combination with wheat, rye, or triticale flour, soy flour could be used in the following proportions: three cups wheat (or rye or triticale) flour to half a cup of soy flour. That combination will produce a light bread with an exceptional protein content. Make sure your kitchen is always stocked with some soy flour and soy oil (refer to page 143).

TEMPEH: Developed in Indonesia, tempeh is prepared from fermented soybeans and then wrapped in banana leaves; the result is a "cheese" with a very distinct taste.

NOTE: Nutrient amounts are listed as milligrams (mg) per 100 grams (g), unless otherwise stated.

Legumes	Main Nutrients, Antioxidants, and Phytonutrients	Aids Which Body Systems
Carob	alkaline, pectin, fiber, calcium, potassium, zinc, iron, carbohydrates	digestive, muscular
Chickpeas	protein, fiber, folate, iron, copper, manganese, potassium, molybdenum	blood , circulatory
Green Beans	folate, potassium, fiber, vitamin A, plant hormones, vitamin K	circulatory, digestive
Kidney Beans	protein, calcium, carbohydrates, fiber, potassium, folate, iron, molybdenum, magnesium, copper	elimination, digestive, growth, blood
Lentils	protein, carbohydrates, fiber, iron, phosphorus, molybdenum	digestive, blood
Lima Beans	protein, magnesium, carbohydrates, phosphorus, iron, molybdenum, fiber, folate, copper, manganese	nervous, blood, elimination, cellular
Mung Beans	protein, fiber, iron, magnesium, folate, potassium, carbohydrates	blood, elimination
Peas	fiber, iron, magnesium, folate, copper, protein, vitamin K	nervous, blood
Peanut	biotin, protein, vitamin B3, folate, magnesium, phosphorus, fiber, manganese, vitamin B5, copper	nervous, muscular, growth
Soybeans	protein, lecithin, fiber, genisten, molybdenum, iron, magnesium, phosphorus, folate, vitamin K, omega-6, omega-3	growth, circulatory, blood, nervous

RECOMMENDATIONS FOR DAILY CARBOHYDRATE INTAKE FROM LEGUMES		Adult Male	Adult Female	Teenager	Child
Total Daily Carbohydrate Intake (based on typical guidelines)		340 g	280 g	400 g	270 g
1. *UNH* recommendation: 20% of carbohydrate intake from legumes		68 g	56 g	80 g	54 g
Note the carb content of common legumes	100 g (3–4 oz) raw legumes*	approx. 12 g of carbohydrate			
	100 g cooked legumes*	approx. 20 g of carbohydrate			
2. U.S. MyPlate and DRIs		3 servings	2 servings	3 servings	2 servings
3. Australian Guide to Healthy Eating		80 g	80 g	80 g	75 g

RECOMMENDATIONS FOR DAILY PROTEIN INTAKE FROM LEGUMES		Adult Male	Adult Female	Teenager	Child
Total Daily Protein Intake (based on typical guidelines)		218 g	170 g	220 g	160 g
1. *UNH* recommendation: 15% of protein intake from legumes		32 g	25 g	33 g	24 g
Note the protein content of common legumes	100 g (3–4 oz) raw legumes*	approx. 4 g of protein			
	100 g cooked legumes*	approx. 8 g of protein			
2. U.S. MyPlate and DRIs		2 servings	1 serving	2 servings	1 serving
3. Australian Guide to Healthy Eating		80 g	80 g	80 g	75 g

UNH = Ultimate Nutrition for Health
DRIs = Dietary Reference Intakes
* 80–100 g of fresh or cooked legumes is equivalent to approx. ½ cup.

For thousands of years fruits have been carefully cultivated to improve quality and increase the varieties available from around the world. These days, we can be thankful and feel fortunate to have such a wide selection of delicious fruits to choose from. Our predecessors would truly have been awed to visit the produce section of a modern-day supermarket.

To ensure maximum nutrition, the human diet needs fresh fruits. On average, 20% of the daily food supply is best obtained as fresh fruits.

Fruits provide an alkaline balance to the blood, which is most beneficial for healing.

Fruits assist in the proper elimination of toxins and body waste, essential for maintenance of daily health.

Fruits are the most refreshing food, especially during hot weather. Store most fruits in the fridge to supply extra crunch and freshness. Fruits are the best foods to enjoy after a complete fast or whenever you need a "mini fast" to offset the effects of those complex protein meals.

The human digestive system is well suited to fruits. The length of the digestive tract is about 12–14 times the height of the body, which is a ratio similar to that of most fruit-eating animals. (The herbivore's digestive tract is approximately 20 times the length of the body, the carnivore's about five times.) Because our complex digestive system is well adapted to fruits, we can expect to obtain maximum nutritional benefit from the proper combination of fruits.

There are four main fruit groups: sweet fruits, sub-acid fruits, acid fruits, and melons. For more on this topic, see page 209. For information on combining other foods with fruits, refer to page 208.

Fruits provide a unique abundance of fruit sugar, termed fructose, which is an ideal source of natural energy. They also provide a variety of minerals and vitamins to assist in the utilization of their fructose content, as well as numerous other positive benefits for health and healing.

Fresh fruits are the easiest food to digest, especially when eaten either on their own or in a fruit salad.

Fruits, with their colorful natural packaging, are also the best "portable" foods. They are ready to go.

Most fruits are best when picked ripe directly from the tree, bush, vine, or plant. However, many people live a long way from the nearest fruit tree. The supermarket, farmer's market, and local fruit stand do their best to supply fruits as fresh as possible.

All fruits afford a unique combination of some of the essential human nutrients. The following pages point out the main nutrient benefits of 32 different fruits. Use this information to reap specific health and healing benefits.

To name just one benefit, fruits are excellent sources of antioxidants. We need all the anticancer and disease-prevention resources we can get, and there are many antioxidants that are only available from fresh fruits—all in the greatest array of unique, sweet flavors and amazing textures.

Welcome to the fruit kingdom. Let fruits provide you with their exceptional health benefits. It would be a dull world indeed without fruits.

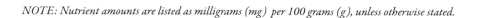

NOTE: Nutrient amounts are listed as milligrams (mg) per 100 grams (g), unless otherwise stated.

APPLES – *Malus domestica*

Apples are of great benefit to the digestive system. Their excellent supply of pectin and malic acid both stimulate the digestive system and cleanse it by eliminating toxins from the small intestine. Whenever you have a weak digestive system, let the apple give you strength. For digestive problems, steam a green granny smith apple. Then progress to fresh ripe apples. If you can "stomach" the apple, you're on your way to recovery.

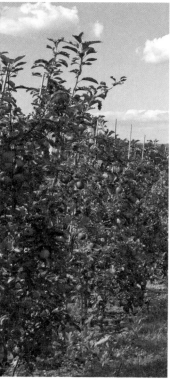

Pectin is a soluble fiber; apples contain 0.78 g per 100 g. Pectin slows digestion and moderates the rise in blood sugar. Because apples have a low glycemic index (36), they are an ideal food for hyperactive children or diabetics. Pectin also reduces the amount of cholesterol produced by the liver, and it may lower blood cholesterol levels and reduce the risk of heart disease. Pectin is especially concentrated in the apple peel. Pectin removes toxins from the digestive tract by supplying a substance called *galacturonic acid*. Pectin promotes proper protein digestion, as it prevents digested proteins in the small intestine from spoiling.

The malic acid content of apples prevents liver disorders and promotes better digestion. Apples' alkaline elements increase the flow of saliva, which boosts carbohydrate digestion.

Red apples contain anthocyanins, which are powerful antioxidants. All apples contain flavonoid antioxdants, such as catechins and quercetin. One study showed a decrease in mental deterioration due to flavonoids, and another study concluded that flavonoids protect against the effects of tobacco carcinogens in cases of bladder cancer.

Apples, the richest fruit source of the flavonoid quercetin, were found to protect against lung cancer and reduce the risk of thrombiotic strokes. The bioavailability of quercetin in apples is among the best; *even a day after eating an apple,* the level of quercetin in the blood is still considered effective. A National Cancer Institute report stated that quercetin helps to prevent the growth of prostate cancer cells.

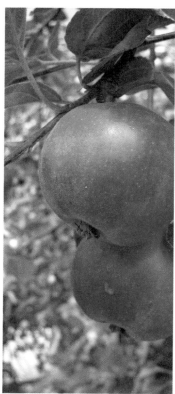

Research has shown that the phytochemicals in the apple skin restrict the growth of colon cancer cells by 43%; however, you have to get your "apple a day" quota to reap those benefits, and the average consumption of apples is one every five days. Additional apple research has discovered the following benefits: a reduction in type 2 diabetes, reduced incidence of asthma, and reduction of cholesterol from consuming apples and apple juice, due to the supply of phytonutrients.

A study at the University of California showed that eating two apples a day, or drinking apple juice, reduced the oxidation of cholesterol and the buildup of arterial plaque. The risk from pulmonary disease in smokers was also reduced by half.

Apples provide potassium (110 mg), vitamin A (90 mg), and trace amounts of vitamins B1, B2, and B3, as well as biotin, folate, vitamin C, and vitamin E (0.71 mg).

Keep red and golden-delicious apples in the fridge for a cool, crisp crunch, and try juicing your own apples. Apple juice is great when combined with pineapple juice.

NOTE: DV amounts listed refer to the daily value for women 25–50 years; refer to DRI charts on pages 95–96 for adult male and child values.

GLYCEMIC INDEX:	TOTAL CALORIES PER 100 G (dried):	CALORIES FROM		
		CARB: 300	PROTEIN: 26	FAT: 39
56	365	82%	7%	11%

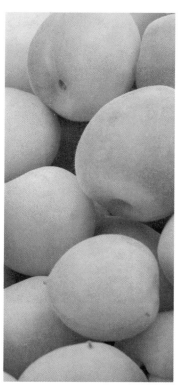

APRICOTS – *Prunus armeniaca*

Apricots provide an excellent supply of carotene (2,985 IU) with the majority in the form of beta-carotene (1,696 mcg), beta cryptoxanthin (161 mcg), and lutein and zeaxanthin (138 mcg). Fresh and dried apricots are of great benefit for the respiratory system. Beta-carotene, a precursor to vitamin A, protects the lungs and respiratory system from infections. It is also vital for healing damaged skin, and it promotes the life of the skin cell through its antioxidant effect on free radicals. The potassium content of fresh apricots is very good at 400 mg. Dried apricots supply 1,510 mg. The combination of potassium and carotene makes apricots a healing food. Potassium repairs muscle and improves blood circulation and blood condition.

Apricots' good supply of silicon promotes skin rejuvenation and cleanses the blood. Apricots are ideal for the blood, skin, and eyes. The supply of lutein, zeaxanthin, and silicon protects against lens deterioration. The potassium in apricots promotes nerve transmission to the brain and retards the process of aging.

Apricots supply copper (0.4 mg) and they are a good source of the trace mineral molybdenum, required for elimination of body waste.

Apricots provide antioxidants from their excellent supply of flavonoids. There are two main types of dried apricots: sun-dried and sulfur-dried. Sulfur-dried apricots are treated with sulfur dioxide, which may be a problem for asthmatics. Sun-dried apricots provide the maximum nutritional value. A safe food for children, they are ideal as a teething aid and energy source. Apricots, fresh and dried, are waiting to be appreciated.

GLYCEMIC INDEX: VERY LOW	TOTAL CALORIES PER 100 G:	CALORIES FROM		
		CARB: 31	PROTEIN: 7	FAT: 123
	160	19%	4%	77%

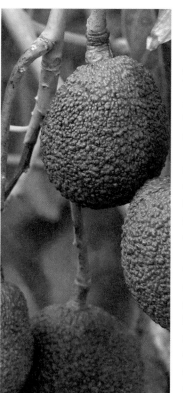

AVOCADO – *Persea americana*

The avocado is the fruit of a tree that belongs to the Laurel family (*Lauraceae*). The Aztecs originally cultivated the avocado. Now there are numerous varieties throughout the world. The hass and fuerte are the most common ones; the gwen, bacon, pinkerton, zutano, and reed are other varieties.

Avocados provide a small amount of the essential fatty acid omega-3. The fact that avocado is eaten raw promotes maximum benefits. About 77% of the avocado is in the form of lipids: 70% are monounsaturated, 12% polyunsaturated, and 15% saturated. The rich oleic acid content is beneficial for reduction of blood cholesterol. Furthermore, avocados contain lecithin, which further reduces blood cholesterol levels. For more information on avocado oil, refer to page 140.

The avocado is a good source of potassium (485–600 mg), a heat-sensitive nutrient vital for the heart muscles. Avocados' very good supply of chlorine (645 mg) and sulfur (505 mg) assists digestion of the fats as well as promoting body cleansing. Avocados are a safe food for diabetics, with a zero glycemic index and that good supply of potassium. The folate content (58 mcg) helps prevent cardiovascular disease. The magnesium (29–45 mg) and phosphorus (52 mg) in avocado are nourishing to the nervous system. The avocado contains no cholesterol and is not a fattening food because the monounsaturated fats are easily used by the body for energy. Few foods can spread so many amazing benefits as the outstanding avocado. Treat your body to an avocado dip today or on your next picnic!

NOTE: Nutrient amounts are listed as milligrams (mg) per 100 grams (g), unless otherwise stated.

GLYCEMIC INDEX: 55	TOTAL CALORIES PER 100 G: 89	CALORIES FROM		
		CARB: 83 93%	PROTEIN: 4 4%	FAT: 3 3%

BANANA – *Musa* spp.

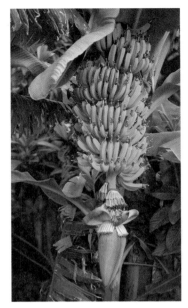

Bananas are big in carbohydrate value. They contain only 89 calories and 0.3 g of fat per 100 g; therefore, you can eat them all day long and never put on weight. Due to the fact that bananas are mainly eaten raw, the full value of the potassium content (370 mg, or 467 mg in the average banana) is available, providing great benefit for the muscular system, the heart muscles, and the skeletal system. Potassium-rich foods counteract the problems with excess intake of salt, such as the loss of calcium from the bones. Bananas are rich in potassium and low in organic sodium (1 mg), thereby promoting an alkaline condition in the blood, which is essential for healing and proper calcium metabolism.

Bananas contain serotonin and norepinephrine, natural hormones that can help to reduce depression. Furthermore, bananas have a moderate glycemic index.

If you are an active person, the banana will easily support your energy requirements and help keep your body flexible and running smoothly. For children, the banana smoothie is a naturally sweet supplier of protein and other nutrients. Get your share of the banana's benefits midmorning, before the chip cravings begin.

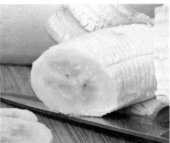

Bananas aid the digestive system due to their pectin content, plus they supply iron (0.7 mg), chlorine (270 mg), sulfur (120 mg), and bromine (0.54 mg), all essential for the glandular and blood system. You have to hand it to bananas, they really offer the sweetest energy. A cavendish banana—the most common variety—with a hint of green near the stem is best for digestion. Lady finger bananas (also known as baby bananas) need to be fully ripe for the best taste and texture.

If you have a digestive problem or lack energy and can't put your finger on the problem, ask yourself, "Have I had a banana recently?"

GLYCEMIC INDEX: <65	TOTAL CALORIES PER 100 G: 56	CALORIES FROM		
		CARB: 52 93%	PROTEIN: 3 5%	FAT: 1 2%

BERRIES – *Rubus ulmifolius, R. loganobaccus*

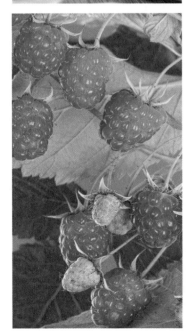

Berries of the *Rubus* family include blackberry, boysenberry, dewberry, cloudberry, loganberry, raspberry, and wineberry. The raspberry and loganberry are the most popular commercially grown Rubus berries. Red berries contain the phytochemicals lycopene and anthocyanins. Lycopene is a very potent antioxidant, and it helps protect the skin against damage from sunlight. Berries colored blue, purple, and black contain antioxidants such as anthocyanins and phenolics. In a list of the top antioxidant foods, measured in units known as as the *oxygen radical absorbance capacity* (ORAC), blackberries measured 2,036 per 100 g; raspberries 1,220; and blueberries 2,400—far more than any vegetable. For example, spinach, at 1,260, measures highest of the common vegetables; broccoli comes in at 890. Berries are a potent source of valuable antioxidant benefits. They reduce the risk of various types of cancer, improve the health of the circulatory system, and reduce the problems of excess cholesterol. Buy or grow beautiful berries. (Refer to page 58 for the strawberry.) Try berries and ice cream for a cool and fabulous party dessert!

NOTE: DV amounts listed refer to the daily value for women 25–50 years; refer to DRI charts on pages 95–96 for adult male and child values.

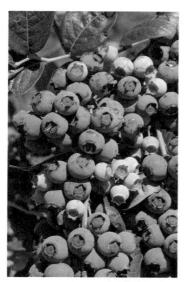

GLYCEMIC INDEX:	TOTAL CALORIES PER 100 G:	CALORIES FROM		
		CARB: 52	PROTEIN: 3	FAT: 1
<65	56	93%	5%	2%

BLUEBERRIES – *Vaccinium* spp.

Blueberries, cranberries, and bilberries all belong to the family *Vaccinium*. They all contain a remarkable supply of antioxidants—more specifically phytonutrients or anthocyanins—which are housed in the fruits' blue-red pigments. These substances promote a reduction of free radicals that can damage cell structure, causing conditions such as heart disease, glaucoma, and cataracts.

Blueberries protect the brain from oxidative stress, possibly retarding the onset of such conditions as dementia. Another antioxidant in blueberries is ellagic acid, which has the ability to inhibit the formation of cancer; this in combination with their good supply of vitamin C gives blueberries a true-blue value. Cranberries provide antibiotic qualities against E. coli, combat urinary infections, and protect against dental plaque and tooth decay. The bilberry is a great food for the eyes; it is usually taken as a concentrated extract and may afford benefit in cases of glaucoma, cataracts, and diabetes. Try blueberry jam with pancakes and cream for a simple and nourishing breakfast or brunch. Three cheers for the beaut blueberry!

GLYCEMIC INDEX:	TOTAL CALORIES PER 100 G:	CALORIES FROM		
		CARB: 30	PROTEIN: 3	FAT: 2
65	34	85%	9%	6%

CANTALOUPE – *Cucumis melo*

Cantaloupe, or rockmelon as we call it in Australia, belongs to the same family as pumpkin, cucumber, and zucchini, the *Cucurbitaceae*. Cantaloupe are a very good source of vitamin A (3,382 IU), nearly all of it in the form of the precursor beta-carotene (2,020 mcg). This is a vital nutrient for the optic system and in particular for protection from cataracts. The beta-carotene content combined with cantaloupe's good supply of vitamin C (37 mg) gives the fruit antioxidant power that has the potential to activate white blood cells against infections and bad bacteria. A fully ripened cantaloupe provides a very sweet meal, making it ideal as a breakfast entrée on a hot summer's day. The potassium content (267 mg) is fully available since the fruit is eaten raw. Potassium promotes muscle power and healthy heart function.

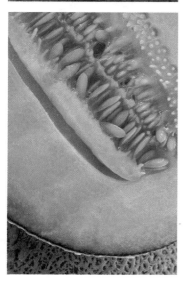

Cantaloupe offers an excellent supply of the trace mineral bromine, which is present in the bloodstream and other bodily tissues and is vital for the glandular system—in particular, prior to and during menopause. A decrease in bromine levels occurs with age, and the bromine levels in the pituitary gland need to be replenished in order to avoid emotional disorders, depression, and premenstrual tension. A regular dose of bromine may offset emotional depression in men experiencing a "midlife crisis." Bromine is not considered an essential mineral, but its benefits are, so keep your emotional life "rock solid" with a regular supply of rockmelon, the food for a peaceful, balanced life!

Cantaloupe also provides folate (21 mcg), ideal for those people who don't like their greens. Cantaloupes are best eaten alone, before a main meal; otherwise they can ferment in the stomach. Melons require hardly any digestion so give them the right of way in the busy traffic of your complex digestive system. Cantaloupes are the ideal food for the elderly, as they are very easy to chew and provide an abundance of life-promoting health benefits. Choose a fully ripened fruit for complete flavor. Roll out the cantaloupe and feel on top of the world at the start of a day. (See page 53 for other melons.)

NOTE: Nutrient amounts are listed as milligrams (mg) per 100 grams (g), unless otherwise stated.

GLYCEMIC INDEX: 22	TOTAL CALORIES PER 100 G: 63	CALORIES FROM		
		CARB: 58 91%	PROTEIN: 4 6%	FAT: 2 3%

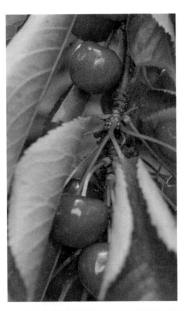

CHERRIES – *Prunus avium, P. cerasus*

Cherries provide a very low glycemic index, making them an ideal fruit for diabetics and hyperactive children. Not only are they much better than candy; they're also the candy look-alike of the fruit world! Cherries are packed with painkilling power due to their supply of anthocyanins, which are housed in the fruit's pigments. A quantity of 20 cherries supplies about 25 mg anthocyanins. Anthocyanins retard the enzymes that cause tissue inflammation and are as effective as aspirin or ibuprofen in cases of headache, gout, or arthritis. Cherries also contain the flavonoids isoqueritrin and queritrin plus the plant phenolic ellagic acid, a potent anticarcinogenic and antimutagenic compound. In addition, cherries are packed with perillyl alcohol, which stunts the growth of cancer cells and flushes them out of the body. Cherries provide significant amounts of melatonin, produced by the pineal gland to promote sleep. Cherries are a blood builder, and they supply vitamin A (213 IU) and potassium (220 mg). If cherries seem expensive, it's because the trees take years to grow, the fruit is hand picked, and they have a very short summer season. As they say, you get what you pay for. Have a good night's sleep, reduce pain, and cherish the cheerful cherry.

GLYCEMIC INDEX: 50	TOTAL CALORIES PER 100 G: 63	CALORIES FROM		
		CARB: 55 87%	PROTEIN: 5 8%	FAT: 3 5%

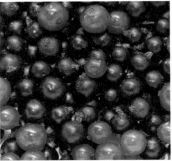

CURRANTS – *Ribes nigrum/R. americanum*

Currants are available in red, black, or white varieties. They aren't very common in the United States, where restrictions have been placed on growing them because they are a host for a plant disease called white pine blister rust. In countries where currants are popular, blackcurrants are the most common. They provide the maximum vitamin C content, with 155–215 mg. White and red currants provide 41–81 mg; dried currants provide 3 mg. The recommended dietary intake of vitamin C for adults is 30–40 mg per day; 60 mg during pregnancy. Blackcurrants are the third-best food source of natural vitamin C, a nutrient that you need every day. Vitamin C's benefits for the immune system and other bodily systems are numerous. (Refer to page 164 for details.) It is an antioxidant, so it protects tissues from free-radical damage. It promotes fat metabolism and is vital for the eyes, teeth, and bones. A handful of blackcurrants will provide an incredible boost to your immune system. Blackcurrant syrup can be a good provider of vitamin C and possibly of the other benefits afforded by this fruit, but check the label for additives.

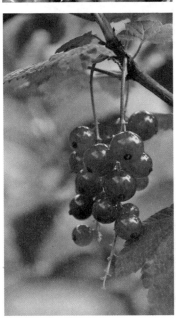

Besides vitamin C, blackcurrants provide exceptional amounts of other antioxidants. They supply nearly double the amount of anthocyanins and polyphenols as blueberries. Anthocyanins are very effective in locating free radicals and destroying their functioning. They also reduce the risk of cholesterol particles attaching to arterial walls, a condition that can eventually lead to high blood pressure and strokes. Blackcurrants are also an excellent source of flavonoids, and they supply a fair amount of iron (2.3 mg), calcium (87 mg, dried), vitamin A (230 IU), carotenes, and potassium (322 mg). For smokers, blackcurrant in fruit or syrup form is very beneficial. Dried blackcurrants are a great sweet treat. Include blackcurrants in your diet to tap into their pure antioxidant power.

NOTE: DV amounts listed refer to the daily value for women 25–50 years; refer to DRI charts on pages 95–96 for adult male and child values.

GLYCEMIC INDEX: 103	TOTAL CALORIES PER 100 G: 282	CALORIES FROM		
		CARB: 270 96%	PROTEIN: 8 3%	FAT: 3 1%

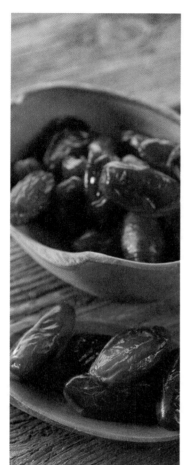

DATES – *Phoenix dactylifera*

Fresh and dried dates are a compact energy food with 75% carbohydrate content and 8 g of fiber—that's bulky. If you lack energy and need a quick snack, dates will boost your whole body. They provide the muscular system with 650–730 mg of potassium, which improves blood circulation, prevents hardening of the arteries, and assists healing. They also supply 1 mg of iron. Both minerals help to utilize oxygen and normalize heart-muscle action.

Dates are a fair source of magnesium (43 mg), calcium (39 mg), and phosphorus (62 mg), all essential for bone strength, healthy nerves, and brain function. Dates provide complete protein in small amounts (2 g). There is no doubt that you could survive in the wilderness with fresh dates for a long time, as they provide energy and a wide variety of nutrients.

The very high glycemic index of dates needs to be considered. They can be beneficial in cases of low blood sugar, or for "instant energy" after a physical or mental workout. Approximately 90% of all glucose (blood sugar) is required for efficient brain functioning. However, for diabetics, dates are best avoided. Ideally, dip dates into tahini for a magnificent snack with a lower glycemic index than dates alone.

Dates are known to strengthen the muscles of the uterus during pregnancy, and they are an ideal snack during lactation because they alleviate depression. Dates also supply copper (0.29 mg) and manganese (0.30 mg). Dates provide 2.8% total mineral content, nearly top of the list of all foods. Dates are usually sold as sun-dried, but fresh dates are best. Dates were given to warriors to stimulate their muscles due to their enormous supply of potassium; nowadays, they are a great food for hikers and backpackers. Try some fresh dates next chance you get. They are the super sweet!

GLYCEMIC INDEX: 61	TOTAL CALORIES PER 100 G: 249	CALORIES FROM		
		CARB: 230 93%	PROTEIN: 11 4%	FAT: 8 3%

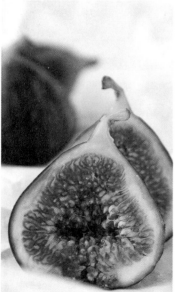

FIGS – *Ficus carica*

Figs provide more minerals than dates, with a far lower GI index. Figs are the best fruit source of calcium (dried, 162 mg; fresh, 35 mg). For a calcium-rich treat, dip figs into tahini. Figs also provide an abundance of potassium (680 mg), which improves calcium balance; people whose diet includes added salt need extra potassium.

A small serving of figs supplies nearly half the day's essential dietary fiber. Research has shown that high-fiber foods reduce the appetite and may assist weight loss. Figs can be baked into cookies, and they make an ideal mid-morning snack with a cup of tea.

Figs supply a good amount of organic iron (2.2 mg), manganese (0.38 mg), and copper (0.30 mg)—a great combination of minerals for building blood and for protection against fatigue, especially since figs also contain a good supply of carbohydrates. Figs supply magnesium (58 mg), phosphorus (67 mg), and silicon (240 mg). If you're feeling teary or weary, call figs to the rescue. Potassium provides muscle power to overcome the obstacles of the tasks ahead of you, and chlorine (100 mg) and sulfur (270 mg) will ensure that your inner state is also tended to. Fresh figs are a most delightful fruit. Forget fatigue with figs!

NOTE: Nutrient amounts are listed as milligrams (mg) per 100 grams (g), unless otherwise stated.

GLYCEMIC INDEX: 25	TOTAL CALORIES PER 100 G: 39	CALORIES FROM		
		CARB: 36 92%	PROTEIN: 2 5%	FAT: 1 3%

GRAPEFRUIT – *Citrus paradisi*

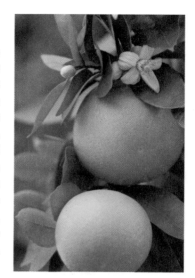

Grapefruit are the second-largest largest citrus fruit (after pomelo), with pale yellow, pink, or ruby flesh. Their bitterness comes from the phytochemical liminoid. Choose very ripe grapefruit for less bitterness. To dull the bitter taste, drizzle a little honey on the fresh fruit, or blend the juice with strawberry juice. Liminoids afford some health benefits: They promote the formation of a detoxifying enzyme, glutathione-S-transferase, that inhibits tumor formation, especially in cases of oral, pancreatic, colon, or stomach cancer. Grapefruit also contains lycopene, a plant pigment that provides similar antitumor and antioxidant activity to fight against atherosclerosis, cataracts, arthritis, and other diseases caused by oxidative stress. Grapefruit contains salicylic acid, which dissolves inorganic calcium, a cause of arthritis. Grapefruit reduces body acidity and protects against kidney stone development. Grapefruit is a good source of vitamin C (38 mg). It supplies biotin (3 mcg), which promotes fat reduction, a bonus when paired with grapefruit's naturally low calorie count and its supply of vitamin B5 (0.28 mg). Grapefruit are a great fruit to reduce body weight and acidity, and to protect against tumors.

GLYCEMIC INDEX: 46	TOTAL CALORIES PER 100 G: 67	CALORIES FROM		
		CARB: 62 93%	PROTEIN: 3 4%	FAT: 2 3%

GRAPES – *Vitis rotundifolia, V. labrusca, V. vinifera*

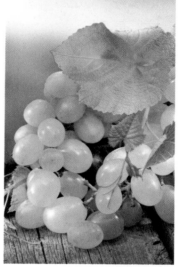

Grapes are one of the most commonly cultivated fruits, mainly for the wine industry, with numerous varieties that rarely reach the local supermarket. Table grapes, the kind that are sold for eating, come in blue, red, purple, green, and yellow varieties.

Fresh grapes afford numerous benefits for the blood system. If you need a natural blood boost, eat a bunch of grapes every day for a week, or drink a freshly pressed glass of grape juice daily. The manganese content (0.8 mg) from one cup of grapes supplies 20% of the daily requirement. Manganese is vital for red blood cell development and for memory; it is especially important during lactation. Grapes also supply tartaric acid, which stimulates the intestines. Red, blue, and purple grapes contain saponin, a glucose-based compound that reduces inflammation and also helps lower cholesterol by reducing oxidation. Furthermore, grapes contain the antioxidant quercetin (see the entry for apples, page 44, for a description of quercetin's benefits).

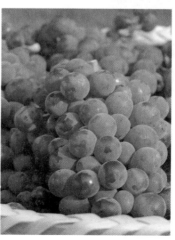

The skin of grapes contains transresveratrol, a natural antibiotic that fights prostate and lung cancer. It inhibits carcinogens from binding to cell receptors, thereby helping to stop the spread of cancer. In addition, it may promote longevity and decrease the risk of heart disease. Grape skin also contains phenolic compounds; these inhibit enzymes that cause blood vessels to constrict and reduce the supply of oxygen to the heart. Grapes increase the body's production of nitric oxide, an antioxidant that protects against blood-clot formation in arteries and reduces oxidation of blood plasma and cholesterol. Grapes also increase blood levels of vitamin E.

Grapes are in season for just a few months, so take advantage of grape season to boost your blood and protect your immune system. Grape juice provides concentrated benefits. Make your own fresh grape juice regularly, and when grapes are out of season, try good-quality grape juice from the store. A "glass of red before bed" will provide a good night's sleep in addition to grapes' natural antibiotic qualities. Grapes are great, mate!

NOTE: DV amounts listed refer to the daily value for women 25–50 years; refer to DRI charts on pages 95–96 for adult male and child values.

GLYCEMIC INDEX:	TOTAL CALORIES PER 100 G:	CALORIES FROM		
<50	68	CARB: 51 75%	PROTEIN: 9 13%	FAT: 8 12%

GUAVA – *Psidium guajava*

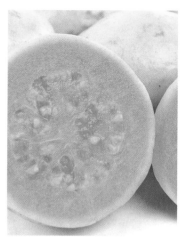

The guava comes in two varieties: green or "apple" (the most common variety in the United States) and red or "strawberry." It has been named gold medalist in one survey that measured four nutrients—vitamin C, carotenoids, folate, and potassium—plus fiber. The guava heads the list with a score of over 400, far greater than any other fruit. Watermelon comes in second, with less than half the value of guava.

There is no doubt that the vitamin C content of fresh guavas is excellent, with over 200 mg per 100 g, about four times that of oranges. Aside from the very hot red peppers, the guava is the richest natural source of vitamin C—and how many hot peppers can you eat in one day? If you are a smoker, you need to replenish vitamin C every few hours, because each cigarette removes about 30 mg of vitamin C from the body. Eating a boxful every week might be the best advice till you quit smoking. The contraceptive pill and antibiotics also deplete vitamin C. If you spend time looking at a computer screen or television, then extra vitamin C is required just to prevent eyestrain. The lens of the eye is dependant on a regular supply of vitamin C—at least twice daily. Keep your eyes open for guavas in season and treat your body to the most abundant supply of vitamin C that nature can provide.

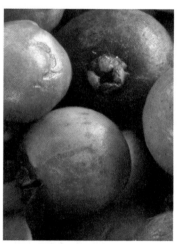

Vitamin C is also considered the antistress vitamin, mainly because it is stored in the adrenal glands, where it can be accessed in case of an emergency, a shock to the system, an unexpected noise, or bad news. The adrenal glands produce the hormone adrenaline, which is involved in digestion, glucose production, regulating heart rate, the nervous system, and dealing with conditions of stress, fear, and excitement.

Guava also provides a fair amount of vitamin A precursors (625 IU), nearly all in the form of lutein and zeaxanthin (5,000 mcg), which are vital for protection from ultraviolet radiation, especially in the eyes.

Even one guava a day can give your eyes great protection, especially for folks over fifty who view the computer or TV for hours a day. Guava is the tropical fruit to set your sights on!

GLYCEMIC INDEX:	TOTAL CALORIES PER 100 G:	CALORIES FROM		
52	61	CARB: 54 88%	PROTEIN: 3 5%	FAT: 4 7%

KIWI – *Actinidia chinensis/A. deliciosa*

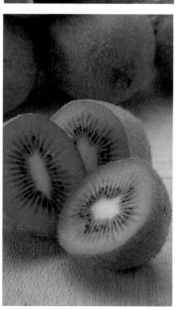

Kiwi, also called kiwifruit or gooseberry, are best known for their distinctive appearance when sliced for fruit salads or desserts. The kiwifruit is a fair source of vitamin A (175 IU) and an excellent source of vitamin C (75–97 mg)—even better than oranges. It is a great alternative for people who dislike citrus fruits. One kiwifruit can provide twice the daily vitamin C requirement for adults. Let the kiwifruit balance and protect your immune system.

Kiwi also provide the trace mineral copper (0.16 mg), a fair iron content (0.41 mg), a good supply of potassium (330 mg), and a small amount of calcium (26 mg). Kiwifruit contain phytonutrients that protect the development of new cells from oxidative stress—an action also provided by vitamin C. For children, kiwifruit have proved beneficial in cases of respiratory problems such as night-coughing and wheezing. Try kiwifruit in your next tropical fruit salad, or try a juice combination of apple and kiwi. The kiwi, when consumed regularly, can be an ideal natural remedy for a child's cough.

NOTE: Nutrient amounts are listed as milligrams (mg) per 100 grams (g), unless otherwise stated.

GLYCEMIC INDEX: <20	TOTAL CALORIES PER 100 G: 29	CALORIES FROM		
		CARB: 23 77%	PROTEIN: 4 13%	FAT: 3 10%

LEMONS AND LIMES – *Citrus limon, C. aurantifolia*

Both lemons and limes are full of citric acid, about 6% by weight. One benefit of citric acid is that it preserves vitamin C activity. Many people reach for a lemon or lime when they have a cold, sore throat, or congestion. Lots of cold medicines contain lemon or lime extracts, but without a doubt a freshly squeezed lemon will provide the maximum benefit. Citric acid relieves congestion, and the sulfur content (125 mg) of these fruits is a bonus because it dissolves mucus in the respiratory system, cleanses the body of toxins, and has an antiseptic and cleansing effect for the digestive system. The vitamin C content (50–75 mg) of lemons and limes, in combination with sulfur, is a great bonus during times of fever.

Lemons and limes provide an alkaline balance to the stomach, because the potassium carbonate they contain forms to neutralize stomach acids. In regions where cholera, typhoid, and diptheria are prevalent, lemons and limes, taken daily, have proved beneficial in preventing the contraction of those conditions. Lemons can also help prevent some forms of cancer due to their powerful detoxifying and antioxidant abilities. Lemons and limes reduce uric acid in conditions such as gout, rheumatism, and gallstones. The juice of these fruits can destroy over 90% of bacteria in seafood within 15 minutes.

If you need a quick, cheap detox, squeeze a lemon or lime, add water, and be on the way to recovery.

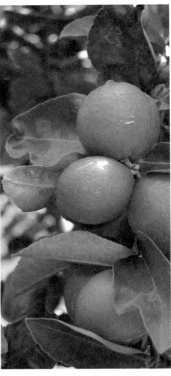

GLYCEMIC INDEX: 55	TOTAL CALORIES PER 100 G: 65	CALORIES FROM		
		CARB: 61 94%	PROTEIN: 2 3%	FAT: 2 3%

MANGO – *Mangifera indica*

Most people need no convincing to eat a fresh, ripe mango, the golden tropical treat. Their health benefits are worth discovering. The most obvious is its rich content of beta-carotene (445 mcg), a precursor to vitamin A, meaning it is converted to vitamin A in the body. Beta-carotene is required for growth, strong bones and teeth, healthy skin and hair, and healthy eyes. One large mango will provide an average adult with the total vitamin A required for a day. Vitamin A can be stored in the liver; however, the body utilizes these stores, especially during times of infection and viruses. Pregnancy, lactation, and the contraceptive pill also deplete reserves of vitamin A.

Mango is also a good source of the mineral chlorine, which is vital for normal blood pressure, purifying the blood, bodily cleansing, and assisting in the digestion of protein foods. Slices of mango make an ideal predinner appetizer or breakfast starter, and mango makes a most delicious fresh juice when combined with orange, strawberry, and pineapple. It provides a rich flavor for any meal or dessert: Try mango sauce on baked fish, or fresh mango with ice cream — mmm, dreamy!

Mango provides fair amounts of vitamin C (28–35 mg), potassium (156 mg), magnesium (9–18 mg), and a very low fat content (0.2 g)—all for a minimal 65 calories. The beta-carotene content, combined with the vitamin C and chlorine content, will provide a cleansing and antioxidant effect on the blood system. As a bonus, your skin will treasure the mango's balance of nutrients. The magnificent mango is the ideal fruit for any celebration.

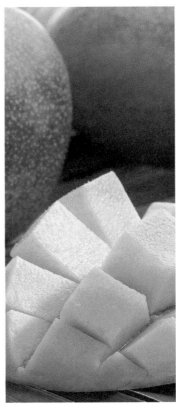

NOTE: DV amounts listed refer to the daily value for women 25–50 years; refer to DRI charts on pages 95–96 for adult male and child values.

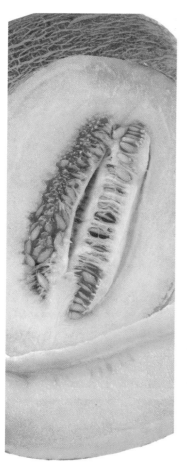

GLYCEMIC INDEX: 72	TOTAL CALORIES PER 100 G: 30	CALORIES FROM		
		CARB: 27 90%	PROTEIN: 2 7%	FAT: 1 3%

MELONS – *Cucumis melo*

Melons, the biggest fruit, come in an enormous assortment of varieties. You've got the canary, crenshaw, galia, honeydew, muskmelon, Santa Claus, cantaloupe, and watermelon. (See page 47 for cantaloupe and page 59 for watermelon.) One of the main features of melons is the alkaline balance they provide in the diet. Most foods are acid forming, but ideally 75% of the diet needs to be based on alkaline foods. Relax with a big slice of melon and balance your body with alkaline benefits. Melons are here to rescue the body; it cannot heal properly if the blood is always in an acidic state. Melons are about 90% natural mineral water. They need no digestion in the stomach so if they are eaten after a meal the problems of flatulence and intestinal aches can easily develop. There is no point in eating melon if it ferments in the digestive system and destroys the valuable supply of nutrients. Eat melons before consuming other foods.

Melons are an excellent source of the trace mineral bromine, which is most valuable for the health of the glandular system. Bromine is one of the "unknown" minerals, generally speaking; however, a constant supply is required in the bloodstream and is controlled by the pituitary gland, the master gland. Bromine is vital for regulating emotions. It is especially required as we get older and in particular during menopause for women. It can also help regulate men's emotions during mid-life crises. Let the melon balance your emotions.

Melons are very low in calories, and therefore ideal for anyone who likes to eat big without putting on weight. Try a "melon fast" once a week during summer and notice the new life the enzymes in melons will give you. Cooked foods provide no enzymes; by contrast, melons are full of enzymes and are also a fair source of vitamin C, potassium, and vitamin A. Melons provide a mighty spark to a dull diet.

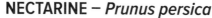

GLYCEMIC INDEX: 54	TOTAL CALORIES PER 100 G: 44	CALORIES FROM		
		CARB: 38 84%	PROTEIN: 4 9%	FAT: 3 7%

NECTARINE – *Prunus persica*

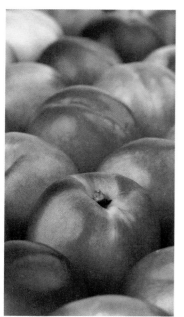

The nectarine is like a cousin to the peach; in fact, there is only one genetic difference: the gene that gives the outer skin of peaches a velvety texture. Generally speaking, the nectarine has the same nutritional value as the peach. The potassium content of the nectarine is 200 mg; the peach supplies 190 mg. The benefits of potassium are for general body healing, movement of oxygen into the brain, regulating the body's water balance, and elimination of blood impurities via the kidneys. Potassium is an alkaline mineral and is often destroyed by heat and cooking. Furthermore, excess salt, alcohol, and caffeine all deplete potassium from the body, so it is easy to see that the average diet may need more fresh foods containing potassium. The nectarine is a delightful choice. Nectarines are also a real bonus for the respiratory system, with 332 IU vitamin A, in the form of beta cryptoxanthin (67 mcg) and beta-carotene (162 mcg). The supply of lutein and zeaxanthin (130 mcg) is most important for the health of the optic system, especially the retina and lens.

Slice a nectarine into your next fruit salad. They also make a delightful snack with almonds.

NOTE: Nutrient amounts are listed as milligrams (mg) per 100 grams (g), unless otherwise stated.

GLYCEMIC INDEX:	TOTAL CALORIES PER 100 G:	CALORIES FROM		
		CARB: 23	PROTEIN: 3	FAT: 89
<5	115	20%	3%	77%

OLIVES – *Olea europaea*

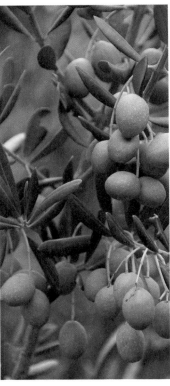

Black and green olives both consist of about 80% fat content with the majority of oil being monounsaturated (9 g). They contain minimal amounts of polyunsaturated (1 g) and saturated (1 g) fats. Refer to pages 131–135 for details on olive oil.

Olives straight from the tree are very bitter as they contain oleuropein, which is mostly concentrated in the olive skin. To remove this compound, olives need to be processed; otherwise they are inedible. Green olives are picked as an unripened fruit; black olives are usually allowed to fully ripen on the tree. To harvest olives they are shaken off the tree and usually collected on large sheets. There are four different processes for olive preparation and they all require many months of soaking (and, with *water-cured* olives, numerous stages of rinsing). Most olives are processed in a *brine or salt solution* for one to six months, the same length of time as oil-cured olives. Green olives are soaked in a solution of lye, thoroughly washed, and then placed in brine. Black olives go straight into the brine, which promotes lactic acid fermentation, and they are later treated with lye to remove the oleuropein. All these steps make olives the most processed fruit.

Olives' high sodium content (800–2000 mg) can be a problem, especially for people with heart problems or circulatory problems. Olives supply some calcium (60 mg), potassium (55 mg), iron (1.6 mg), and vitamin A (400 IU), plus trace amounts of other minerals. Olives are an ideal addition to pizza, and any time you need a salt flavor for a salad or other dish, a few olives is all it takes. No need for the salt shaker. Enjoy olives once in a while, and use olive oil regularly on your salads.

GLYCEMIC INDEX:	TOTAL CALORIES PER 100 G:	CALORIES FROM		
		CARB: 36	PROTEIN: 2	FAT: 1
58	39	92%	5%	3%

PAPAYA – *Carica papaya*

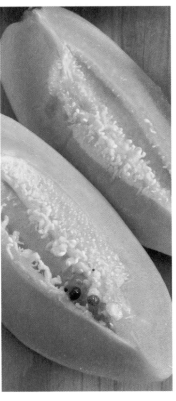

The incredible-tasting papaya is one of the best all-around healing foods. This golden fruit contains numerous active enzymes that are most valuable for the digestive system. In particular, the enzyme papain is beneficial as an aid to digest proteins. If you have a weak stomach, the ripe, golden papaya will be the easiest food to digest.

Papaya is an almost unique food source of two enzymes: carpain, which is beneficial for the heart, and fibrin, for blood clotting. Papain and the enzyme chymopapain are both of great benefit for the healing of burns and the reduction of inflammation. Papaya also supplies vitamin E (1 mg) and has an excellent vitamin C content (62 mg). It provides a fair amount of vitamin A (1,095 IU), in the form of beta cryptoxanthin (761 mcg), beta-carotene (276 mcg), and lutein and zeaxanthin (75 mcg). Because lutein is heat sensitive, the papaya, which is consumed raw, provides the full benefit. The optic system is well rewarded with papya's excellent supply of vitamin C, lutein, and zeaxanthin. If you need to prevent eye deterioration, papaya is pleased to participate. The high beta cryptoxanthin content may help in the healing of colon cancer and lung cancer.

Papaya is the perfect food for the elderly and for young children as it is very easy to digest—no chewing required—and it provides a wealth of healing and digestive benefits. Papaya and its skin can be placed directly on wounds for healing, or try papaya gel or ointment for any skin damage. If your body needs healing, tap into the proven benefits of papaya power.

NOTE: DV amounts listed refer to the daily value for women 25–50 years; refer to DRI charts on pages 95–96 for adult male and child values.

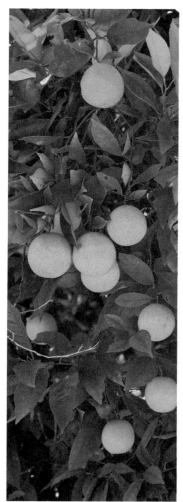

ORANGES – *Citrus sinensis*

Fresh oranges are the most convenient form of fruit drink available today. Slice an orange in half and you have an instant nature drink for two. The benefits of freshly squeezed orange juice are far above those of commercially prepared substitutes. Most commercial orange juice consists of water added to orange concentrate. Why pay extra for added water and for artificial preservatives, added sugar, coloring, and fancy packaging? Instead, have a freshly squeezed juice and obtain all the benefits. Even a package labeled 100% juice, in accordance with regulations, can be processed to extend its shelf life and may contain aromas other additives, without having to say so on the container. The vitamin C content (53 mg) of fresh oranges is the fruit's best known nutritional benefit, but does vitamin C, the most easily destroyed vitamin, survive being processed into juice? Does it stay intact once the commercial container has been opened at home? Not really.

The bioflavonoid rutin (sometimes called vitamin P) is also abundant in fresh oranges, but is found in only very limited amounts in orange juice. In fact, unstrained juice contains only about 10% of the vitamin P value of a whole orange. Vitamin P, located in the white pith of citrus fruits and in peppers, is essential for strong blood capillaries, protection from varicose veins, and the efficient functioning of vitamin C. Now it becomes clear why processed juices are not ideal to rely on for your daily vitamin C requirement. Buy in-season oranges next time they are available and make a freshly squeezed orange juice daily. Ideally, use organic or home-grown oranges; they are superior in flavor as they do not contain the artificial dye, citrus red number 2, that is injected into some commercial oranges to obtain a uniform orange color. A glass of fresh organic orange juice is full of natural life.

Oranges are one of the best fruit source of the mineral calcium (40 mg), which, in combination with the mineral phosphorus (20 mg), is beneficial for protection from infections and viruses. Oranges are beneficial for the maintenance of healthy skin and hair, as vitamin P and C work together to produce collagen, the substance that joins skin tissues.

Oranges supply magnesium (10 mg), which, in addition to the citric acid, vitamin C, and enzymes, gives this fruit its revitalizing power. A glass of freshly squeezed orange juice is a great way to start the day. If you smoke, drink alcohol, or tend to be nervous, orange juice will provide a good natural balance, in addition to the extra vitamin C you need daily to counteract the negative effects of those habits.

Oranges provide a good source of phytonutrients, including one that is unique to oranges, hesperidin. In animal studies, it has proved effective in lowering blood cholesterol and blood pressure; plus it provides anti-inflammatory effects. It, too, is located in the white pith or pulp of the whole orange. The fiber content of a whole orange provides 10–15% of the daily dietary requirement, helping to reduce cholesterol and protect against colon cancer by attaching to cancer-causing elements in the digestive system.

The mandarin orange is often the forgotten fruit in most health and nutrition books, but it provides a delicious and unique flavor with a great supply of vitamin P and all the benefits of the orange. The mandarin makes a delightful juice when combined with strawberries. Give the mandarin a quick peel next time it's in season. Oranges and mandarins are conveniently portable treasures of precious phytonutrients and antioxidants.

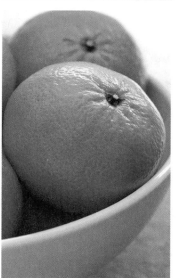

ORANGES

NOTE: Nutrient amounts are listed as milligrams (mg) per 100 grams (g), unless otherwise stated.

GLYCEMIC INDEX: 42	TOTAL CALORIES PER 100 G: 39	CALORIES FROM		
		CARB: 34 87%	PROTEIN: 3 8%	FAT: 2 5%

PEACHES – *Prunus persica*

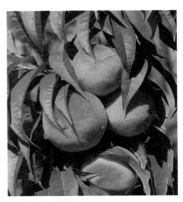

Peaches, a most delicate and delicious fruit, are a valuable source of vitamin A (300–500 IU) in the form of beta-carotene (162 mcg), beta cryptoxanthin (67 mcg), and lutein and zeaxanthin (91 mcg). Fresh peaches are an excellent food for healthy skin due partly to the carotene content but mainly due to their good supply of the mineral sulfur, one of the most important cleansing minerals. Sulfur foods prevent infection, such as acne, and they improve the complexion by cleansing the body of acid poisons and by cleansing the blood.

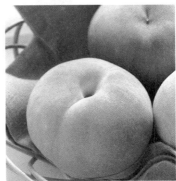

Peaches contain antioxidants such as polyphenols, flavonols, procyanidins, and hydro-cinnamic acid. They provide an alkaline balance to the blood and assist in the cleansing of the kidneys and bladder. The triple combination of carotene, sulfur, and polyphenols in peaches is ideal for prevention from infections such as bronchitis and gastritis. The potassium content (190–210 mg) is fair and helps remove blood impurities via the kidneys. Peaches don't provide much vitamin C (7 mg), but their small supply of vitamin E (1.2 IU), in combination with the other nutrients mentioned, gives them the ability to be a skin-rejuvenating food. Peaches supply more vitamin E than cashews, macadamias, or coconuts. For the maximum vitamin E snack treat, enjoy a handful of almonds with a fresh, ripe peach. The combo is out of this world in both flavor and vitamin E content, as almonds are a big "E" food (50 IU).

Try a fruit salad with peaches, nectarines, strawberries, and mango. Fresh peaches in season are worth their weight in flavor; plus, you receive a bonus of a rejuvenated complexion. Reach for a peach as a real treat!

GLYCEMIC INDEX: 38	TOTAL CALORIES PER 100 G: 58	CALORIES FROM		
		CARB: 56 96%	PROTEIN: 1 2%	FAT: 1 2%

PEARS – *Pyrus communis*

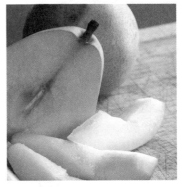

There are over 50 varieties of common pear throughout the world, and they come in the colors green, yellow, red, or brown. The best-known varieties in the United States are anjou, bartlett, bosc, comice, and concorde.

Raw pears, in particular, provide a very good fiber content: One pear supplies 20% of daily fiber. This abundance of fruit fiber is delicate on the digestive system when compared to wheat bran, a common high-fiber food. The fiber in pears can bind with toxins in the colon and reduce their effectiveness, thereby helping to protect against colon cancer. In addition, pears supply a fair amount of the trace mineral copper (0.12 mg). Copper has proved to be deficient in people with colon cancer, and a low copper intake can increase free-radical production within the colon. The combination of copper and fiber makes this fruit a top preventive for people prone to colon cancer.

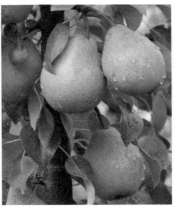

Pears, especially when nice and ripe, are a very simple food to digest. Steamed or poached pears are ideal for babies, children, and the elderly. Pears also combine well with apples. Pears supply potassium (120 mg), iron (0.25 mg), and a good amount of silicon, which is vital for protection from development of cancerous tissue and for body cleansing. The folate (7.5 mg) in pears also helps, in combination with fiber, to protect from gastrointestinal disorders, constipation, and diarrhea. If you have problems "down below," reach for a pear and keep the bad bugs at bay. Pears, with their fabulous fiber benefits, are waiting to attack the enemy!

NOTE: DV amounts listed refer to the daily value for women 25–50 years; refer to DRI charts on pages 95–96 for adult male and child values.

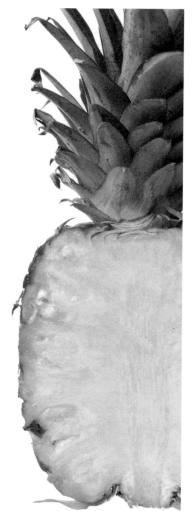

PINEAPPLE – *Ananas comosus*

Pineapples are a versatile fruit for numerous recipes. One of their main health benefits is for the respiratory system due to the good supply of the cleansing minerals chlorine and sulfur, both of which are best obtained from fresh foods because they are heat sensitive. Sulfur protects against accumulation of mucus in the respiratory system and digestive system. Chlorine (30–46 mg) reduces congestion and bronchial problems. Both minerals provide relief from bronchitis and even tuberculosis. Fresh pineapple will cleanse the respiratory system when taken regularly—fresh juice is best. The fair vitamin A content (56 IU) protects against respiratory infections, and the fair vitamin C content (36 mg) also protects against infections. The pineapple is a great choice when the common cold or cough is going around the workplace.

Pineapples are the best fruit source of the mineral manganese (1.7 mg), often termed the "memory mineral" because it helps to nourish the nervous system and brain. It is also valuable for lactating mothers because it stimulates gland secretions that promote the development of breast milk. Freshly made pineapple juice is one of the best drinks for women, especially those with menstrual problems. Manganese is destroyed by processing; however, wheat germ and bran are also excellent sources.

Pineapples are a natural blood thinner, which can prevent the development of blood clots; for this reason, drink pineapple juice before and during long flights. Pineapples must be restricted for people with liver or kidney disease or hemophilia. Pineapples are a unique provider of bromelain, an enzyme that promotes protein digestion. The natural anti-inflammatory properties of bromelain are equally important, especially for conditions such as gout and rheumatoid arthritis.

Pineapple will balance your blood's acid–alkaline levels due to its great supply of bromelain, and it will also promote hormone production, particularly for the pancreas, which produces amylase (to process uncooked starch), lipase (which converts fats), and trypsin (for protein conversion). To obtain the maximum bromelain value, eat fresh pineapple alone, between meals, or as a fresh breakfast juice. In addition, pineapple's supply of organic acids—citric, malic, and tartaric—promotes digestion. Malic acid stimulates the production of digestive enzymes. Pineapples supply fair amounts of iron (0.5 mg), copper (0.07 mg), selenium (0.6 mg), and zinc (0.25 mg). When consumed fresh, in the form of juice, the pineapple is good at reducing fever, especially during midwinter virus season. Canned pineapple provides only a small portion of the benefits; both sulfur and chlorine are depleted by the canning process, as is vitamin C, and often syrup or sugar is added. Pineapple is a favorite pizza topping, and because it promotes digestion of protein, fat, and carbohydrate, it makes sense to put pineapple on pizza, which is a "busy" meal to digest. The pineapple's silicon content (11–70 mg) assists body cleansing and blood and skin cell development. Finally, pineapples have antioxidant power because manganese is a key ingredient in the production of enzymes that defend our cells from free radical damage.

Pineapples purify and protect!

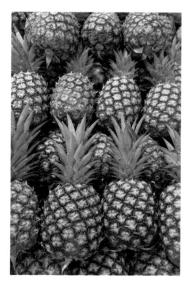

GLYCEMIC INDEX: 39	TOTAL CALORIES PER 100 G: 46	CALORIES FROM		
		CARB: 41 92%	PROTEIN: 2 4%	FAT: 2 4%

PLUMS AND PRUNES – *Prunus domestica*

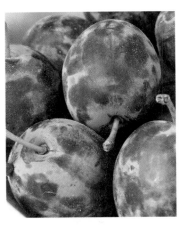

Plums and dried plums, or prunes, are packed with phytonutrients affording great anti-oxidant power, especially protection from free radicals as a result of cooked fats. Prunes in particular are the greatest antioxidant food based on the ORAC comparison, one measure of the total antioxidant potential of a food. Prunes were top of the list with 5,770 ORAC units per 100 g, more than double that of blueberries (2,400) and plums (949). (Due to the dehydrated weight of prunes, they measure higher, so blueberries are actually top of the list.)

Plums contain neochlorgenic and chlorogenic acid, or phenols that can protect against the free radicals known as superoxide anion radicals. The phenols contained in plums and prunes have also shown to be effective in neutralizing the free radicals that can damage the fats within the structure of brain cells. Plum sauce is a good addition to those heavy fat-based meals, as it provides antioxidant power to help protect from cholesterol and excess triglycerides. Plums provide vitamin A (345 IU), trace amounts of iron (0.1 mg), copper (0.04 mg), manganese (0.04 mg), and a fair supply of potassium (157 mg). Plums supply 9 mg of vitamin C and a fair supply of lutein and zeaxanthin (73 mg) and beta-carotene, all benefiting the optic system.

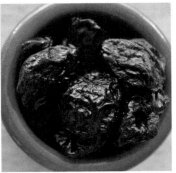

Prunes are a compact energy food with a low glycemic index (39). Prunes are well known as a natural laxative: The high level of sorbitol, a sugar alcohol, plus the high potassium content (810 mg) and fiber content are the main laxative factors. Prunes and plums are packed with power to protect against fatty oxidation problems and to promote proper elimination.

GLYCEMIC INDEX: 40	TOTAL CALORIES PER 100 G: 32	CALORIES FROM		
		CARB: 27 85%	PROTEIN: 2 6%	FAT: 3 9%

STRAWBERRIES – *Fragaria ananassa*

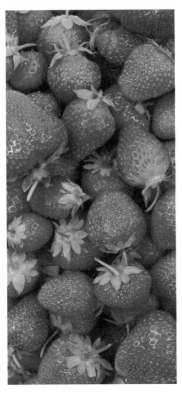

Strawberries are a worldwide favorite, especially when served with cream. Strawberries contain vitamin P, also known as rutin, which is a valuable blood thinner, increases the strength of blood vessels, and promotes circulation. Fresh strawberries eaten regularly will promote reduced blood pressure and improved eyesight and possibly prevent the development of glaucoma.

Strawberries are a good food for the blood due to the fair iron content (1 mg). In addition, the sulfur content promotes blood cleansing, while the manganese (0.28 mg) and copper (0.37 mg) content help build blood cells. The combination of strawberries' silicon content, sulfur content, and excellent vitamin C (57 mg) content make them a skin and beauty treatment; for the price of one facial, you can purchase about 20 small baskets of the delightful red berry! Strawberries are full of antioxidants such as antho-cyanins that give them their bright red color. They protect the body's cells by preventing oxygen damage. Strawberries are anti-inflammatory due to the ability of phenols such as anthocyanin and ellagitannins to reduce the activity of enzymes that cause inflammation.

Strawberries supply vitamins K and F (another term for essential fatty acids), potassium (153 mg), and folate (24 mcg). A regular intake of strawberries will do wonders for the skin and eyes, will strengthen and protect the immune system, and will help to make some of the millions of blood cells your body relies on. Strawberries are ready for your next transfusion!

NOTE: DV amounts listed refer to the daily value for women 25–50 years; refer to DRI charts on pages 95–96 for adult male and child values.

GLYCEMIC INDEX: 38	TOTAL CALORIES PER 100 G: 18	CALORIES FROM		
		CARB: 14 78%	PROTEIN: 2 11%	FAT: 2 11%

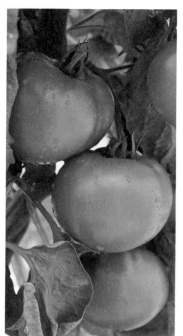

TOMATO – *Solanum lycopersicum*

Tomatoes, an acid fruit, provide citric acid (0.38 mg), malic acid, and oxalic acid in small amounts. The tomato is the best food source of natural chlorine (1,800 mg). Chlorine has numerous functions: it stimulates the liver to filter out waste products, it stimulates the production of gastric juices for protein digestion, and it assists weight reduction by maintaining correct fluid-level retention of body cells and reducing excess blood fat. Organic chlorine is a heat-sensitive mineral, so these benefits do not extend to cooked tomatoes; however, with fresh tomato juice, the cleansing power is red hot.

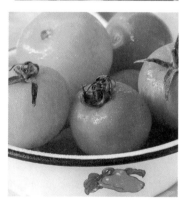

One major benefit obtained from both cooked and fresh tomatoes is the excellent supply of lycopene (2,570 mcg), a carotenoid and one of the precursors to vitamin A. Lycopene has proven to be protective against cancers of the breast, prostate, and lung, due to its antioxidant power and protection of white blood cells.

Tomatoes may also protect against stomach and colon cancer if taken on a regular basis. Tomatoes protect against sun damage, as lycopene is part of the skin's adipose tissue protective structure. Tomatoes are a very good source of sulfur (500 mg). Also an acid mineral that is heat sensitive, sulfur assists the liver in secreting bile, and it has a cleansing and antiseptic effect on the digestive system, bloodstream, and skin. Other minerals well supplied by the tomato are the heat-sensitive potassium (244 mg) and silicon (175 mg). The vitamin C content (23 mg) is fair, the very low calorie count (18) is ideal for weight watchers, and the low glycemic index (38) makes tomatoes safe for nearly everybody. The raw tomato will provide all the benefits; the cooked tomato or sauce will provide the lycopene, and that is a bonus for numerous cooked meals, pizzas, and pasta sauces.

Tomatoes provide a fair supply of vitamin K (8 mcg) and vitamin E (1 mg), and a good supply of biotin (1.5 mcg). One tomato can supply nearly half the daily requirement of biotin, which is vital for energy exertion and the prevention of cramps (also a benefit provided by tomatoes' good potassium content). The tomato is one of the easiest fruits to grow at home. A tomato a day can help you play!

GLYCEMIC INDEX: 72	TOTAL CALORIES PER 100 G: 30	CALORIES FROM		
		CARB: 27 90%	PROTEIN: 2 7%	FAT: 1 3%

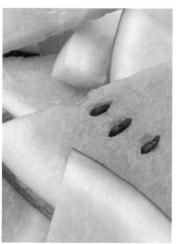

WATERMELON – *Citrullus lanatus*

Watermelons are the greatest fruit for both their large size and the summer satisfaction they provide. Chill them in big red slices and serve just before the children ask for a soft drink. For women, melons are the ideal food for emotional balance due to the super supply of bromine, which is required by the pituitary gland to control the glandular system. In countries where melons are consumed regularly, depression and menopausal problems are uncommon. The melon can also help men through a midlife crisis, and its relaxing power may even help children slow down. The GI is high but the carbohydrate content is low. Watermelon promotes cleansing of the kidneys. It is low in most nutrients except vitamin A (590 IU) and lycopene (its content of 4,532 mcg is nearly twice that of tomatoes). Melons are a great antioxidant, alkalinizer, balancer, and relaxant. Have a great summer holiday, and don't forget the melon!

NOTE: Nutrient amounts are listed as milligrams (mg) per 100 grams (g), unless otherwise stated.

Fruits	Main Nutrients, Antioxidants, and Phytonutrients	Aids Which Body Systems
Apples	alkaline, pectin, malic acid, antioxidants, quercetin	digestive
Apricots	beta-carotene, potassium, lutein, zeaxanthin, silicon, molybdenum	respiratory
Avocado	omega-3, lecithin, potassium, folate, phosphorus, magnesium	circulatory
Banana	potassium, serotonin, norepinephrine, pectin, chlorine, sulfur	muscular
Berries	lycopene, anthocyanins, phenolics, ellagic acid, vitamin C, vitamin P	immune
Cantaloupe	vitamin A, vitamin C, potassium, bromine, folate	skin
Cherries	anthocyanins, isoquercetin, quercetin, ellagic acid, perillyl alcohol, melatonin, vitamin A, potassium	immune
Currants	vitamin C, anthocyanin, vitamin A, potassium	immune
Dates	fiber, potassium, iron, magnesium, calcium, phosphorus, copper	muscular
Figs	calcium, potassium, fiber, iron, manganese, copper, magnesium, phosphorus, silicon, chlorine, sulfur	blood
Grapefruit	liminoids, lycopene, salicyclic acid, vitamin C, biotin, B5	joint
Grapes	manganese, saponin, trans-resveratrol, phenolic compounds	blood
Guava	vitamin C, lutein, zeaxanthin	immune
Kiwi	vitamin C, vitamin A, copper, iron, potassium, phytonutrients	respiratory
Lemon/lime	citric acid, sulfur, vitamin C, antioxidants	respiratory
Mandarin oranges	vitamin P, vitamin C, citric acid, calcium, phosphorus, magnesium, phytonutrients, fiber	immune, respiratory
Mango	beta-carotene, chlorine, vitamin C, potassium	respiratory
Melons	alkaline, bromine, vitamin C, potassium, vitamin A, enzymes	glandular
Nectarine	potassium, beta cryptoxanthin, beta-carotene, lutein, zeaxanthin	respiratory
Olives	added sodium, calcium, potassium, iron, vitamin A, oleic acid	none
Papayas	papain, carpain, chymopapain, vitamin C, beta-cryptoxanthin, beta-carotene, lutein, zeaxanthin	immune, repair, skin
Peaches	beta-carotene, beta-cryptoxanthin, lutein, zeaxanthin, sulfur	skin, elimination
Pears	fiber, copper, potassium, silicon, folate	elimination
Pineapple	chlorine, sulfur, manganese, bromelain, vitamin C, copper, selenium, zinc	respiratory, blood
Plums	phytonutrients, phenols, vitamin A, copper, manganese, beta-carotene	immune, brain
Strawberries	vitamin P, vitamin C, iron, sulfur, copper, silicon, antioxidants, phenols, vitamin K, potassium, folate	circulatory, blood, skin, immune
Tomato	chlorine, lycopene, sulfur, potassium, silicon, vitamin C, biotin	immune, skin
Watermelon	bromine, lycopene, vitamin C, vitamin A, alkaline	glandular, urinary

RECOMMENDATIONS FOR DAILY CARBOHYDRATE INTAKE FROM FRUITS		Adult Male	Adult Female	Teenager	Child
Total Daily Carbohydrate Intake (based on typical guidelines)		340 g	280 g	400 g	270 g
1. *UNH* recommendation: 15% of carbohydrate intake from fruit		51 g	42 g	60 g	40 g
Note the carbohydrate content of common fruits	100 g (3–4 oz) fresh fruit*	approx. 12 g of carbohydrate			
	100 g dried fruit	approx. 65 g of carbohydrate			
1. *UNH* recommendation: 5% of carbohydrate intake from fruit juice		17 g	14 g	20 g	13 g
Note the carbohydrate content of fruit juice	100 g fruit juice**	approx. 10 g of carbohydrate			
2. U.S. MyPlate and DRIs***		3 servings	2 servings	3 servings	2 servings
3. Australian Guide to Healthy Eating***		2 servings	2 servings	3 servings	1 serving

UNH = Ultimate Nutrition for Health; DRIs = Dietary Reference Intakes

* 100 g of fresh fruit is equivalent to any one of the following: approx. 1 small apple, 3 apricots, 1 small banana, 1 cup of berries, 12 dried dates, ½ grapefruit, 1 cup of grapes, 1½ kiwi, ½ mango, 1 small orange, 1 peach , or 1 tomato.

** 100 g of fruit juice = ½ glass (approx. 100 ml)

***1 serving is equivalent to: 1 medium piece of fruit (apple, banana, orange, or pear), 2 small pieces of fruit (apricot, kiwi, plums [150 g]), 1 cup of diced canned fruit (150 g), 4 dried apricots, or ½ cup (125 ml) fruit juice.

The vegetable kingdom provides incredible benefits in a full range of colors and an extraordinary variety of flavors, textures, shapes, and sizes. Nutritionally speaking, we would be lost without vegetables, as a major portion of the essential minerals and vitamins are derived from fresh vegetables. Fresh vegetables are a great provider of the heat-sensitive nutrients that are required for body cleansing and for numerous body system functions.

Throughout this section, the benefits of 25 vegetables are detailed. Armed with this information, you might be encouraged to reap their matchless nutritional rewards.

Some vegetables need cooking, especially the starchy ones: artichoke, parsnips, potatoes, sweet potatoes, pumpkin, and turnips. Cooking opens up the concentrated starch structure of foods, allowing easier digestion. This enables larger quantities of the food to be eaten, thereby providing longer-lasting energy.

Vegetables are very low in calories and have almost zero fat content; on their own they are not a fattening food. Some vegetables provide powerful protective action against free radicals. They are really essential in this era of fast fried foods, as they strengthen the immune system and counteract oxidization.

Another nearly unique benefit of some vegetables is the supply of chlorophyll. Chlorophyll has a structure nearly identical to human blood. It is based on a magnesium atom and blood is based on an iron atom—apart from that, the two substances are identical. Green leafy vegetables will help to regenerate your blood system. Green, fresh vegetables are great blood builders, blood cleansers, and body system activators.

Vegetables are a wonderful source of organic mineral water as the average vegetable contains over 70% water: the potato is 80% water, spinach and lettuce are 90% water. These days it is vital to obtain pure water plus organic mineral water from vegetables to supply the daily water and nutrient requirements, without the addition of the *inorganic* chlorine and fluoride that are contained in some city water supplies. Many vegetables provide organic chlorine and fluoride to provide protection against infection and tooth decay.

The ideal daily diet requires 70% fresh foods, and 75% alkaline foods. Eating a garden salad is one simple way to gain these benefits. Most vegetables are alkaline, but dairy, meat, fish, cheese, and eggs are very acid forming. Vegetables can provide the healing balance to the diet because an alkaline blood balance promotes natural healing.

Vegetables may provide only a small amount of complete protein, but combined with grains or legumes, they help to increase a meal's protein value. Plus they add a lot of flavor and color to grain and legume meals.

Vegetables are meal-makers. Even with the most common meals, a few vegetables are usually added to the plate to make it look nice. Eat those veggies, because they provide a valuable supply of nutrients that are lacking from cooked animal foods. The home garden can supply an abundance of the essential basic vegetables.

Vegetables are just waiting for an invitation to your next lunch, evening meal, or banquet!

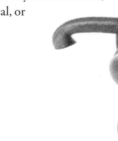

NOTE: Nutrient amounts are listed as milligrams (mg) per 100 grams (g), unless otherwise stated.

GLYCEMIC INDEX: VERY LOW	TOTAL CALORIES PER 100 G: 54	CALORIES FROM		
		CARB: 38 70%	PROTEIN: 8 15%	FAT: 8 15%

ARTICHOKE – *Cynara cardunculus, Helianthus tuberosus*

There are two main types of artichoke: the globe artichoke and the Jerusalem artichoke. They have varying nutritional values: The globe artichoke contains 54 calories per 100 g compared to 76 calories for the Jerusalem artichoke. The main common nutrient is potassium: The globe has 370 mg, the Jerusalem 429 mg. The sodium content of the globe artichoke is 94 mg; the Jerusalem supplies only 4 mg. They both supply about 77 mg of phosphorus. The iron content of Jerusalem artichoke is very good at 3.4 mg, while the globe supplies only 1.6 mg. The vitamin A content of the globe is far better at 185 IU, compared to 20 IU for the Jerusalem. Artichokes have basically no protein and a very low fat content. Over 80% of the calories come from carbohydrate. They are a good source of dietary fiber. One medium globe artichoke provides over 20% daily dietary fiber, ideal for meals with chicken or meat.

Clinical trials with artichokes and their active ingredients, cynaropicrin and cynarin, showed that patients experienced a reduction in cholesterol and low density lipids and an increase in the beneficial high density lipids. Artichokes provide a stabilizing effect for the metabolism due to the supply of valuable oils. Artichokes are beneficial for the liver as they stimulate liver cell regeneration. They also assist in the reduction of water retention, a condition known as edema. The raw artichoke contains the enzyme inulase, which assists with conversion of the starch content. Artichokes have been used in cases of diabetes and may also benefit in cases of atherosclerosis.

Artichokes are really worth the effort.

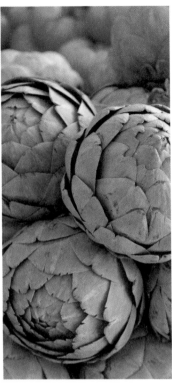

GLYCEMIC INDEX: VERY LOW	TOTAL CALORIES PER 100 G: 20	CALORIES FROM		
		CARB: 14 70%	PROTEIN: 5 25%	FAT: 1 5%

ASPARAGUS – *Asparagus officinalis*

Asparagus, a member of the lily family (*Liliaceae*), has been recognized for centuries for its distinctive flavor and therapeutic qualities. There are three main types: the green spears, blanched white (grown underground), and the French asparagus with a blue-violet color and stronger flavor. The main benefit of asparagus comes from the alkaloid *asparagine,* which stimulates the cleansing of the kidneys and bladder. The strong smell associated with asparagus once the urine passes is due to the alkaloid residue. Asparagus is a very good source of *silicon* (950 mg), for healthy hair; this, in combination with the minerals sulfur (536 mg) and chlorine (510 mg), also makes it ideal for skin cleansing. However, canned or overcooked asparagus may not do the trick as both chlorine and sulfur are heat-sensitive nutrients. Blanch only the stems in boiling water for two minutes, then "dip the tips" in the boiling water for a second, and serve for the full flavor and benefits. Asparagus supplies good amounts of natural fluoride for the eyesight and bromine for the glandular system. Asparagus also contains glutathione, an anticarcinogen, and rutin (vitamin P) to strengthen the blood vessels. For a "land food" asparagus is a good source of iodine, which promotes correct thyroid metabolism. Asparagus, canned and fresh, is a very good source of folate (120 mcg), vital for the nerves and brain and during pregnancy. It also provides vitamin A (900 IU), plus isoleucine for the glands. Asparagus may seem a luxury, but when it is in season grab a bunch to cleanse the urinary system and help balance the wonderful glandular system.

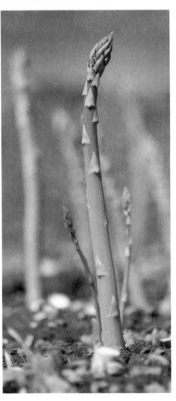

NOTE: DV amounts listed refer to the daily value for women 25–50 years; refer to DRI charts on pages 95–96 for adult male and child values.

GLYCEMIC INDEX: VERY LOW	TOTAL CALORIES PER 100 G: 42	CALORIES FROM		
		CARB: 37 88%	PROTEIN: 4 10%	FAT: 1 2%

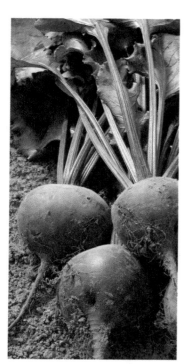

BEETS – *Beta vulgaris*

Beets have been considered a nutritional food since the early Roman and Greek times for reduction of fevers and for the blood. Even though the iron content is only fair at 0.91 mg, it is in an easily assimilated form due to the content of vitamin C (4.9 mg) and of the minerals manganese (0.34 mg) and copper (0.007 mg).

The supply of organic sodium (72 mg) and potassium (325 mg) is one reason for the blood-cleansing abilities of beets and, in particular, of fresh beet juice.

The cleansing power of beets continues with the excellent supply of chlorine (295 mg) and sulfur (50 mg). Both are heat sensitive, so canned beets may not be the way to go for body cleansing. Sulfur *cleanses the digestive system* and protects against infections. Chlorine *purifies the blood, the skin, and the glandular system.*

Beets should be obtained fresh and grated or juiced for maximum benefits. A juice made from a combination of carrot (120 ml), beet (50 ml), and parsley (10 ml) juices is the tonic for women with menstruation or menopause problems. Try freshly grated beets with your next salad. Other recognized benefits of beets include the following: cleanses the lymphatic system, thereby also helping the immune system; has *anticarcinogenic properties;* cleanses the kidneys; aids digestion; restores health in people with general weakness, sexual weakness, prostate troubles, and liver disorders.

Canned beets do not contribute all these benefits. Let the bright, bold, and raw beet be part of your health-restoration program.

GLYCEMIC INDEX: VERY LOW	TOTAL CALORIES PER 100 G: 34	CALORIES FROM		
		CARB: 24 70%	PROTEIN: 7 21%	FAT: 3 9%

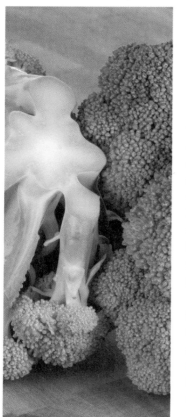

BROCCOLI – *Brassica oleracea*

Broccoli is a good source of both vitamin A (1,500 IU) and vitamin C (94 mg). Vitamin C is heat sensitive. Therefore, prolonged cooking of broccoli is not advised. Overcooking will also "stink out" the kitchen, due to the loss of nutrients such as sulfur, thereby reducing the health benefits. To prepare broccoli, place only the stems in water, and lightly steam the vegetable for two minutes, with the lid on. Add small florets of raw broccoli to a fresh garden salad for maximum benefits. Broccoli is a good source of calcium (103 mg) and phosphorus (78 mg), both valuable for the building and maintenance of strong bones. It also provides magnesium (24 mg), which, together with vitamins A and C, promotes efficient metabolism of the calcium and phosphorus. Broccoli supplies good amounts of iron (1.1 mg), another nutrient enhanced by its vitamin C content. Research has shown that broccoli has anticancer properties due to the abundance of vitamins A and C and of selenium (3 mg), which affords both anticancer and antiviral properties.

Broccoli contains *indole-3-carbinol,* which the body converts into an *antiandrogen* that can inhibit the growth of prostate cancer cells. Broccoli also contains the potent compound *sulforaphane,* which is able to destroy the *Helicobacter pylori* bacterium, which causes most stomach ulcers and cancers and which is not destroyed by common antibiotics. Broccoli is a very good source of chromium, which protects against adult-onset (type 2) diabetes by boosting the activity of insulin in glucose-intolerant people. Broccoli may also lower blood cholesterol due to its supply of *calcium pectate.*

Finally, broccoli gives a beneficial antibacterial boost.

NOTE: Nutrient amounts are listed as milligrams (mg) per 100 grams (g), unless otherwise stated.

GLYCEMIC INDEX: VERY LOW	TOTAL CALORIES PER 100 G: 43	CALORIES FROM		
		CARB: 32 74%	PROTEIN: 8 19%	FAT: 3 7%

BRUSSELS SPROUTS – *Brassica oleracea gemmifera*

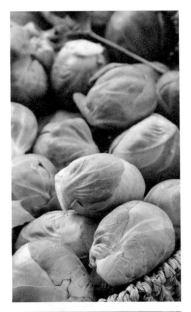

The "small cabbage," named after the capital of Belgium, is a very good source of the mineral sulfur, which has a cleansing and antiseptic effect on the digestive system, bloodstream, and skin cells. Sulfur foods are essential for maintenance of healthy skin, nails, and hair because they are a rich source of keratin, a protein substance that is also part of insulin. Brussels sprouts should not be boiled, as sulfur is heat sensitive. They can be lightly steamed or finely chopped and added to a fresh garden salad. The strong taste of raw Brussels sprouts comes from their high sulfur content. Sulfur foods also promote the digestion of protein foods. Brussels sprouts contain the nitrogen compounds known as indoles, which, in combination with the content of vitamin C (85 mg) and vitamin A (750 IU), provide a cancer-inhibiting factor. Brussels sprouts provide selenium (2 mcg) and a fair amount of potassium (386 mg); both help to protect against cancer. Brussels sprouts are a good source of magnesium (23 mg), iron (1.3 mg), and folate (61 mcg); plus they provide a valuable amount of dietary fiber (4 g) with a low calorie value and a fair amount of vegetable protein. They also contain *isothiocyanates* that can suppress the growth of tumors. Roll out the big benefits of the tiny Brussels sprout.

GLYCEMIC INDEX: VERY LOW	TOTAL CALORIES PER 100 G: 24	CALORIES FROM		
		CARB: 19 80%	PROTEIN: 4 16%	FAT: 1 4%

CABBAGE – *Brassica oleracea capitata*

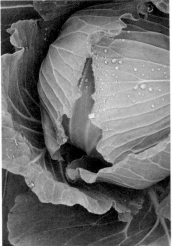

Cabbages are an excellent source of the two cleansing minerals chlorine (1,045 mg) and sulfur (1,710 mg). Both work as a team in expelling waste matter and cleansing the blood, and they also tend to reduce excess body weight. A deficiency of chlorine foods can lead to poor liver function and various types of congestion such as sinusitis. Regular consumption of fresh cabbage, in the form of coleslaw or finely chopped and added to a salad, is most beneficial for protection from the common cold and other viruses. Try the taste of homemade cabbage rolls and rice on a winter's night—but be aware that the more the cabbage is cooked, the more the chlorine and sulfur benefits disperse.

There are numerous varieties of cabbage; green, bok choy, red, napa, and savoy are the main types. The common green cabbage supplies the best chlorine and sulfur content. If for nothing more than the supply of those two nutrients, cabbage would be an excellent food, but there's more! Cabbages are a good source of chlorophyll, the green magic medicine, and a unique source of a substance that has been proven to heal peptic ulcers (sometimes called vitamin U). It is likely that the sulfur content also helps, as *sulforaphane* destroys the *Helicobacter pylori* bacterium that causes stomach ulcers. Medicinal tonic doses of raw cabbage juice in 13 ulcer patients, over ten days, provided a 100% success rate. To avoid the discomfort of an ulcer and the bitter taste of a tonic, enjoy the flavor of coleslaw regularly.

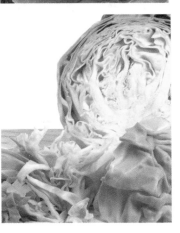

Cabbage is the main ingredient in *sauerkraut*, a product of German ingenuity. Sauerkraut, formed from fermented cabbage leaves, supplies an abundance of vital enzymes. Cabbage is a good source of bromine for glandular functioning, vital during menopause, and it is very low in calories and has a very low fat content. Add a low-cal citrus dressing and dig in!

NOTE: DV amounts listed refer to the daily value for women 25–50 years; refer to DRI charts on pages 95–96 for adult male and child values.

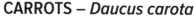

GLYCEMIC INDEX: 6	TOTAL CALORIES PER 100 G: 41	CALORIES FROM		
		CARB: 36 88%	PROTEIN: 3 7%	FAT: 2 5%

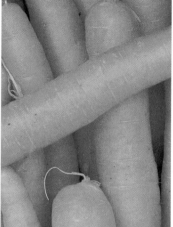

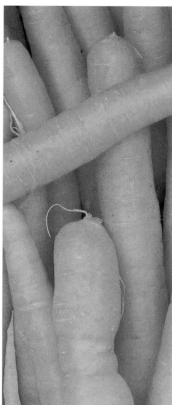

CARROTS – *Daucus carota*

Carrots were used by the Greeks and Romans as medicine, and they are now the most widely cultivated vegetable. The numerous varieties and colors include the white, purple, red, yellow, and, the "king of carotene," the orange carrot. There are two main types of carotene, both available in carrots: beta-carotene (5,774 mcg) and alpha-carotene (2,817 mcg). There are two types of vitamin A: preformed vitamin A (retinol), obtained from animal origin, and provitamin-A (carotene), from plant origin. Carrots are the best vegetable source of carotene, which the body converts into vitamin A. (Diabetics may be unable to convert carotene into vitamin A. Intake of retinol from animal origin—e.g., as cod liver oil—may be essential for diabetics, especially in times of illness.)

Carotene has unique protective and healing abilities. Alpha-carotene may be more powerful than beta-carotene in inhibiting tumor growths; one study showed it to be ten times more potent. Most research has focused on beta-carotene, which shows benefits in the treatment of lung and pancreatic cancer. Supplements of beta-carotene are not advised; it is best to obtain the natural balance from carrots, which contain not only alpha- and beta-carotene but also active enzymes. Cooked carrots provide more usable carotene than raw carrots. The exception is raw carrot juice; both cooking and juicing open up the carotene starch structure. Carrots provide so much carotene, however, that eating raw carrots will still supply ample amounts—plus affording the full benefit of numerous heat-sensitive nutrients. These are also available in fresh carrot juice. In summary, the carrot's exceptionally rich supply of carotene and natural phytochemicals boosts the immune system, improves eyesight, heals wounds, reduces high blood pressure, cleanses the liver, improves skin condition, reduces acne, reduces mucus, prevents jaundice, promotes skin protection from sunshine, protects against ulcers, and generally prevents the development and reduces the duration of infections, viruses, and colds.

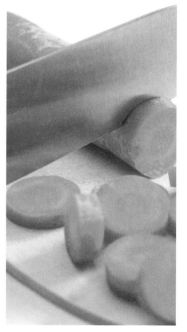

Carrots' sulfur (445 mg) and chlorine (318 mg) content is the main reason for the remarkable liver-cleansing abilities of fresh carrot juice. Cooking increases the carotene value but greatly decreases the sulfur, chlorine, and potassium content (341 mg). Skin cleansing is easy with fresh carrot juice; in addition, the supply of silicon (166 mg) also promotes a good complexion. As to whether an "excess" intake of carrot juice causes orange skin, the answer is no. It is the elimination of toxins from the liver that can cause skin to discolor, or the inability of the body to process carotene properly. Excess consumption of any food is a problem, however, so limit your carrot juice intake to no more than three times a week of the following quantities: children 120 ml (four fluid ounces), adults 240 ml (eight fluid ounces). Vitamin A is a fat-soluble vitamin, so it is not required every day. If you need exceptional healing, drink some wheatgrass juice on the other days, or mix carrot with beet or celery juice.

Cooked carrots provide a vital balance to meat meals, so don't leave them off the plate. They are a great food for children as carrots are the sweetest vegetable; add a little honey to mashed carrots for babies. For nursing moms, carrot juice promotes lactation.

Carrots provide iron (0.5 mg), copper (0.05 mg), manganese (0.15 mg), and selenium, a natural antioxidant, especially in combination with the abundant supply of alpha- and beta-carotene.

Carrots are the root of all natural healing!

CARROTS

NOTE: Nutrient amounts are listed as milligrams (mg) per 100 grams (g), unless otherwise stated.

GLYCEMIC INDEX: VERY LOW	TOTAL CALORIES PER 100 G: 40	CALORIES FROM		
		CARB: 37 93%	PROTEIN: 3 7%	FAT: 0 0%

CAPSICUM (BELL PEPPERS) – *Capsicum annuum*

Bell peppers, referred to as capsicum in some parts of the world, are the best vegetable source of precious vitamin C. The red bell pepper supplies 204 mg, the green bell pepper 128 mg. The benefits of obtaining your vitamin C naturally, as opposed to taking it in tablet form, cannot be overstated. The action of vitamin C is dependant on a supply of *bioflavonoids,* which are contained in the white part (pith) of the fruit or vegetable. A vitamin C supplement may supply no bioflavonoids, thereby greatly retarding the action of vitamin C. Foods that naturally contain vitamin C also supply an abundance of enzymes that promote the vitamin's numerous functions. The supplement tablet is the expensive way to get what only nature can provide in correct balance for human nutrition. Remember to enjoy a couple of bell peppers every week to prevent numerous health problems. (Cooked peppers afford fewer benefits because vitamin C is heat sensitive.)

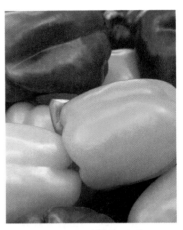

Peppers are an excellent source of vitamin P, or bioflavonoids, which is vital for increasing the strength of the capillaries. A deficiency of this nutrient can lead to varicose veins, arteriosclerosis, arthritis, and rheumatism. They are also a very good source of vitamin A (red: 4,450 IU, green: 420 IU). Peppers add color to your salads — red, orange, yellow, and green slices of vitamins C, A, and P. Children enjoy the variety of colors. A crisp, cool bell pepper is one way to provide nutritional benefits without the citrus acid tang that some children and adults cannot tolerate.

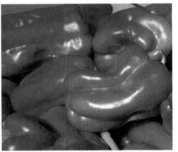

Bell peppers supply low amounts of minerals. Think of them as a huge vitamin C, A, P tablet.

GLYCEMIC INDEX: 30	TOTAL CALORIES PER 100 G: 25	CALORIES FROM		
		CARB: 19 76%	PROTEIN: 5 20%	FAT: 1 4%

CAULIFLOWER – *Brassica oleracea*

Cauliflower is the pure white vegetable. In addition to its excellent supply of sulfur (1,186 mg) and chlorine (310 mg) when eaten raw, the other nutrient benefits are vitamin C (78 mg) and potassium (206 mg). If you can handle the taste of fresh cauliflower florets in a salad, you will gain maximum cleansing benefits from cauliflower. Sulfur reduces body toxins, prevents the development of infections, cleanses the digestive system, and protects against stomach ulcers. The combination of sulfur and silicon (337 mg) gives cauliflower the power to promote hair growth, improve skin condition, promote blood hemoglobin development, improve blood circulation, and protect against the formation of arthritic conditions. To ensure a reasonable supply of sulfur and chlorine,when cooking cauliflower, lightly steam the whole head with the stalk immersed in simmering water for five minutes. Cauliflower *au gratin* (with cheese) is very popular. Place the steamed cauliflower heads in a baking dish, sprinkle with grated Parmesan and cheddar, and bake for ten minutes in a preheated oven. With the cheese topping, it's big in calcium and protein, ideal for growing children. Serve with dark-colored foods (mushrooms, spinach, carrots), but avoid combining with rice, pumpkin, or potatoes — too much starch, too little color, too little flavor. Cauliflower also supplies vitamins K, C, A, folate, and biotin. Let the "power of the cauliflower" loose once in a while.

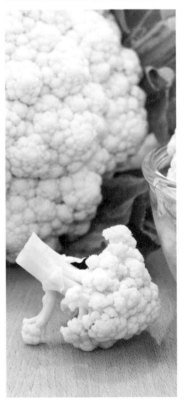

DV amounts listed refer to DRI charts on pages 95–96 for adult male and child values.

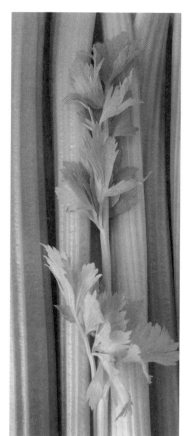

CELERY – *Apium graveolens*

Celery has a long history of therapeutic benefits, and with more research the benefits increase. In ancient Rome, celery was used to offset hangovers. The Greeks found it beneficial for gallstones, liver problems, and constipation. During the seventeenth century, Italian gardeners converted celery from a very bitter food to a variety that is now mass produced; they blanched the plant by covering the stems with soil to decrease the bitterness.

The two main active ingredients in celery that provide its unique taste and smell are sedanolide and 3-n-butylphthalide; they are responsible for the plant's antitumor and cholesterol-lowering properties. In addition, compounds known as pthalides relax the muscles that line the blood vessels, thereby decreasing blood pressure. In addition, celery prevents hardened arteries and edema, and can naturally thin the blood, helping to prevent clotting. Pthalides also lower the production of hormones known as catecholamines, decreasing nervous stress.

Celery is a very good source of vitamin A in the form of beta-carotene (324 mg) and the relatively unknown lutein and zeaxanthin (340 mcg), all members of the carotenoid family. This combination gives celery the status of being a good food for the eyes, as these substances, the only carotenoids naturally occurring in the lens of the human eye, protect against phototoxic blue light and ultraviolet radiation, as well as against age-related increases in lens density and cataract formation.

It is fairly well known that celery is the richest vegetable source of organic sodium (96–126 mg), which keeps calcium soluble within the bloodstream and body cells. In fact, every cell in the body is covered by a solution of saline water. Commercial salt is not completely water soluble, but celery sodium is totally soluble. Refined foods, white bread in particular, contain inorganic calcium that can accumulate over years, leading to arthritis or the depositing of calcium around bones and joints. Celery has the power to address the calcium imbalance before it causes long-term damage.

Celery also provides protection from cancer due to the ingredient acetylenic, which has been shown to stop the growth of cancer cells. In addition, the phenolic acids contained in celery block the action of the prostaglandin hormones, which encourage the growth of cancerous tumors and which contribute to the pain of arthritis and rheumatism. Celery is also a diuretic, and it promotes virility.

As you can see, celery, eaten raw or consumed as a fresh juice, is abundant in benefits. Especially during hot summer days, celery juice will replace lost sodium, protecting against muscle cramps. Enjoying celery soup in winter can provide many of these benefits as the nutrients in celery are for the most part not heat sensitive.

Celery is a good food for diabetics as it stimulates the pancreas to produce insulin, promoting carbohydrate digestion. It provides excellent amounts of chlorine (1,780 mg), sulfur (650 mg), silicon (430 mg), and bromine (17 mg). It is the weight watchers' dream food, with only 18 calories per 100 g. Eat a whole bunch and fill up but not out!

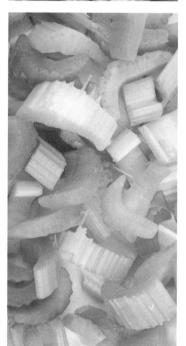

CELERY

NOTE: Nutrient amounts are listed as milligrams (mg) per 100 grams (g), unless otherwise stated.

GLYCEMIC INDEX: VERY LOW	TOTAL CALORIES PER 100 G: 15	CALORIES FROM		
		CARB: 12 80%	PROTEIN: 2 13%	FAT: 1 7%

CUCUMBER – *Cucumis sativus*

Cucumber is an excellent source of the mineral silicon, containing 800 mg per 100 g. Very few foods contain silicon; however, it is a major nutrient, often forgotten in general human health. With the increase in cases of osteoporosis and osteoarthritis, silicon may eventually be recognized for its vital role in the proper construction of bones. Cucumber supplies 16 times more silicon than wheat or wheat bran. There's a lot to be said about the cucumber sandwich; it provides strength to the bones and promotes hair growth, as hair is made primarily of silicon. (Lettuce provides the best silicon supply.) There is no recommended dietary intake for silicon, but you can be assured it is required.

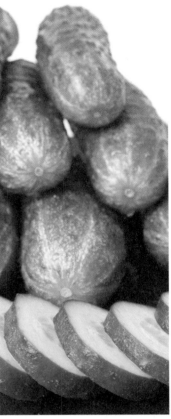

Cucumber is full of water (95%), making it ideal for hot days. If you peel the cucumber, most of the silicon disappears, but the sulfur (690 mg) and chlorine (660 mg) remain. Sulfur and silicon both promote healthy skin; the cucumber facial is not just for fun. This vegetable really does provide cooling and beneficial qualities, whether taken internally or externally. The chlorine in cucumber promotes rejuvenation of skin tissues and cleansing of the blood, and promotes digestion of fats and proteins. An appetizer of cucumber and yogurt is an ideal choice before a meal.

Cucumbers contain the enzyme erepsin, which is required to convert peptides into amino acids. Cucumber is an excellent diuretic and helps to prevent kidney stones, high blood pressure, and rheumatism.

Cucumber can reduce excess uric acid in the blood, often a direct result of overindulgence in meat and chocolate. Cucumbers are a good source of fiber, and the seeds provide numerous nutrients such as vitamin E. Keep cool, clean, and content with cucumber!

GLYCEMIC INDEX: VERY LOW	TOTAL CALORIES PER 100 G: 24	CALORIES FROM		
		CARB: 20 84%	PROTEIN: 2 8%	FAT: 2 8%

EGGPLANT – *Solanum melongena*

Eggplant, also known as aubergine, is most commonly purple, but white and variegated varieties are also available. The eggplant provides very little flavor on its own so it requires French cooking or Italian ingenuity or Turkish talent to make it a delight. Herbs, lemon juice, butter, and a sprinkle of cheese usually do the trick, as do olive oil, garlic, tomatoes, and black pepper. The nutritional value of eggplant is fairly basic apart from the good chlorine (670 mg) and sulfur (445 mg) content. Chlorine stimulates protein digestion in the stomach. It also cleanses the body of excess fats, a feature that may be essential when cheese is added to the eggplant. The sulfur content promotes carbohydrate digestion and cleanses the digestive system. Eggplant provides 3 g of dietary fiber per 100 g, about 14% of total daily requirement (chicken and meat, by contrast, supply none). If you have never cooked eggplant before, find a good recipe or ask a friend who knows how to cook for some help—that's the best way to begin.

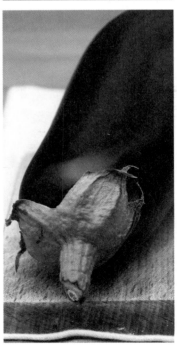

Eggplants provide valuable phytosterols (7 mg), which boost the immune system. Eggplant soak up the oils during the cooking process so use a cold-pressed flaxseed or walnut oil to get a big dose of the essential omega-3. Eggplants are ready to oblige!

NOTE: DV amounts listed refer to the daily value for women 25–50 years; refer to DRI charts on pages 95–96 for adult male and child values.

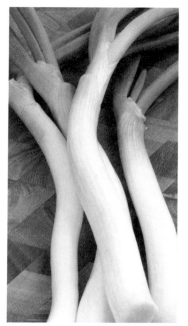

GLYCEMIC INDEX: VERY LOW	TOTAL CALORIES PER 100 G: 61	CALORIES FROM		
		CARB: 54 88%	PROTEIN: 4 7%	FAT: 3 5%

LEEKS – *Allium ampeloprasum*

Leeks, the long and straight member of the onion family, are the ideal winter option in a cream of leek soup. Don't worry about the high fat content of cream; sulfur compounds supplied by leeks promote the secretion of bile, thereby assisting in the digestion of fats. Leeks supply *cycloallin,* which has the ability to dissolve blood clots that form on the inside of blood vessels. Even cooking does not affect this special ingredient. Cycloallin also helps to dissolve fibrin from inflamed joints. The excellent carotene content (1,667 IU) of leeks, comprising beta-carotene (1,000 mcg) and lutein and zeaxanthin (1,900 mg), promotes healthy eyesight and protects against some forms of cancer. Regular onions do not supply the carotenoids; the leek is the only "onion" source of these substances and must therefore be considered the most valuable. Leeks have a natural antiseptic quality due to their supply of sulfur and of allyl disulfate and cycloallin. Insulin is a sulfur compound, making leeks a safe food for most diabetics. Leeks provide a fair source of organic iron (2 mg), copper, folate, vitamin B6, and vitamin K.

Leeks are the sweet onion. Added them to any salad or quiche.

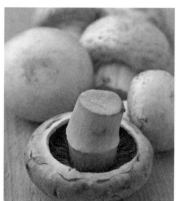

GLYCEMIC INDEX: VERY LOW	TOTAL CALORIES PER 100 G: 22	CALORIES FROM		
		CARB: 11 50%	PROTEIN: 8 36%	FAT: 3 14%

MUSHROOMS – *Agaricus campestris, A. bisporus*

Mushrooms grow in the dark, in a world of their own, and they are full of unique nutritional benefits. The number of available varieties is extraordinary, but some are poisonous, so be sure to obtain mushrooms from a reputable source. Such varieties as the portobello, button, cup, flat, porcini or cap mushroom, truffles, chanterelle, maitake, shiitake, reishi, and the common white or brown mushroom provide varied benefits. The maitake mushroom contains adaptogen, which helps the body adapt to stress and promotes normal metabolism. It also contains polysaccharides that inhibit the growth of cancerous cells, destroy HIV, and promote the activity of the immune system's T-helper cells. It may assist in cases of hepatitis, high blood pressure, and chronic fatigue syndrome. The shiitake mushroom contains the polysaccharide lentinan, which strengthens T-cell formation. The reishi and shiitake mushrooms have antitumor properties and may assist in the treatment of some cancers. In Japan, shiitake mushroom extract is licensed as an anticancer drug.

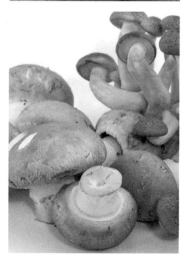

Generally speaking, mushrooms are termed probiotic: They strengthen the immune system, balance the body, and provide natural resistance to disease. They contain host defense potentiators (HDP), which enhance the immune system. They also provide antiviral, analgesic, antioxidant, and anti-inflammatory benefits. Mushrooms are a good source of potassium (400 mg on average), which promotes healing and improved blood circulation. They contain no vitamin A and very little calcium or iron, but they supply fair amounts of phosphorus for the nerves and brain. Mushrooms are low in calories and supply a little complete protein. They absorb a lot of oil when fried so take it easy. Fresh mushrooms contain 90% water and are a good source of the amino acid lysine.

Mushrooms' natural medicinal properties are still being discovered.

NOTE: Nutrient amounts are listed as milligrams (mg) per 100 grams (g), unless otherwise stated.

GLYCEMIC INDEX: <11	TOTAL CALORIES PER 100 G: 15	CALORIES FROM		
		CARB: 10 72%	PROTEIN: 3 21%	FAT: 1 7%

LETTUCE – *Lactuca sativa*

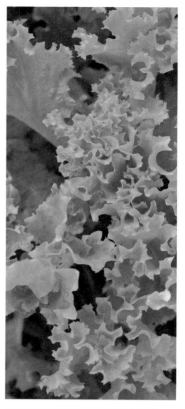

Lettuce is rarely cooked, which means it provides an abundance of essential human nutrients. Different varieties of lettuce are growing in popularity, including iceberg, romaine, butter or Boston, and looseleaf (red and green), to mention a few of the more common types. Generally speaking they all supply the same dominant nutrients.

The supply of chlorophyll from the green lettuce leaves provides an excellent source of healing benefits (see page 112 for more on chlorophyll). Lettuce may be the only source of living chlorophyll that some people eat; a simple sandwich that is loaded with lots of green lettuce leaves is a bonus for the blood, brain, and nervous system. In addition, the very good supply of vitamin K (24–125 mcg) is essential for blood coagulation. Aspirin, X rays, and radiation all deplete vitamin K from the human body, and frozen foods supply no vitamin K. Let lettuce keep your blood in active defense mode!

Another major benefit of lettuce is its excellent supply of the mineral silicon (500–2,400 mg). Iceberg lettuce is the richest source, and the same applies for vitamin A (1,900 IU), in the form of the precursors beta-carotene (3,484 mcg) and lutein and zeaxanthin (2,312 mcg). Silicon and vitamin A are vital for healthy skin and rejuvenation, and vitamin A affords protection from cancer and optic deterioration. Silicon is vital for skin repair and, in particular, for hair growth. This, combined with lettuce's chlorophyll content, means it is possibly the only food that can restore hair loss. A tonic serving (120 ml) of lettuce juice mixed with carrot juice (50 ml), taken three times a week, will give the body the essential elements required to make hair. Meat, bread, fish, and processed foods provide no silicon or chlorophyll. Keep ahead of things by eating lettuce preventively, especially if you are likely, genetically speaking, to go thin on top. A regular serving of fresh lettuce will feed the hair, but the juice will be more easily absorbed, providing greater quantity and quality.

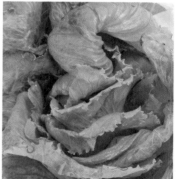

Lettuce also provides a good source of folate (30–130 mcg), required for production of red blood cells in the bone marrow, for brain function, and for a healthy nervous system. A prolonged deficiency of folate may trigger the onset of leukemia, especially in children; because they grow so fast, they need ample folate to manufacture blood cells. During pregnancy, a daily folate intake of 400 mcg is required for the development of the fetus. Green vegetables are a vital source of folate, so take to heart to the old saying: "If you don't eat your greens, you're not getting dessert!"

Lettuce's supplies of chlorine (500–1,380 mg) and sulfur (580–680 mg) are really top quality. These are heat-sensitive nutrients, but luckily, in lettuce (usually eaten uncooked), the benefits are fully available; they include purifying the blood, cleansing the body of toxins, preventing infections, and many more. Keratin, a major component of hair and skin in addition to silicon, contains sulfur.

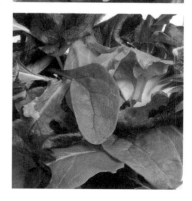

Lettuce is a fair source of organic iron (0.5–2 mg), plus trace amounts of copper (0.03 mg), manganese (0.6 mg), and vitamin C (6–24 mg), all required in combination for blood development. The potassium supply (247 mg) exceeds the sodium supply (8 mg), a vital balance in these days of excess salt consumption in the form of processed food and drink. Next time you think about lunch, crunch into a fresh salad!

NOTE: DV amounts listed refer to the daily value for women 25–50 years; refer to DRI charts on pages 95–96 for adult male and child values.

ONIONS – *Allium cepa*

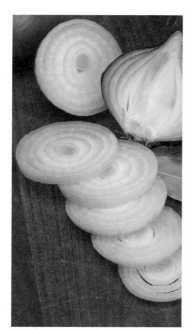

Onions, onions, onions! There are over three hundred varieties, of which the most widely consumed are the common yellow, red, and white onions, plus shallots and leeks. They all provide similar benefits. Onions are not eaten in large quantities, and they are fairly low in the main nutrients: calcium (22 mg), iron (0.5 mg), and phosphorus (27 mg). Their pungent flavor is the major benefit they bring to cooking; as you may know, you can caramelize onions on the stove top or in the oven with very little added oil. Onions contain natural antiseptic oils such as allyl disulfate and cycloallin. Research has shown that cycloallin has the unique ability to perform fibrinolysis: that is, to dissolve blood clots that can form inside blood vessels—in particular, in the veins. Another study suggested that cycloallin may also dissolve the fibrin formed around damaged or inflamed joints, as with arthritis. The good news is that cooking doesn't destroy the cycloallin in onions.

Other research has revealed that the substance quercetin, which is well supplied by onions, has numerous beneficial properties. Quercetin is a water-soluble pigment, a flavonoid. It provides antihistamine and anti-inflammatory qualities. It is also classed as a phytoestrogen and was shown to inhibit breast cancer cells in test tube research. Quercetin is a potent antioxidant, protecting against heart disease. It is also valuable for diabetics as it inhibits the enzyme that causes accumulation of a substance called sorbitol, a factor in the deterioration of the eyes, kidneys, and nerves in diabetics. Onions have a very low glycemic index and are therefore safe and ideal for most diabetics to include in their diets. Onions supply a fair amount of potassium (144 mg), but really it is the trace substances plus the sulfur oil content that give onions their mighty power. By providing internal cleansing, they keep those nasty internal toxins at bay (similar to how they keep people at a distance after you've eaten them!). Onions are also recognized to protect against and relieve prostatitis, reduce blood sugar, balance blood pressure, and reduce sinusitis, colds, and infections. Onion oil is often used for treatment of earaches and catarrh (inflammation of the mucus membranes).

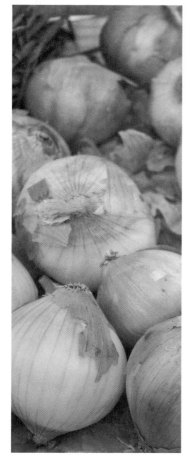

Onions promote beneficial bacteria in the lower intestine and cleansing of the respiratory system. Onions are great, but beware of eating them with added fats, especially when they're served with barbecue or sausages—pile your plate with onions, but hold off on all that saturated fat and cholesterol. A baked or roasted onion is ideal and full of mild flavor. Also try onion bread or French onion soup. So many recipes call for onion—stews, soups, pizza, salad—that you're well advised to keep a few in your pantry. Chives, a member of the onion family, are another great kitchen companion. You can grow them in containers even if you live in a high-rise apartment, and they add charm to numerous snacks and entrées. If you have a problem with onion breath, chew some fresh parsley or mint to restore your confidence.

The trace mineral molybdenum, required for fat metabolism, is supplied by onions. Onions also provide trace amounts of the antioxidant selenium (6 mcg), folate (19 mcg), and vitamin C (8 mg). They provide very little vitamin A (40 IU) or fiber (0.6 g). Last but not least, onions provide fructans as part of their carbohydrate structure. Fructans increase bifidobacteria and decrease detrimental bacteria in the intestines, reduce toxins, prevent constipation, reduce cholesterol, and lower blood pressure.

Peel an onion for unique and unreal benefits!

ONIONS

NOTE: Nutrient amounts are listed as milligrams (mg) per 100 grams (g), unless otherwise stated.

GLYCEMIC INDEX: 52	TOTAL CALORIES PER 100 G: 75	CALORIES FROM		
		CARB: 69 92%	PROTEIN: 3 4%	FAT: 3 4%

PARSNIPS – *Pastinaca sativa*

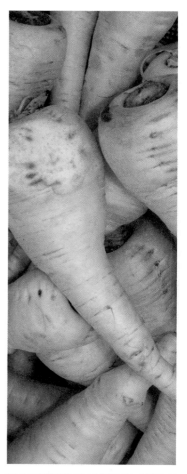

The parsnip is one of the underestimated vegetables: it may seem pale in appearance but it can pack a punch, nutritionally speaking. It is traditionally an essential ingredient of the meat-and-vegetable pie known as the British pasty (although very few commercial pasties include the parsnip). The potassium content (541 mg) of the parsnip exceeds that of the banana (370 mg) and the potato (407 mg). Potassium is the foundation mineral of all muscular tissues. In addition, potassium and phosphorus (77 mg) combined are vital for the transportation of oxygen into the brain. The only problem is that potassium is fairly heat sensitive—over 30% can be destroyed by excess cooking—therefore, continue to rely on bananas for pure potassium power.

The mineral silicon (800 mg), by contrast, is not heat sensitive, and parsnips are nearly second highest to lettuce in this essential mineral for the skin, hair, and nails. Parsnips are a rich source of organic chlorine (1,040 mg), containing twice the content of lettuce and nearly 1,000 times that of meat, grains, or cheese. The cause of numerous common ailments, especially of the respiratory and glandular system, is a lack of body cleansing, problems alleviated by these minerals. Sulfur (960 mg) is also abundant in parsnip, and is part of the reason for its unique flavor. Give your body a chance to do some spring cleaning: dig into parsnips!

The high glycemic index of parsnips (90) needs to be considered; balance the GI by roasting or baking parsnips and serving them with a cream sauce, or mashing them with milk and butter, or adding a cream sauce, onions, and maybe mushrooms. Parsnips' rich supply of cleansing nutrients can offset the added fats, as chlorine rids the body of excess fats, assists the liver, and cleanses the blood. Sulfur has a cleansing and antiseptic effect on the digestive system and also promotes fat metabolism.

Be smart: Don't forget the parsnip on your next shopping trip!

GLYCEMIC INDEX: VERY LOW	TOTAL CALORIES PER 100 G: 43	CALORIES FROM		
		CARB: 29 67%	PROTEIN: 5 12%	FAT: 9 21%

PEPPERS (CHILI) – *Capsicum annuum, C. frutescens*

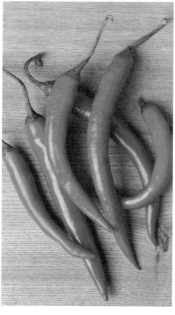

Chili peppers are small, bright, and potent. They range in color from green to yellow to cream to purple to red. And there's no way of telling, until you try one, how hot a chili is! Because chili peppers are consumed in minute amounts compared to other foods, their nutritional value is minimal; however, the benefits afforded by the supply of nutrients is remarkable. Approximately half the vitamin A content of fresh sweet red chilies (4,450 IU), hot red chilies (21,600 IU), hot green chilies (770 IU), and sweet green chilies (420 IU) is in the form of beta-carotene, the balance in the form of lutein and zeaxanthin. In addition, the rich supply of vitamin C (hot red 369 mg; hot green 235 mg) makes chili peppers a great food for the eyes—when taken internally, that is. Keep your hands away from your eyes and other sensitive areas when preparing peppers! Vitamins A and C are the main nutrients in chilies. Chilies are very low in most minerals except potassium (300 mg on average). Besides vitamins A and C, two special substances in peppers are capsaicin and resiniferatoxin. These both proved effective, in research, at killing a majority of skin cancer cells, causing them to self-destruct due to oxygen starvation. A little chili pepper goes a long way to heat up a dish—can you handle it?

NOTE: DV amounts listed refer to the daily value for women 25–50 years; refer to DRI charts on pages 95–96 for adult male and child values.

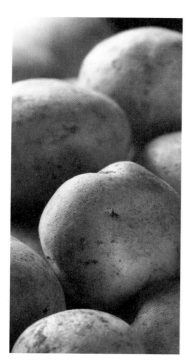

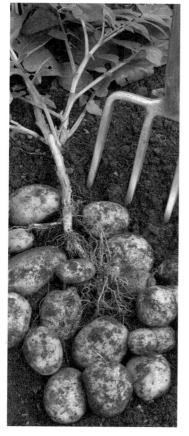

POTATOES – *Solanum tuberosum*

Potatoes are the greatest "down to earth" food; apart from the nutrients they afford, they seem to get you back on track, especially after a juice fast or a hectic day at the office. However, this refers only to the full potato, not to the ubiquitous packaged chips. The oversupply and overconsumption of potato chips and fast-food fries needs to be mentioned, as they are detrimental foods. They provide no health benefits, and they rob the pocketbook while robbing the body of the chance to eat proper food. In addition, the free radicals produced by heating the cooking oil used for frying chips is a major factor in the development of cancer, and the added salt contributes to heart disease. Chips and French fries supply 300 to 500 calories per 100 g; compare that to a baked potato, which supplies no oil and only 100 calories. That's a huge difference. Chips are popular due to their fat content combined with the additives that make them taste good and that provide quick, crunchy energy. They're also cheap. Children love chips, but next time you're at the store pick up some honey cashews or a sesame bar and get real food value.

Potatoes are a fair source of carbohydrate (17 g), which, depending on their preparation, can be good or bad. The fact that baked potatoes have a very high glycemic index of around 93, on their own, is cause for concern. The way to decrease the GI is to serve baked potatoes with mushrooms, onions, broccoli, cabbage, and a dab of butter, sour cream, or cheese sauce. Because meat supplies no carbohydrate and potatoes supply a fair amount, it is okay to have a serving of lean meat and veggies with your baked potato. Another way to lower the GI of potatoes is to prepare mashed potatoes, but they are still moderately high GI so it is best to add the veggies mentioned above for a balanced meal and a reduced GI. Potatoes absorb fat, so if you're going to fry potatoes or add oil to the cooking process, cut the potato pieces as big as possible (into wedges or steak-cut frieds) and use the oil only once. Use safflower, sunflower, or olive oil for frying, to reduce the free radical problem. Thin French fries absorb the most oil and have a GI of 75; potato chips have a moderate GI of 54, due to the abundance of oil.

Potatoes supply low amounts of complete protein, but it adds up considerably when fish or cheese is added to make a fulfilling meal. A meal of fish and chips is ideal for vacations, as long as children eat a good serving of fish before filling up on soft drinks and chips.

The potato has very few nutrient benefits apart from a good supply of potassium (400–500 mg), and fair amounts of vitamin C (10–20 mg), sulfur (289 mg), chlorine (155 mg), silicon (88 mg), phosphorus (53 mg), and iron (0.06 mg). That combination was enough to keep a generation of Irish people from starving in the early nineteenth century!

The numerous varieties of potatoes are worth discovering for their unique variations in flavor and texture and their use in specific recipes. All around the world, the potato is used in local dishes; it's the food of nations. It supplies a little of this and a little of that, and great quantities can be consumed to provide a storehouse of energy. In Ireland, during the potato famine, each person ate an average of 7.5 pounds (3.5 kg) of potates a day for years! Potatoes supply no vitamin A and only a small amount of vitamin C, so add a carrot or a slice of bell pepper, and top them with a yeast extract gravy for the B vitamins. Enjoy the apple of the earth!

POTATOES

NOTE: Nutrient amounts are listed as milligrams (mg) per 100 grams (g), unless otherwise stated.

GLYCEMIC INDEX: 75	TOTAL CALORIES PER 100 G: 26	CALORIES FROM		
		CARB: 23 88%	PROTEIN: 2 8%	FAT: 1 4%

PUMPKINS / WINTER SQUASH – *Cucurbita pepo*

Winter squash (referred to as pumpkins in Australian English) are related to the melon family, the *Cucurbitaceae,* all of which seem to spread easily throughout home gardens and entire fields. For full flavor, the flesh of winter squash needs to be a bright orange, which also indicates a maximum supply of vitamin A and carotenoids (1,600–7,000 IU). Over 50% of the carotene is in the form of beta-carotene (3,100 mcg), with beta-cryptoxanthin a close second at 2,145 mcg, and, third, lutein and zeaxanthin (1,500 mcg).

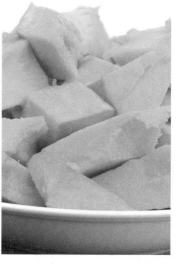

Winter squash and pumpkins are the ultimate food source of beta-cryptoxanthin; research has shown a direct benefit of this nutrient to the respiratory system—in particular, the lungs. For smokers and those exposed to secondhand smoke, a decreased blood serum level of beta-cryptoxanthin was found. Carotenoids in general are vital to the respiratory system, and beta-carotene also provides well-known antioxidant properties, as mentioned with carrots. However, carrots only supply 78 mcg of beta-cryptoxanthin, most vegetables contain none, and a few tropical fruits supply moderate amounts. Winter squash can therefore be considered the "king of cryptoxanthin." As a kind gesture to any smokers you know (yourself included) you can prepare a meal fit for royalty. Enjoy pumpkin scones or cookies for an afternoon snack; butternut squash soup as an appetizer; roasted winter squash for a main course; and for dessert, a luscious pumpkin pie. The addition of cream or butter to the soup, pie, or scones will improve the absorption of the beta-cryptoxanthin. As with all carotenoids, they are fat soluble, so the addition of dietary fat increases their absorption in the digestive tract.

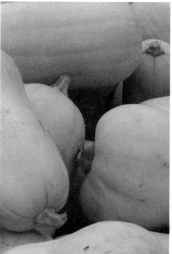

Winter squash are low in calcium (21 mg) and other minerals except potassium (340 mg), silicon, iron (1 mg), and chlorine. They are a great food for the eyes, skin, and hair, and during the winter, when they're in season, they provide plenty of energy with a moderately high GI (75). Add a dab of butter to the mash or cream to the soup to smooth the effect on blood sugar levels.

Although the smoking habit has unfortunately spread around the world, the benefits of this kingly vegetable can prevail.

GLYCEMIC INDEX: VERY LOW	TOTAL CALORIES PER 100 G: 16	CALORIES FROM		
		CARB: 13 81%	PROTEIN: 2 13%	FAT: 1 6%

RADISHES – *Raphanus sativus*

Radishes take up little space in this book, and that's all they need on your plate. They are a great promoter of digestive juices, as they are a very good source of organic chlorine (1,000 mg), which is ideal for stimulating the supply of protein-digestive enzymes in the stomach through the release of *pepsinogen*. Chlorine is heat sensitive, so it's beneficial that radishes are usually consumed raw. Chlorine is also great for reducing mucus; in addition, radishes supply a volatile ether oil that increases mucus elimination and has proved beneficial in cases of tuberculosis, coughs, and bronchitis. Radishes supply sulfur (715 mg), ideal for people with weak bile secretion to assist with fat digestion. The strong taste of radishes is due to their chlorine and sulfur content. Buy them young and freshly harvested, whenever possible; they are much sweeter that way.

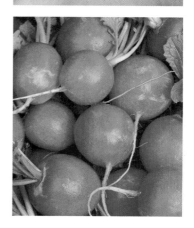

NOTE: DV amounts listed refer to the daily value for women 25–50 years; refer to DRI charts on pages 95–96 for adult male and child values.

GLYCEMIC INDEX: <20	TOTAL CALORIES PER 100 G: 23	CALORIES FROM		
		CARB: 13 57%	PROTEIN: 7 30%	FAT: 3 13%

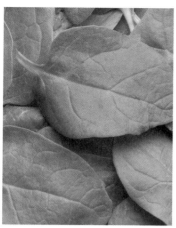

SPINACH (AND OTHER GREENS) – *Spinacia oleracea*

Spinach always gets a mention in health books, but let's not forget some of the other important leafy greens, such as Swiss chard *(Beta vulgaris)* and kale (*Brassica oleracea acephala*). Swiss chard is a distant cousin to spinach, and kale is technically a member of the cabbage family. They all provide a valuable supply of chlorophyll when eaten raw—and "true spinach" (*Spinacia oleracea*) is the easiest to eat raw.

Spinach and chard (but not kale) supply fair amounts of oxalic acid (0.97 g per 100 g), which is often considered a problem. Oxalic acid is a necessary component of blood (288 mcg per 100 ml) and is produced by the body. The immune system requires oxalic acid to protect against disease. Such factors as citric acid additives and alcohol increase the blood's oxalic acid levels. A prolonged deficiency of vitamin B6 can increase oxalic buildup in the kidneys. If spinach is eaten raw, the oxalic acid content is of no concern; it remains in an organic form, assists in the absorption of calcium, and is required for *peristalsis,* the involuntary movement of food through the esophagus. When these leafy greens are cooked, however, the oxalic acid they contain can "lock calcium" and be one cause of kidney stones. Inadequate water intake is another cause. The magnesium in spinach (79 mg) increases the solubility of oxalic acid. If you eat cooked spinach once a week, no worries, but if you eat chocolate regularly, drink very little water, consume alcohol in excess, and eat a lot of meat, with salt, you increase the risk of stone formation and poor calcium absorption.

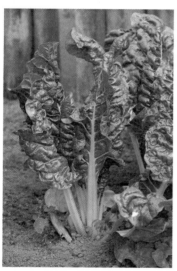

Spinach, chard, and kale are excellent sources of the carotenoids lutein and zeaxanthin (8,800–11,000 mcg), which are vital for the eyes of adults, as well as beta-carotene, which supplies anticancer properties. Spinach is an excellent source of potassium (558 mg), the "muscle mineral"—Popeye was right! It has a fair iron content (3 mg), a very rich folate content (194 mg), and an abundant vitamin K content (483 mg), but remember that freezing destroys vitamin K, so raw is best and very lightly steamed is okay. Spinach is a great health-restoring food.

GLYCEMIC INDEX: 54	TOTAL CALORIES PER 100 G: 249	CALORIES FROM		
		CARB: 233 94%	PROTEIN: 12 5%	FAT: 4 1%

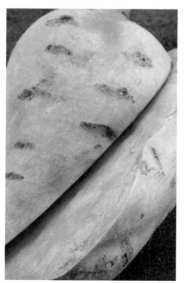

SWEET POTATO – *Ipomoea batatas*

Sweet potatoes are not yams, and they're not related to the potato. They do grow from a vine, and they form the underground tuberous part of the plant, same as potatoes. The sweet potato has a much lower glycemic index (54) than the regular potato, and that's a great start, especially as it is packed with carbohydrate value (95%) and has no fat content. It's a good food for anyone who is overweight or athletic; plus it provides dietary fiber.

Sweet potatoes are a pure beta-carotene food (8,728 mg) with a bit of vitamin C (38 mg)—less when cooked—and a fair supply of potassium (337 mg). They contain a dash of iron (1 mg), magnesium (25 mg), phosphorus (47 mg), folate (14 mcg), and vitamin E (0.4 mg). And there's no doubt that sweet potatoes are one of the sweetest vegetables. They contain the full range of plant sugars: sucrose (2,170 mg), glucose (1,010 mg), and fructose (710 mg), but these are "safe sugars" with a moderate GI for a stable increase in blood sugar and energy. The beta-carotene value gives the sweet potato a special title: the sweetest anticancer vegetable. So put it on your plate and tantalize your palate.

NOTE: Nutrient amounts are listed as milligrams (mg) per 100 grams (g), unless otherwise stated.

GLYCEMIC INDEX: 75	TOTAL CALORIES PER 100 G: 28	CALORIES FROM		
		CARB: 25 86%	PROTEIN: 3 10%	FAT: 1 4%

TURNIPS – *Brassica rapa*

Turnips (sometimes called white turnips) belong to the wallflower family: They rarely get up to dance. Their closest partner is the rutabaga, or yellow turnip (*Brassica napus,* called a swede in Australian and British English), a hybrid of broccoli and turnip. Compared to the amazing broccoli, turnips and swedes have no carotene character, not even a bit of beta-. Neither has any significant nutritional features: They always look chubby even though they carry no fat content, they provide very little calcium (30 mg), and they have very little "muscle tone" (potassium, 191 mg). They often taste a dash salty due to their organic sodium content of 67 mg, and that's a good thing because their blood count is really low in iron (0 mg) and their nerves are shaking with minimal magnesium (11 mg) and phosphorus (27 mg). Maybe it's that small bit of vitamin C (21 mg) that gives them a tiny spark of life. You can, however, eat as many as you like, without worrying about calories.

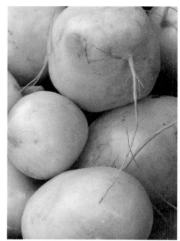

GLYCEMIC INDEX: VERY LOW	TOTAL CALORIES PER 100 G: 43	CALORIES FROM		
		CARB: 33 82%	PROTEIN: 5 13%	FAT: 2 5%

ZUCCHINI – *Cucurbita pepo*

Zucchini, a variety of summer squash with a delicate, water-based flavor, provide nutritional benefits that are similar to the yellow or crookneck squash, a member of the same family. Compared to winter squash, zucchini afford only a fairly basic supply of nutrients. Also known as the French courgette or Italian zucchini, they are occasionally served at the best restaurants. They are best eaten whole and lightly steamed or quickly fried, to retain their delicate flavor and moisture content. The zucchini supplies a small amount of vitamin A (323 IU), plus a good supply of potassium (200–400 mg), phosphorus (29 mg), calcium (27 mg), iron (0.3 mg), and vitamin C (19 mg).

Zucchini are a carbohydrate food with a low starch content and a trace of fiber (1 g); therefore, they need only a slight amount of heat—whether steaming, baking, grilling, or frying—to soften them. Zucchini also supply a small amount of complete protein (3 g). Serve lightly steamed, topped with cheese, on a bed of rice with cashew nuts for a simple, complete-protein meal. If you are on a weight-loss program, steamed zucchini with rice and a few raw cashews (which contain the lowest fat content of all nuts at 47 g per 100 g) can provide a large meal with very few calories, a low fat content, and a fair supply of complete protein. Grated zucchini make an excellent addition to burgers. Or try grilling zucchini, cut in half lengthwise and brushed with olive oil, on the barbecue; they're full of flavor due to the added fats.

Zucchini are the fastest-growing garden vegetable, famous for growing to huge sizes seemingly overnight after a rainstorm. If you grow them, you'll need to come up with creative ways to serve and eat them. Zucchini, along with most green leafy vegetables, supply folate (61 mcg). So serve a fresh salad or coleslaw along with plenty of grilled zucchini at your next cookout, and you'll be set to fight those nasty free radicals.

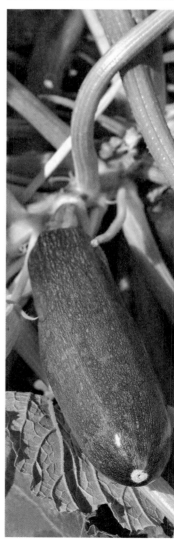

NOTE: DV amounts listed refer to the daily value for women 25–50 years; refer to DRI charts on pages 95–96 for adult male and child values.

Vegetables	Main Health Benefits, and Main Nutrients, Antioxidants, and Phytonutrients	Aids Which Body Systems
Artichoke	fiber, stabilize the metabolism, beneficial for the liver, potassium	digestive
Asparagus	asparagines, fluoride, bromine, glutathione, rutin, folate, sulfur, chlorine	urinary, glandular
Beet	chlorine, sulfur, manganese, sodium, potassium, copper, iron	blood, glandular
Broccoli	vitamin A, vitamin C, calcium, indole-3-carbinol, sulforane, chromium	immune, glandular
Brussels sprouts	sulfur, indoles, vitamin C, vitamin A, selenium, potassium, folate, fiber	digestive
Cabbage	vitamin A, vitamin C, potassium, bromine, folate	skin
Carrots	anthocyanins, isoquercetin, quercetin, ellagic acid, perillyl alcohol, melatonin, vitamin A, potassium	immune
Capsicum (bell pepper)	vitamin C, anthocyanin, vitamin A, potassium	immune
Cauliflower	fiber, potassium, iron, magnesium, calcium, phosphorus, copper	muscular
Celery	calcium, potassium, fiber, iron, manganese, copper, magnesium, phosphorus, silicon, chlorine, sulfur	blood
Cucumber	liminoids, lycopene, salicyclic acid, vitamin C, biotin, B5	joint
Eggplant	manganese, saponin, trans-resveratrol, phenolic compounds	joint
Leek	vitamin C, lutein, zeaxanthin	immune
Mushrooms	vitamin C, vitamin A, copper, iron, potassium, phytonutrients	respiratory
Lettuce	citric acid, sulfur, vitamin C, antioxidants	immune
Onions	beta-carotene, chlorine, vitamin C, potassium	respiratory
Parsnips	alkaline, bromine, vitamin C, potassium, vitamin A, enzymes	glandular
Peppers (chili)	potassium, beta-cryptoxanthin, beta-carotene, lutein, zeaxanthin	respiratory
Potato	added sodium, calcium, potassium, iron, vitamin A, oleic acid	none
Pumpkin (winter squash)	papain, carpain, chymopapain, vitamin C, beta-cryptoxanthin, beta-carotene, lutein, zeaxanthin	immune, repair, skin
Radish	vitamin P, vitamin C, citric acid, calcium, phosphorus, magnesium, phyto-nutrients, fiber	immune, respiratory
Spinach	beta-carotene, beta-cryptoxanthin, lutein, zeaxanthin, sulfur	skin, elimination
Sweet potato	fiber, copper, potassium, silicon, folate	elimination
Turnips	chlorine, sulfur, manganese, bromelain, vitamin C, copper, selenium, zinc	respiratory, blood
Zucchini	phytonutrients, phenols, vitamin A, copper, manganese, carotene	immune, brain

RECOMMENDATIONS FOR DAILY CARBOHYDRATE INTAKE FROM VEGETABLES		Adult Male	Adult Female	Teenager	Child
Total Daily Carbohydrate Intake (based on typical guidelines)		340 g	280 g	400 g	270 g
1. *UNH* recommendation: 15% of carbohydrate intake from vegetables, in the following proportions:		51 g	42 g	60 g	40 g
65% starch vegetables	100 g* (3–4 oz) contains approx. 14 g of carbohydrate				
10% leafy salad vegetables	100 g* contains approx. 3 g of carbohydrate				
25% brassica vegetables	100 g* contains approx. 5 g of carbohydrate				
1. *UNH* recommendation: 5% of carbohydrate intake from vegetable juice		17 g	14 g	20 g	13 g
	100 g vegetable juice** contains approx. 9 g of carbohydrate				
2. U.S. MyPlate and DRIs		an abundance of vegetables			
3. Australian Guide to Healthy Eating***		5 servings	5 servings	3–4 servings	2 servings

UNH = Ultimate Nutrition for Health; DRIs = Dietary Reference Intakes

* 100 g is equivalent to any one of the following: 1 medium potato, 1 medium bowl of salad vegetables, or 1 full cup of cooked brassica vegetables, ½ cup raw cauliflower, or 1 small carrot, ½ cup raw spinach, 2 scoops mashed pumpkin, 3 cups shredded lettuce, 3 pieces celery—9 in long, 4 florets broccoli, or ½ a large parsnip.

** 100 g of vegetable juice = ½ glass (approx. 100 ml)

*** 1 serving is equivalent to: ½ cup cooked vegetables (75 g), 1 cup salad vegetables, or 1 small potato.

The use of herbs for their medicinal properties is a specialized field, and only fully trained practitioners can provide accurate advice and diagnosis. The information on herbs in the following pages is provided as a basic guide to some common herbs and how they're used for healing. This guide is not intended to be used for any treatment or diagnosis, or to determine dosage. Obtaining both medical and naturopathic advice is always recommended.

By maintaining a natural-food diet and overall healthy lifestyle you can be sure of reaching your maximum health potential. Many herbs are part of the common diet and provide well-recognized benefits, but under some conditions, such as during pregnancy, they may be unsuitable for consumption. For this reason, proper advice is required to ensure they are used safely.

Herbs have a long history of providing benefits, and it is safe to use some time-tested herbs, such as garlic, parsley, ginger, and mint, on a regular basis during most times in life. Herbs are often used simply to add flavor to meals, but they can also provide numerous health benefits. Pages 78–80 describe some of the most common herbs in more detail. When considering the intake of a new herb, always check with a medical practitioner, as some herbs may react with common medications.

Herbs have been used for healing for eons. When properly diagnosed, a health condition may gain great improvement from the addition of properly prepared herbal tonics or infusions. Give the herb kingdom a chance to add spice to your life and promote maximum healing power.

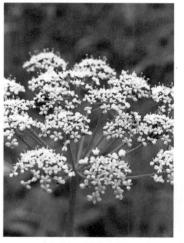

ANISE – *Pimpinella anisum*

Anise produces seeds that contain a special oil, anethole. It is this substance that provides the herb's main benefits, as either a tea infusion or an oil. It is commonly used in cough medicines and lozenges. The tiny seeds, when used in cooking, promote the digestion of fatty foods as they provide the B vitamin choline. For babies with colic, regular use of anise tea by the nursing mother may relieve the condition. Anise oil may also be used in formula milk to relieve colic. Anise tea promotes lactation and purifies the digestive system. Anise tea is beneficial for a weak digestive system; it helps to balance acidity and relieve stomach cramps. Anise oil in a vaporizer helps in cases of bronchitis, emphysema, laryngitis, and persistent cough. Anise oil mixed with milk may promote sleep and relieve cases of insomnia. Anise seeds are ideal to add to fish, pork, or veal dishes and to sauces. The oil is used in liqueurs, such as anisette. Anise oil and seeds are valuable digestive aids.

BASIL – *Ocimum basilicum*

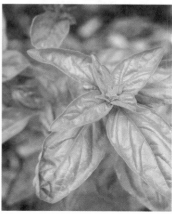

The delightfully flavored basil provides the flavonoids vicenin and orientin, which protect cells from the effects of free radicals and radiation. The variety of oils, which are extracted from the leaves, provide the main benefits. They contain the compounds cineole, eugenol, estragole, limonene, myrcene, and sabinene. The oils provide a powerful antibacterial effect, even against some bacteria that are resistant to the action of antibiotics. Basil oil also provides anti-inflammatory action, as eugenol blocks the activity of an enzyme that causes inflammation. Basil promotes appetite and relieves headaches, stomach cramps, and constipation.

Basil is the chef's best man!

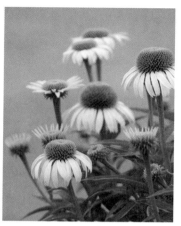

ECHINACEA – *Echinacea angustifolia, E. pallida, E. purpurea*

Echinacea increases the body's ability to produce white blood cells, which are required especially during times of infections, viruses, and colds. It is an excellent blood cleanser, removing toxins from the blood and improving filtration and drainage of the lymphatic system, which collects toxins before they enter the blood system. Echinacea is a natural antibiotic and may provide relief from tonsillitis and respiratory and bladder infections. It is also used to reduce fever. Externally, echinacea may relieve psoriasis, eczema, arthritis, and burns. It may help in cases of an enlarged or weak prostate. Extracts of echinacea root may provide relief from chemotherapy symptoms and from yeast infections. Echinacea is not recommended for children under two years, or during pregnancy or lactation. In addition, diabetics and people with autoimmune diseases, tuberculosis, leukemia, multiple sclerosis, or collagen disease should not use echinacea.

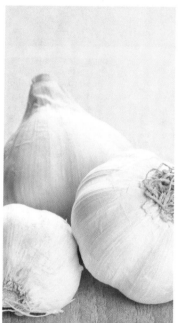

GARLIC – *Allium sativum*

Garlic has been the champion of herbs since the beginning of time. The Egyptian slaves refused to work when garlic was not provided. Garlic is the best source of sulfur compounds—e.g., allicin—which provide powerful antibacterial, antibiotic, antiviral and anti-infection action. Garlic reduces the activity of inflammations that cause the spread of common colds and viruses. Allicin compounds protect against colon cancer and may stop the growth of bacteria that cause stomach cancer. The substance ajoene, another sulfur compound found in garlic, may help reduce skin cancer. Regular use of garlic may provide protective benefits for diabetics due to increased antioxidant levels and reduced triglycerides, insulin, and blood pressure. Garlic also contains allyl disulfate, which provides antiseptic power and antiviral activity. Fresh (raw) garlic is the best source of these sulfur oils, as excess cooking destroys sulfur compounds. Regular use of garlic cleanses the body of toxins. Garlic is the ideal herb for relief of respiratory disorders, bronchitis, dysentery, cholera, typhoid fever, and intestinal worms. It can also help to reduce blood pressure and improve circulation and heart action. Odorless garlic capsules taken regularly may provide a fair amount of protection. Garlic is the one essential herb in any kitchen; consuming a clove every few days is the ideal way to stay healthy, fit, and active and to protect against any nasties that want a free ride. Give garlic a go for any ailment; it provides pure white healing power.

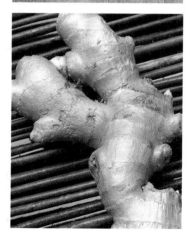

GINGER – *Zingiber officinale*

Ginger may provide relief from inflammation due to the supply of compounds known as gingerols. Such conditions as osteo- and rheumatoid arthritis and swollen joints may be relieved with regular use of the ginger root. Gingerols reduce the production of nitric acid, which causes free radical damage. Ginger may provide protection from motion sickness, sea sickness, and nausea during pregnancy. Ginger boosts the immune system, relaxes digestion, provides antioxidant power, and promotes sweating.

NOTE: Nutrient amounts are listed as milligrams (mg) per 100 grams (g), unless otherwise stated.

GINSENG – *Panax ginseng, P. quinquefolius*

Ginseng comes in two main varieties: Oriental and American. However, true ginseng is obtained from the Chinese or Korean plant. Chinese ginseng contains the active ingredient, panax, which stimulates the entire body, relieves fatigue, improves circulation, nourishes the blood, reduces blood sugar levels, and promotes normal blood pressure. It is not recommended for ailments with inflammation, during menstruation, or times of fever.

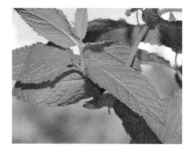

MINT – *Mentha piperita*

Peppermint contains a phytonutrient termed perillyl alcohol, which may help retard tumors of the pancreas, liver, and mammary glands. Peppermint oil in a vaporizer may protect against various bacteria and fungi. Peppermint also contains rosmarinic acid for improved respiration and relief of asthma. Peppermint tea promotes digestion and helps to relieve conditions of indigestion, irritable bowel syndrome, nervousness, insomnia, migraine, headaches, coughs, and heartburn.

PARSLEY – *Petroselinum crispum*

Parsley is rich in vitamin A (8,500 IU) and vitamin C (172 mg). Both of these give it the power to prevent colds and viruses due to the supply of water-soluble vitamin C, fat-soluble vitamin A, and antioxidants. In addition, the rich supply of iron (6.2 mg) provides protection from colds. Dishes such as tabouli provide maximum parsley power, or try a few sprigs with a carrot or celery juice for a real rush of benefits. Parsley contains special oils such as myristicin that may retard tumor development, especially in the lungs. Parsley provides protection against carcinogens in cigarette smoke and other environmental pollutants. Another benefit of parsley comes from the supply of flavonoids such as apiin, which promotes digestion, and especially luteolin, which protects against the effects of free radical damage, or oxygen damage to cells that can be caused by cooked oils. Try a tabouli salad and feel at ease about the free radicals. Parsley is food for blood building due to the content of iron, folate, magnesium, manganese, and copper. Parsley may help to relieve bladder infections, improve digestion, promote lactation, and alleviate menstruation. When infused and applied to eyes, parsley relieves conjunctivitis. Avoid using parsley in cases of kidney inflammation, and avoid the seeds and large quantities of the leaves during pregnancy. Parsley is a potent herb.

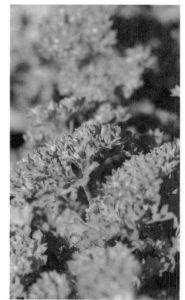

PEPPER – *Piper nigrum*

Black, green, and white pepper are derived from the same plant: they are the pepper berry at varying stages of ripening. Black pepper is fully ripe and promotes maximum benefits such as activating digestion and stimulating protein-digestive enzymes and fat breakdown. Pepper also provides antioxidant and antibacterial action and protects against flatulence. Pepper promotes sweating and diuretic functions. It's a great spice to add.

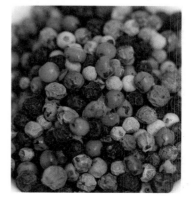

The table and glossary on pages 81–84 are provided as a basic guide to the most common herbs and their association with healing, their effect on body and mind, and their basic use and preparation.

This guide is not intended to be used for any personal application or to recommend dosages. Medical and naturopathic advice is always recommended. The purpose of the table is to provide a view of the additional benefits for healing that Nature has provided, in addition to the wide range of natural foods and a wonderful environment.

NOTE: DV amounts listed refer to the daily value for women 25–50 years; refer to DRI charts on pages 95–96 for adult male and child values.

Naturopaths are trained to recognize illness and prescribe the proper dosage of herbs. Often a combination of herbs is provided in tonic, drop, or emollient form. Some herbs may cause problems when combined with prescription medications. Check with a reputable naturopath. Finally, always remember that natural foods provide all the nutrients to keep healthy.

It is interesting to be aware of the effects of herbs and spices that you may use regularly, if only in the kitchen. Some herbs have been used successfully for thousands of years for healing, and today most herbs have well-recognized functions.

THE MOST COMMON HERBS AND THEIR USES

Herb	Uses
ACACIA *Acacia senegal*	Coughs, colds, sore throat, catarrh, diarrhea, dysentery. Dissolved in water.
ADDER'S TONGUE *Ezythronium americanum*	Emetic, antiscrofulous, emollient. Fresh leaves crushed into poultice with cider.
AGAVE *Agave americana*	Disinfectant, laxative, diuretic, diseased liver, jaundice. Boil plant.
ALFALFA *Medicego sativa*	Appetizer, diuretic, tonic, bowel problems, peptic ulcers. Use fresh leaves, make tea.
ALOE *Aloe vera*	Sunburn, wrinkles, insect bites, cuts, wounds. Break leaves to extract juice, use direct from plant.
ALPINE CRANBERRY *Vaccinium vitis idaea*	Gout, rheumatism, diarrhea, disinfectant. Boil leaves into tonic or eat berries.
ALTHEA *Althea officinalis*	Demulcent, emollient, diuretic, burns, carbuncles, wounds, gargle, coughs, whooping cough, bronchitis, catarrh. Steep leaves, flowers, or root in boiled water.
AMARANTH *Amaranthus hypochondriacus*	Astringent, gargle, throat irritations, dysentery, diarrhea. Infuse leaves in water, drink the infusion.
AMERICAN CENTAURY *Sabatia angularis*	Indigestion, dyspepsia, tonic. Steep in boiling water, using leaves.
AMERICAN IVY *Parthenocissus quinquefolio*	Astringent, coughs, colds, tonic. Use bark and twigs chopped into cold water.
ANGELICA *Angelica archangelica*	Tonic, appetizer, carminative, diuretic, flatulence, headaches, colic, fever, stomach and intestinal problems. Infuse crushed seeds in boiling water.
ANISE *Pimpinella anisum*	Digestion, flatulence, colic, eye wash, cramps and spasms, insomnia, purifier, lactation. Crush seeds and steep in boiling water, strain, drink hot.
ARNICA *Arnica montana*	Wounds, bruises. Diluted infusion from dried flowers.
ARUM *Arum maculatum*	Bronchitis, asthma, catarrh, flatulence, rheumatism, gargle. Dried rootstock only, boiled, cooked, diluted, syrup with honey.
ASARUM *Asarum europaeum*	Diuretic, catarrh, emetic, mucus, eliminative. Use only with medical direction.
BALM *Melissa officinalis*	Nervous disorders, cramps, colic, bronchitis, catarrh, asthma, migraine, toothache, dizziness, melancholy, hysteria, insomnia, insect bites. Use fresh leaves, make tea.
BARBERRY *Berberis rulgans*	Liver ailments, high blood pressure, gargle, pyorrhea. Ripe berries or boil bark of the root into tea.
BASIL *Ocimum basilicum*	Appetizer, stomachic, cramps, vomiting, constipation, whooping cough. Use with meals or make into tea.
BEARBERRY *Arctostaphylos uva-ursi*	Gallstones, cystitis, bronchitis, kidney stones. Make tea from leaves, use small quantities only.
BEAR'S GARLIC *Allium ursinum*	Arteriosclerosis, liver problems, diarrhea, emphysema, bronchitis, high blood pressure. Use as a salad green, soup.
BEDSTRAW *Galium aparine, verum*	Catarrh, diaphoretic, diuretic, epilepsy, dropsy, calmative. Use fresh leaves, steep in warm water.
BENNETT *Geum urbanum*	Diarrhea, gargle, tonic, halitosis. Make decoction with herb or roots in water.
BETONY *Stachys officinalis*	Heartburn, sweating, varicose veins, worms, neurasthenia, sores, cuts. Infuse the flowering herb in water.
BILBERRY *Vaccinium myrtillus*	Fever, antiseptic, astringent, gargle, coughs, vomiting, eyesight. Use berries, or dry and make infusion.
BIRCH *Betula alba, alta*	Astringent, worms, rheumatism, boils, diuretic, anthelmintic. Make decoction with inner bark or leaves in water.
BIRTHROOT *Trillium pendulum*	Antiseptic, tonic, coughs, colds, insect bites and stings. Use roots in a decoction with hot water or milk.
BIRTHWORT *Aristolochia clematitis*	Snakebite, abdominal and menstrual problems, childbirth. Boil roots or fresh plant in water.
BISTORT *Polygonum*	Diarrhea, dysentery, astringent, diuretic. Use roots, boil in water.

(cont'd.)

Herb	Uses
BLACK, RED, & SMOOTH ALDER *Alms glutinosa, alumbra, serrulata*	Lice, scabies, scabs, astringent. Boil inner bark, apply diluted.
BLACK COHOSH *Cimicifuga racemosa*	Hysteria, whooping cough, chorea, sedative, cardiac stimulant, rheumatism, bronchitis. Use roots at the time berries form. Boil in water.
BLACK ROOT *Varonicastrum*	Emetic, cathartic, hepatic. Use root under medical supervision only.
BLAZING STAR *Liatris spicata, squarrosa*	Gonorrhea, snakebite. Use root extracts directly, or boil root in water.
BLIND NETTLE *Lamium album*	Menstrual irregularities, astringent, varicose veins, and gout. Use plant or flowers, infuse in water.
BLOODROOT *Sanguinaria canadensis*	Sedative, tonic, stimulant, eczema, sores. Roots used only under medical supervision.
BLUE COHOSH *Caulophyllum thalictroides*	Colic, childbirth, regulate menstruation, cramps. Roots used only with medical supervision.
BLUE FLAG *Iris versicolor*	Heartburn, gastritis, enteritis, migraine, dropsy. Use boiled roots. For burns and sores use crushed fresh leaves.
BLUE VERVAIN *Verbena hastata*	Tranquilizer, emetic, tonic, fevers and colds, insomnia, worms. Use roots, boil in water. Use leaves to make tea.
BORAGE *Borago officinalis*	Fever, antidote for poisons, pleurisy, lactation. Dried flowers or leaves, steep in cold water.
BOXWOOD *Buxus sempervirens*	Purgative, diaphoretic. Use under medical supervision.
BRIAR HIP *Rosa canina*	Diuretic, kidney stones, gout, rheumatism, eliminates uric acid. Use fruit without seeds, boil in water.
BROOKLIME *Veronica beccabunga*	Anemia, febrifuge. Use fresh juice diluted with water or milk.
BRYONY *Bryonia alba, dioica*	Purgative, constipation, whooping cough. Extracts from root, use under medical supervision only.
BUCHU *Barosma betulina*	Aromatic, stimulant, urinary disorders, stomachic, tonic. Use leaves, steep in water.
BUCK BEAN *Barosma serratifolia*	Fever, migraine, indigestion. Use dried leaves, steep in water.
BUCKTHORN *Rhamnus frangula, cathartica*	Constipation, obesity, dropsy. Use bark from *R. frangula*, use dried bark only.
BURDOCK *Arctium lappa*	Neutralize poisons, stimulate bile, acne. Use leaves/root, boil in water.
BUTTERCUP *Ranunculus acris*	Rheumatism, sciatica, rhinitis. Use fresh plant only with medical supervision.
CALENDULA *Calendula officinalis*	Bruises, sprains, pulled muscles, burns, and sores. Use boiled dried flowers or leaves with lard.
CAMOMILE *Anthemis nobilis*	Aromatic, flatulence, colic, fever, restlessness, sores and wounds, stomach cramps. Use flowers, make tea.
CANNABIS *Cannabis sativa*	Analgesic-hypnotic, antiasthmatic, antibiotic, antiepileptic, antidepressant, antiglaucoma, tranquilizer, euphorigenic, alcohol withdrawal. Flowering top and leaves ingested, inhaled. Note: prohibited plant in most countries.
CARAWAY *Carum carvi*	Stomachic, expectorant, appetizer, menagogue, carminative. Use seeds in cooking, salads, bread.
CARDAMOM *Elettaria cardamomum*	Flatulence, spice, appetizer, stimulant, stomachic. Use as flavor or spice in cooking.
CATNIP *Nepeta cataria*	Stomach upsets, enema, bronchitis, colic, aromatic. Use herb in boiled water, steep quickly, do not boil.
CAYENNE *Capsicum frutescens*	Appetizer, digestive, cramps, bowel pains. Use pepper with meals.
CHERVIL *Anthriscus cerefolium*	Eczema, gout stones, abscesses, dropsy, high blood pressure. Use fresh or dried herb with meals.
CHICKWEED *Stellana media*	Laxative, expectorant. Use herb, boil in water, use as tea/tonic. Can be eaten with salads or vegetable meals.
CHICORY *Cichorium intybus*	Jaundice, spleen problems, bile production, gallstones, mucus. Make tea from leaves.
CHIVE *Allium schoenoprasum*	Appetizer, digestive, anemia. Use fresh leaves.
CLOVE *Caryophyllus aromaticus*	Antiseptic, anodyne, toothache, vomiting, nausea, aphrodisiac. Use buds or oil tincture.
COLTSFOOT *Tussilago farfara*	Respiratory problems, coughs, colds, bronchitis. Steep in warm water. For insect bites, inflammations, burns. Use the crushed leaves in decoction.
COMFREY *Symphytum officinale*	For digestive problems, excess menstruation, use as tea. Use powdered roots for coughs, dysentery, and diarrhea. Use leaves as a poultice for wounds, insect bites, and sores.
CORIANDER *Coriandrum sativum*	Appetizer, aromatic, antispasmodic, used as spice with seeds. Externally, use for relief of rheumatism and pain in the joints, make into poultice.
DANDELION *Taraxacum officinale*	Edema, stimulates bile formation, liver problems. Tonic, stimulant, constipation, gallstones, jaundice, anemia, fever, insomnia, hypochondria. Use plant direct, or steep in boiled water. Also available in herbal drinks.
DILL *Anethum graveolens*	Upset stomach, insomnia, flatulence, lactation, use fruit seeds, steep in boiled water, serve as tea or tonic.

(cont'd.)

EUCALYPTUS *Eucalyptus globulus*	Antiseptic, deodorant, colds, lung disease, sore throat, asthma, bronchitis, pyorrhea, burns, infection, fever. Boil leaves and condense water to get oil. Use diluted as directed.
FENNEL *Foeniculum milgare*	Aromatic, stomach and intestinal disorders, appetite stimulant, colic, abdominal cramps, flatulence, mucus, lactation. Use seeds fresh crushed, steep in boiled water. Use as a spice for any fish meal or fatty meal.
FIGWORT *Scrophularia nodosa*	Scabies, tumors, eczema, rashes, skin problems, bruises. Use plant directly, steep in water.
FLAX *Linum usitatissimum*	Coughs, catarrh, chest and lung problems, make decoction with seeds in boiled water. The oil (linseed) is used for gallstone elimination.
GARDEN VIOLET *Viola odorata*	Respiratory problems, gargle, headaches, whooping cough. Use boiled roots solution.
GINGER *Zingiber officinale*	Stimulant, appetizer, carminative, menstruation relief, colic, digestive. Use root in meals.
GINSENG *Panax schinseng, quinquefolius*	Panacea, stimulant, fever, blood disease, childbirth, vigor, digestive, aphrodisiac, nerves, glands, coughs, colds, chest problems. Use as a tea, oil extract, or dried root only.
GOLDENSEAL *Hydrastis canadensis*	Antiseptic, laxative, diuretic, catarrh, pyorrhea. Use powdered roots in boiled water, cool.
HAWTHORN *Crataegus oxyacantha*	Sedative, high blood pressure, cardiac, arteriosclerosis, nervous heart problems, insomnia. Use flowers, steep in water or make tea from the fruit, boil and strain.
HIBISCUS (MUSKMELLOW) *Hibiscus abelmoschus*	Antispasmodic, itchy skin, nervine, stomachic. Emulsion made from seeds.
HOLLY *Ilex aquifolium, opaca*	Gout, gallstones, bronchitis, arthritis, rheumatism, diuretic. Boil leaves in water. Berries are mildly poisonous.
HOPS *Humulus lupulus*	Sedative, hypnotic, calmative, insomnia, flatulence, intestinal cramps. Steep hop fruit in water, use fresh.
HORSERADISH *Armoracia lapathifolia*	Gout, rheumatism, colitis, coughs, asthma, congestion. Use root extracts, chopped finely in salads.
IRISH MOSS *Chondrus crispus*	Coughs, colds, tuberculosis, mucilaginous. The plant is generally used as a decoction, also in cough lozenges.
JASMINE *Jasminum officinale*	Calming, snake bite. Use flowers, steep in water. The scent is sensual when the plant is in full flower.
JUNIPER *Juniperus communis*	Tonic, antidiuretic, make tea from berries. Also use spice to stimulate appetite. Juniper oil is used for bone/joint pains and as a vapor for bronchitis and lung infection.
KNOTWEED *Polygonum*	Dysentery, bronchitis, enteritis, lung problems, coagulant, peptic ulcers, kidney stones, and gallstones. Use flowering herb, steep in water.
LAVENDER *Lavandula vera*	Sedative, tonic, migraine, stimulant, flatulence, antiseptic, cleansing, nausea. Use leaves prior to flowering, steep in water/infusion.
LICORICE *Glycyrrhiza glabra*	Diuretic, laxative, bronchitis, congestion, peptic ulcers, fever. Use roots infused in water.
LINDEN *Convallaria*	Stomachic, colds, coughs, sore throat. Flowers and leaves in tea.
LOVAGE *Levisticum officinale*	Stimulant, diuretic, stomachic. Should not be used by pregnant women. Roots infusion in water.
MAGNOLIA *Magnolia glauca*	Dysentery, dyspepsia, tonic, tobacco cure, astringent. Use bark decoction.
MALLOW *Malva sylvestris, rotundifolia*	Expectorant, demulcent, emollient, bronchitis, respiratory ailments. Use fresh plant only, make infusion or decoction in water.
MARJORAM *Origanum vulgare, hortensis*	Carminative, stomachic, tonic, coughs, colic, cramps, menstruation, regulation, seasickness, calmative. Use herb and flowers, infuse in water or take as a spice with foods.
MINT *Mentha piperita, spicata* **(peppermint, spearmint, and curled mint)**	Stomachic, tonic, antispasmodic, nerves, coughs, migraine, digestion, heartburn, nausea, cramps, aphrodisiac. Use as tea, leaves only before flowering, pick on a hot sunny day.
MUSTARD *Brassica nigra, hirta*	Digestive, appetizer, bronchitis, pleurisy, antiseptic. Use with foods.
NASTURTIUM *Tropaeolum majus*	Disinfectant, antiseptic, congestion, colds, blood formation, expectorant. Use leaves and flowers to make juice as tonic.
NETTLE *Urtica dioica*	Digestive, lactation, astringent, hemorrhoids, rheumatism, diarrhea. Cook plant, or infusion, or juice tonic.
NUTMEG *Myristica fragrans*	Aromatic, hallucinogenic, flatulence, carminative, use seed ground into powder. Do not eat seeds whole as they are fairly poisonous.
PASSION FLOWER *Passiflora incamata*	Sedative, nerves, diaphoretic. Use as prescribed.
PENNYROYAL *Hedeoma pulegioides*	Colds, nausea, diaphoretic, carminative, menstruation, headache, rashes. Not to be used during pregnancy. Make infusion.
PERIWINKLE *Vinca major, minor*	Sedative, toothache, nerves, hysteria, fits, astringent, menstruation. Use the herb as tea, or chew for toothaches.
PLANTAIN *Plantago*	Coughs, gastritis, respiratory, blood coagulation, worms, sores, cuts, bites, hemorrhoids, toothache. Use and chew root. Make infusion or decoction.

(cont'd.)

POMEGRANATE *Punica granatum*	Diarrhea, astringent, gargle, tapeworm. Use as fruit in moderation.
PRIMROSE *Primula officinalis*	Insomnia, bronchitis, coughs, lung problems, blood cleanser, rheumatism, gout, skin blemishes. Use flowers as infusion, or decoction with roots.
RAGWORT *Senecio aureus*	Menstruation, diuretic. Contains toxic alkaloids.
RED EYEBRIGHT *Euphrasia officinalis*	Eye inflammations, eyewash, coughs, colds, congestion, hay fever. Use fresh herb as infusion.
RHUBARB *Rheum palmatum*	Appetizer, purgative, tonic, laxative. Use in small doses as food, not for pregnancy or lactation periods. Use stem only, leaves contain high oxalic acid content.
ROSE *Rosa* spp.	Headaches, nerve and heart tonic, blood purifier, sores, toothache, use red rose petals. The fruit-hip is a very rich source of vitamin C, use in tea.
ROSEMARY *Rosmarinus officinalis*	Stimulant, liver functioning, digestion and bile production, improves circulation, raises blood pressure. Use as dried herb sparingly, use oil for bruises, eczema, sores, and wounds.
SAGE *Salvia officinalis*	Reduces perspiration, stops flow of mother's milk, nerves, depression, diarrhea, stomach disorders, sore throat, use as infusion. Fresh leaves for insect bites and warts. Crush leaves to extract juice.
SARSAPARILLA *Smilax officinalis*	Tonic, rheumatism, colds, fever, flatulence, blood purifier. Use roots infusion or as a drink.
SASSAFRAS *Sassafras albidum*	Rheumatism, gout, arthritis, antiseptic, diuretic, pain relief, fever, tonic. Use infusion of bark.
SAVORY *Satureja hortensis*	Stomach disorders, cramps, nausea, poor appetite, gargle, aphrodisiac. Use infusion of herb.
SKULLCAP *Scutellaria lateriflora*	Sedative, nerves, diuretic, tonic, insomnia, rheumatism, neuralgia, menstruation. Use plant as infusion.
TARRAGON *Artemisia dracunculus*	Digestion, kidneys, menstruation, insomnia, hypnotic. Use flowering plant as infusion.
THYME *Thymus vulgaris, serpyllum*	Sedative, bronchitis, diarrhea, coughs, colic, antispasmodic, use fresh herb as infusion. Use oil for antiseptic, toothpaste, mouthwash, warts, rheumatism, bruises, sprains. Use a salve for shingles. Use sparingly as an herb in food.
WILD DAISY *Bellis perennis*	Laxative, tonic, purgative, burns, colds, congestion, stomach problems, liver, kidneys. Use as tea or use externally for injuries, stiffness.

GLOSSARY

ACRID • having a hot or biting taste.

ALTERNATIVE • a substance that gradually restores body functions.

ANODYNE • a substance that relieves pain.

ANTHELMINTIC • a substance that removes worms.

ANTIBIOTIC • an agent that fights microorganisms.

ANTIEMETIC • a substance that relieves nausea and vomiting.

ANTISEPTIC • a substance that destroys harmful germs or bacteria.

ANTITUSSIVE • a substance that provides relief to coughing.

APERIENT • a laxative, stimulates bowel.

APHRODISIAC • an agent that increases or stimulates sexual desire or potency.

APPETIZER • promotes the appetite.

AROMATIC • a spicy fragrant herb or extract with pleasant smell.

ASTRINGENT • a substance that contracts skin tissue or reduces discharges and secretions.

BALSAM • extract of certain trees that is a healing or soothing agent.

CALMATIVE • provides a relaxing, calming effect on the body and mind.

CARDIAC • a substance that affects the heart either by stimulating or restoring other functions.

CARMINATIVE • an extract that helps to relieve digestive gas.

CATARRH • inflammation of the respiratory tract, congestion.

CATHARTIC • laxative, relieves bowel.

CHOLAGOGUE • a substance that promotes bile flow.

COAGULANT • promotes clotting of the blood.

DECOCTION • a herbal preparation by simmering in water.

DEMULCENT • soothes inflamed membranes, tissues, mainly mucus membrane.

DEPRESSANT • a substance that decreases nervous function.

DEPURATIVE • an agent that purifies the blood.

DIAPHORETIC • promotes perspiration.

DIGESTIVE • an ingredient that promotes or enhances digestion.

DIURETIC • causes an increase in the secretion of urine.

EMETIC • promotes vomiting.

EMMENAGOGUE • increases menstrual flow.

EMOLLIENT • a substance or lotion that soothes skin.

ERRHINE • a substance that promotes or causes sneezing.

EXPECTORANT • a substance that promotes mucus discharge.

HEMOSTATIC • an ingredient that helps stop bleeding.

HEPATIC • a substance that has an effect on the liver.

NEPHRITIC • a substance or tonic that heals the kidneys.

NERVINE • an agent that produces a calming effect on the nerves.

OXYTOCIC • a substance that stimulates uterine contraction.

PECTORAL • used for heart or chest disorders.

PURGATIVE • a substance that has a strong laxative effect.

SIALOGOGUE • a substance that promotes saliva secretion.

STOMACHIC • an agent that stimulates, heals the stomach.

STRYPTIC • a substance that contracts blood vessels, stops bleeding.

VERMIFUGE • a substance that destroys or expels worms in the intestine.

VULNERARY • an agent that assists in the healing of wounds.

PROTEIN INTRODUCTION

WHAT IS PROTEIN?

Protein is made up of amino acids: organic compounds of carbon, hydrogen, oxygen, and nitrogen.

WHAT ARE AMINO ACIDS?

Amino acids are the individual units that make up complete protein. The human body needs a total of 20 amino acids for growth and life. Eight amino acids are considered "essential amino acids" (for children, the number is nine). The body cannot manufacture these amino acids, so they must be provided in the diet.

WHAT IS COMPLETE PROTEIN?

Complete protein is obtained from foods that contain all eight of the essential amino acids. (But refer to page 90 for a discussion of what are considered "high-quality" protein foods.)

WHAT FOODS SUPPLY COMPLETE PROTEIN?

- grains
- legumes
- nuts
- seeds
- fish
- seafood
- meat
- poultry
- eggs
- dairy products

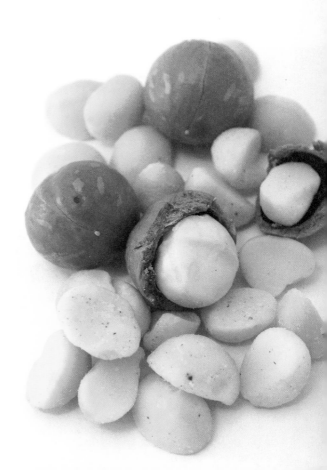

HOW MUCH PROTEIN DO I NEED EVERY DAY?

The table below shows several population groups and the U.S. Recommended Dietary Allowance (RDA) of protein for each group, measured in grams per day, based on what has been determined as a healthy average body weight.

These amounts are presented as a guide and may vary due to physical activity levels, recommended height-to-weight ratios, and, for children, times of rapid growth.

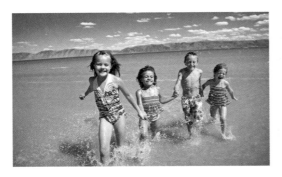
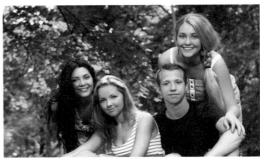

CHILD

	1–3 YEARS	4–8 YEARS	9–13 YEARS (BOY)	9–13 YEARS (GIRL)
DAILY PROTEIN RDA (G)	13	19	34	34

TEENAGER

	14–18 YEARS (BOY)	14–18 YEARS (GIRL)
DAILY PROTEIN RDA (G)	52	46

ADULT MALE

	19–30 YEARS	31–50 YEARS	51–70 YEARS	70+ YEARS
DAILY PROTEIN RDA (G)	56	56	56	56

ADULT FEMALE

	19–70 YEARS	70+ YEARS	PREGNANT 19–50 YEARS	LACTATING 19–50 YEARS
DAILY PROTEIN RDA (G)	46	46	71	71

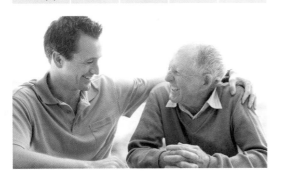
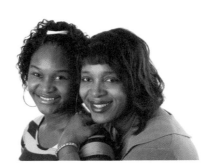

WHAT DOES PROTEIN DO AND HOW DO I OBTAIN THE REQUIRED DAILY PROTEIN?

Protein is required for growth, especially from birth till about age 20–24. Protein is used to make all types of body cells, including bone cells, blood cells, skin cells, and muscle cells. Protein is vital for the repair of body tissues, hormone production, blood clotting, digestion, metabolism, and for the glandular system. Amino acids are considered the building blocks of body cell construction. Protein is a vital component of blood. It also helps control adrenaline production, formation of skin and hair pigment, and regulation of sleep and mood patterns. Protein assists the functions of the kidneys, gallbladder, and nervous system.

If you refer to the table below, it is clear that protein can be obtained from every meal or snack, in portions that add up to provide the Recommended Dietary Allowances (RDAs). Protein foods and meals containing excess saturated fats are more difficult to digest. Protein is digested in the stomach, a process that can take three to five hours. Excess alcohol consumption during meals and eating protein foods with saturated fats may all reduce the protein value of a meal.

BREAKFAST	OATMEAL 13 G	TOAST & EGGS 17 G	YOGURT 8 G	MUESLI & MILK 10 G
MORNING SNACK	CAKE & COOKIES 5 G	PASTRY 6 G	MUFFIN 9 G	COTTAGE CHEESE 15 G
LUNCH	VEGGIE SANDWICH 6 G	150 G ROAST BEEF SANDWICH 13 G	50 G TUNA & SALAD 14 G	PASTA & CHEESE (50 G) 14 G
AFTERNOON SNACK	CHEESE & CRACKERS 18 G	250 G CHOCOLATE MILK 7 G	TEA & MUESLI BAR 8 G	FRUIT & 50 G NUTS 12 G
EVENING MEAL	FISH & CHIPS 17 G	CHICKEN & RICE 25 G	TOFU & VEGETABLES 11 G	VEGETABLES & LEGUMES 11 G
TOTAL DAILY PROTEIN	59 G	68 G	50 G	62 G

The table above is based on 100 g food portions (approximately) unless otherwise stated.

WHAT ARE THE BEST PROTEIN FOODS?

The best protein foods are listed in order in the table on the next page. The protein amounts shown on the next page are based on nutritional information outlined in the table below, which shows the main protein groups, lists an example of each, and also lists seven factors that are very important when evaluating the best protein foods. Let's look at tuna, for example. Tuna contains 30 g of protein (Total Protein Value) per 100 g (3.5 oz) portion. Eighty % of that is usable protein, also referred to as Net Protein Utilization (NPU).

Such factors as saturated fat and cholesterol need to be restricted in the regular diet, due to their link to heart disease and other health problems. Cooking and adding fats to protein foods also increase the health risk problems. The fiber content of food is a beneficial factor.

The best protein foods also contain a good balance of minerals and vitamins. Food such as nuts, seeds, whole grains, and legumes supply an abundance of protein, minerals, vitamins, essential lipids, and trace nutrients.

	Total Protein Value (g/100 g serving)	NPU (%)	Total Fat (g)	Saturated Fat (g)	Cholesterol (mg)	Fiber (g)	Calories
Grains (wheat, whole grain)	15	45%	2	0	0	12	329
Legumes (kidney beans)	24	38%	1	0	0	25	333
Nuts (almonds)	21	50%	49	4	0	12	578
Seeds (sunflower)	23	58%	50	5	0	11	570
Fish (tuna)	30	80%	6	2	49	0	184
Fish (perch)	19	89%	1	0	90	0	91
Meat (lean beef, raw)	18	67%	22	9	81	0	277
Chicken	21	65%	21	6	88	0	300
Eggs (whole)	13	94%	10	3	423	0	143
Cheese (cheddar)	25	70%	33	21	105	0	403
Milk (whole, 3.5%)	3	82%	3	2	10	0	60
Yogurt (plain, whole)	3	82%	3	2	13	0	61

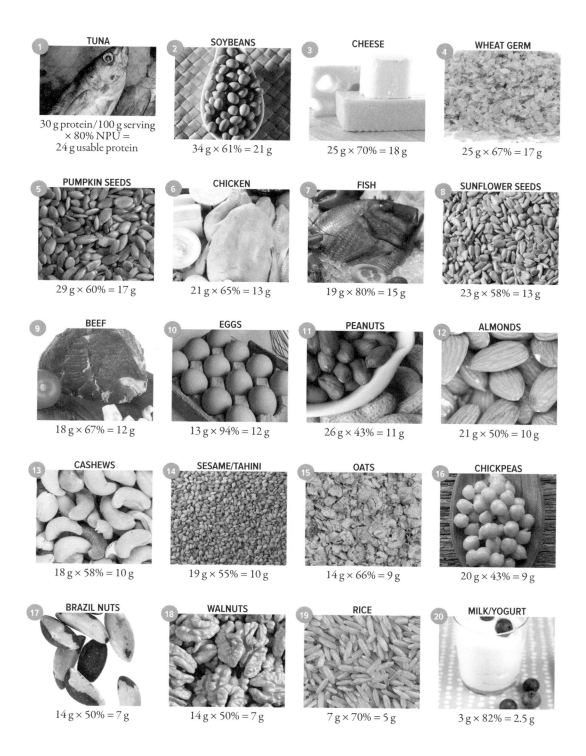

TUNA

30 g protein/100 g serving
× 80% NPU =
24 g usable protein

SOYBEANS

34 g × 61% = 21 g

CHEESE

25 g × 70% = 18 g

WHEAT GERM

25 g × 67% = 17 g

PUMPKIN SEEDS

29 g × 60% = 17 g

CHICKEN

21 g × 65% = 13 g

FISH

19 g × 80% = 15 g

SUNFLOWER SEEDS

23 g × 58% = 13 g

BEEF

18 g × 67% = 12 g

EGGS

13 g × 94% = 12 g

PEANUTS

26 g × 43% = 11 g

ALMONDS

21 g × 50% = 10 g

CASHEWS

18 g × 58% = 10 g

SESAME/TAHINI

19 g × 55% = 10 g

OATS

14 g × 66% = 9 g

CHICKPEAS

20 g × 43% = 9 g

BRAZIL NUTS

14 g × 50% = 7 g

WALNUTS

14 g × 50% = 7 g

RICE

7 g × 70% = 5 g

MILK/YOGURT

3 g × 82% = 2.5 g

NOTE: Nutrient amounts are listed as milligrams (mg) per 100 grams (g), unless otherwise stated.

WHAT TYPE OF PROTEIN DOES THE BODY REQUIRE?

There are a number of factors when evaluating the type of protein the human body requires. For adults, eight essential amino acids are required:

1. ISOLEUCINE   2. LEUCINE   3. LYSINE   4. METHIONINE
5. PHENYLALANINE   6. THREONINE   7. TRYPTOPHAN   8. VALINE

(Children need the eight essential amino acids plus one more: histidine.) As mentioned earlier, these are considered "essential" because the human body cannot manufacture them and therefore must obtain them from foods.

Amino acids are required by the body in a specific ratio, as presented in the table below. No food provides the exact same ratio, but many foods provide a reasonable balance of the essential amino acids. Any food that supplies the eight essential amino acids is termed a complete-protein food. All grains, legumes, nuts, seeds, dairy, meat, poultry, and fish supply the eight essential amino acids. The best protein foods are low in saturated fats and require the least cooking, plus they supply a good amino acid balance. Foods that provide their amino acid balance in a ratio similar to that in the graph are termed "high-quality protein foods." The term net protein utilization (NPU) is used as a measure of protein foods' supply of amino acids, as compared to the *ideal* proportion shown in the graph. By combining foods such as rice and corn or bread and cheese, for example, increased protein value is obtained due to an improved amino acid balance. Proper food combination can improve the digestion of protein foods. Refer to the food combination table and information guide on pages 208–209. Also be aware that excess intake of protein foods can lead to weight gain.

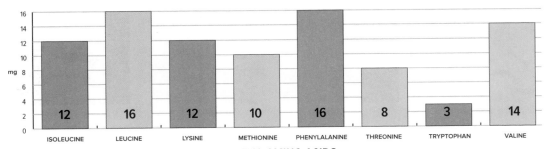

DAILY AMOUNTS REQUIRED OF THE 8 ESSENTIAL AMINO ACIDS

This chart shows the various amounts, in mgs, that the body requires each day of the eight essential amino acids from foods, in order to obtain "complete protein."

WHICH PROTEIN FOODS PROVIDE THE BEST NET PROTEIN UTILIZATION?

The five protein foods listed in the following table have the best net protein utilization (NPU) of all foods. Eggs have the highest value, with 94%.

EGGS	MILK/YOGURT	TUNA	FISH	CHEESE
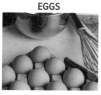	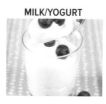	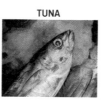	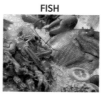	
13 g protein/ 100 g × 94% NPU = 12 g usable protein	3 g × 82% = 3 g	30 g × 80% = 24 g	19 g × 80% = 17 g	25 g × 70% = 18 g

The following table shows that, for eggs, the amino acid methionine is low (401 mg) compared to the required 600 mg for a 100 g serving (two eggs). Therefore, to obtain all of one's daily protein from eggs, a person weighing 60 kg (132 lbs) would need to consume about three eggs. However, it is best to limit egg consumption to about five eggs per week, due to eggs' high cholesterol value. Refer to page 121 for details.

AMINO ACIDS	ISL	LEU	LYS	MET	PHE	THR	TRY	VAL
EGGS (100 G)	850	1126	819	401	739	637	211	950
DAILY REQUIREMENT FOR 60 KG ADULT	720	960	720	600	960	480	180	840
TUNA (100 G)	1,481	2,178	2,556	842	1,074	1,249	290	1,554

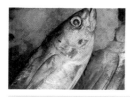

The RDA (Recommended Dietary Allowance) for teenage boys and men is 52–56 g of protein per day. This refers to a food's total protein value—for example, tuna contains 30 g of protein per 100 g serving; eggs contain 13 g protein per 100 g.

TUNA: 30 G PER 100 G (TOTAL PROTEIN VALUE) X 80% NET PROTEIN UTILIZATION = 24 G OF USABLE PROTEIN

To obtain better protein value from a meal, combine the following foods to obtain an increased NPU (and add vegetables whenever possible): bread and cheese, rice and corn, legumes and rice, chicken and rice, eggs and bread, almonds with Brazil nuts and cashews, tahini and bread, milk and cereals, fish and rice.

NOTE: Nutrient amounts are listed as milligrams (mg) per 100 grams (g), unless otherwise stated.

HOW MUCH PROTEIN DO FOODS CONTAIN?

The table below provides a detailed list of the individual amino acid content of the main protein foods, based on mg per 100 g portions.

It is clear that all of the foods listed supply complete protein, as they contain the eight essential amino acids (plus histidine, required for children). To obtain a well-balanced diet and good-quality protein, regularly include whole grains, legumes, rice, fish, eggs, chicken, meat, and cheese with vegetables.

Food Type	Natural Food	HIS	ISL	LEU	LYS	MET	PHE	THR	TRY	VAL
Whole grains	barley	239	545	889	433	184	661	433	160	643
	corn	206	462	1,296	288	186	454	389	61	510
	millet	240	635	1,746	383	270	506	456	248	682
	oats	261	733	1,065	521	209	758	470	183	845
	rice	126	352	646	296	135	377	294	82	524
	rye	276	515	813	494	191	571	448	137	631
	wheat	286	607	939	384	214	691	403	173	648
	wheat germ	687	1,177	1,708	1,534	404	908	1,343	265	1,364
Legumes (beans & peas)	chickpeas	559	1,195	1,538	1,434	276	1,012	739	170	1,025
	kidney beans	658	1,312	1,985	1,715	233	1,275	1,002	214	1,401
	lentils	548	1,316	1,760	1,528	180	1,104	896	216	1,360
	lima beans	669	1,199	1,722	1,378	331	1,222	980	195	1,298
	peanuts	749	1,266	1,872	1,099	271	1,557	828	340	1,532
	soybeans	911	2,054	2,946	2,414	513	1,889	1,504	526	2,005
Nuts	almonds	517	873	1,454	582	259	1,146	610	176	1,124
	Brazil nuts	367	593	1,129	443	941	617	422	187	823
	cashew nuts	415	1,222	1,522	792	353	946	737	471	1,592
	coconut	69	180	269	152	71	174	129	33	212
	hazelnuts	288	853	939	417	139	537	415	211	934
	pecans	273	553	773	435	153	564	389	138	525
	pistachios	507	880	1,520	1,080	370	1,090	610	273	1,340
	walnuts	405	767	1,228	441	306	767	589	175	974
Seeds	pumpkin seeds	711	1,737	2,437	1,411	577	1,749	933	560	1,670
	sesame seeds	441	951	1,679	583	637	1,457	707	331	885
	sunflower seeds	586	1,276	1,736	868	443	1,220	911	343	1,354
Dairy foods	whole egg	1,123	850	1,126	819	401	739	637	211	950
	milk (cow's)	92	233	344	272	86	170	162	40	240
	yogurt	146	214	336	282	78	180	160	37	255
	cheddar cheese	815	1,685	2,437	1,834	650	1,340	929	341	1,974
Tuna	tuna	880	1,481	2,178	2,556	842	1,074	1,249	290	1,554
Beef	beef porterhouse	569	858	1,343	1,433	407	674	724	192	911
Poultry	chicken	593	1,088	1,490	1,810	537	811	877	250	1,012
	turkey	649	1,260	1,836	2,173	664	960	1,014	238	1,187
Lamb	lamb	501	933	1,394	1,457	432	732	824	233	887

The graphs below and on the following page show the information about amino acid requirements in a more visual way. For each essential amino acid, these graphs show the daily requirement, in mg, for individuals of various body weights (50–80 kg). For example, a person weighing 50 kg requires about 600 mg per day of isoleucine. Next, the graph shows how much of that amino acid is obtained from a 100 g serving of various foods. For example, you can see that a 100 g serving of grains doesn't provide the full daily requirement of the amino acid isoleucine for a person of any size, but a serving of legumes does.

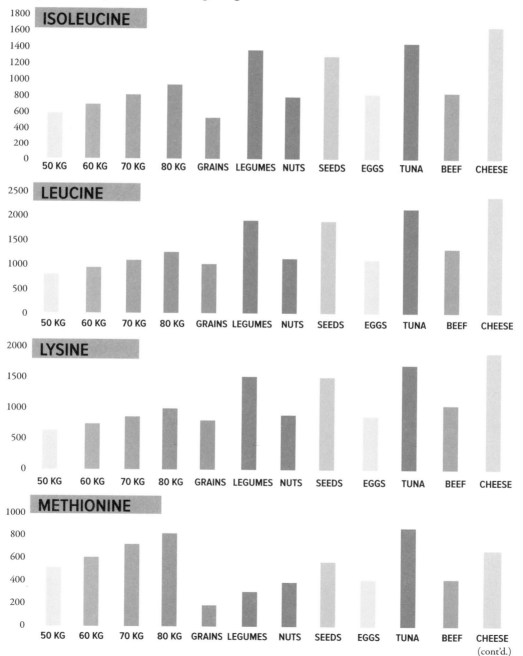

(cont'd.)

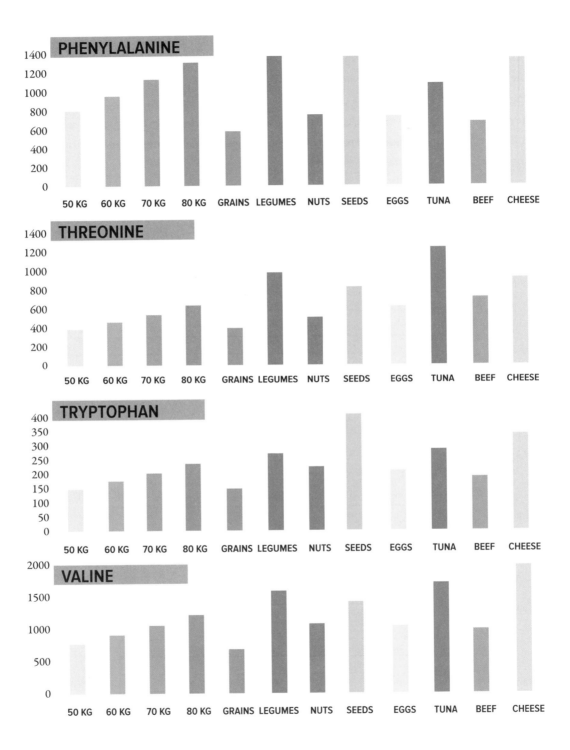

PROTEIN INTRODUCTION

DIETARY REFERENCE INTAKE (DRI) TABLE

The Dietary Reference Intake (DRI) system was introduced in 1997 as a way to broaden the guidelines provided by the Recommended Daily Allowances (RDAs), the familiar nutrtion recommendations we've all been exposed to since childhood. The DRI guidelines include not only the RDAs, but also other categories, such as Adequate Intake (AI), for nutrients that don't have established RDAs. AIs are levels that are believed to be adequate for everyone in the population group.

The DRIs are established by the Institute of Medicine, part of the U.S. National Academy of Sciences. They are used by both the United States and Canada.

Essential Minerals, Protein, and Lipids	VALUE REF.	Young Child		Child				Male Adult				Female Adult					
		1–3 years	4–8 years	9–13 years (boys)	9–13 years (girls)	14–18 years (boys)	14–18 years (girls)	19–30 years	31–50 years	51–70 years	70+ years	19–30 years	31–50 years	51–70 years	70+ years	Pregnant, 19–50 years	Lactating, 19–50 years
Iron (mg)	RDA	7	10	8	8	11	15	8	8	8	8	18	18	8	8	27	9
Copper (mcg)	RDA	340	440	700	700	890	890	900	900	900	900	900	900	900	900	1,000	1,300
Magnesium (mg)	RDA	80	130	240	240	410	360	400	420	420	420	310	320	320	320	360	320
Calcium (mg)	RDA	700	1,000	1,300	1,300	1,300	1,300	1,000	1,000	1,000	1,200	1,000	1,000	1,200	1,200	1,000	1,000
Phosphorus (mg)	RDA	460	500	1,250	1,250	1,250	1,250	700	700	700	700	700	700	700	700	700	700
Selenium (mcg)	RDA	20	30	40	40	55	55	55	55	55	55	55	55	55	55	60	70
Chromium (mcg)	AI	11	15	25	21	35	24	35	35	30	30	25	25	20	20	30	45
Manganese (mg)	AI	1.2	1.5	1.9	1.6	2.2	1.6	2.3	2.3	2.3	2.3	1.8	1.8	1.8	1.8	2.0	2.6
Sodium (g)	AI	1.0	1.2	1.5	1.5	1.5	1.5	1.5	1.5	1.3	1.2	1.5	1.5	1.3	1.2	1.5	1.5
Potassium (g)	AI	3.0	3.8	4.5	4.5	4.7	4.7	4.7	4.7	4.7	4.7	4.7	4.7	4.7	4.7	4.7	5.1
Molybdenum (mcg)	RDA	17	22	34	34	43	43	45	45	45	45	45	45	45	45	50	50
Iodine (mcg)	RDA	90	90	120	120	150	150	150	150	150	150	150	150	150	150	220	290
Fluoride (mg)	AI	0.7	1.0	2.0	2.0	3.0	3.0	4.0	4.0	4.0	4.0	3.0	3.0	3.0	3.0	3.0	3.0
Zinc (mg)	RDA	3	5	8	8	11	9	11	11	11	11	8	8	8	8	11	12
Protein (g)	RDA	13	19	34	34	52	46	56	56	56	56	46	46	46	46	71	71
Linolenic acid (omega-3) (g)	AI	0.7	0.9	1.2	1.0	1.6	1.1	1.6	1.6	1.6	1.6	1.1	1.1	1.1	1.1	1.4	1.3
Linolenic acid (omega-6) (g)	AI	7	10	12	10	16	11	17	17	14	14	12	12	11	11	13	13

(cont'd.)

DIETARY REFERENCE INTAKE (DRI) TABLE (CONT'D.)

The RDAs were originally established in World War II and are updated every five to ten years. The RDA is the daily intake level of a nutrient considered sufficient by the Food and Nutrition Board (now part of the Institute of Medicine) to meet the requirements of 97.5% of healthy individuals in the specific gender and age group. The allowances were meant to provide superior nutrition for civilians and military personnel, so they included a "margin of safety." They are the guidelines used to determine the information that is printed on food labels in the United States and Canada.

Vitamins, Water, and Fiber	VALUE REF.	Young Child		Child				Adult Male				Adult Female					
		1—3 years	4—8 years	9—13 years (boys)	9—13 years (girls)	14—18 years (boys)	14—18 years (girls)	19—30 years	31—50 years	51—70 years	70+ years	19—30 years	31—50 years	51—70 years	70+ years	Pregnant, 19—50 years	Lactating, 19—50 years
Vitamin A (mcg) (Retinol equivalents)	RDA	300	400	600	600	900	700	900	900	900	900	700	700	700	700	770	1,300
Thiamin (mg)	RDA	0.5	0.6	0.9	0.9	1.2	1.0	1.2	1.2	1.2	1.2	1.1	1.1	1.1	1.1	1.4	1.4
Riboflavin (mg)	RDA	0.5	0.6	0.9	0.9	1.3	1.0	1.3	1.3	1.3	1.3	1.1	1.1	1.1	1.1	1.4	1.6
Niacin (mg) (Niacin equivalents)	RDI	6	8	12	12	16	14	16	16	16	16	14	14	14	14	18	17
Panthothenic acid (mg)	AI	2	3	4	4	5	5	5	5	5	5	5	5	5	5	6	7
Vitamin B6 (mg)	RDA	0.5	0.6	1.0	1.0	1.3	1.2	1.3	1.3	1.7	1.7	1.3	1.3	1.5	1.5	1.9	2.0
Biotin (mg)	AI	8	12	20	20	25	25	30	30	30	30	30	30	30	30	30	35
Choline (mg)	AI	200	250	375	375	550	400	550	550	550	550	425	425	425	425	450	550
Total folate (mcg)	RDA	150	200	300	300	400	400	400	400	400	400	400	400	400	400	600	500
Vitamin B12 (mcg)	RDA	0.9	1.2	1.8	1.8	2.4	2.4	2.4	2.4	2.4	2.4	2.4	2.4	2.4	2.4	2.6	2.8
Vitamin C (mg)	RDI	15	25	45	45	75	65	90	90	90	90	75	75	75	75	85	120
Vitamin E (mg) (alpha-tocopherol equivalents)	RDA	6	7	11	11	15	15	15	15	15	15	15	15	15	15	15	19
Vitamin K (mcg)	AI	30	55	60	60	75	75	120	120	120	120	90	90	90	90	90	90
Total water (l/day)*	AI	1.3	1.7	2.4	2.1	3.3	2.3	3.7	3.7	3.7	3.7	2.7	2.7	2.7	2.7	3.0	3.8
Dietary fiber (g)	AI	19	25	31	26	38	26	38	38	30	30	25	25	21	21	28	29

*Total water includes all water contained in food, beverages, and drinking water.

Nuts provide numerous nutritional benefits. The following pages offer a descriptive evaluation of the most common varieties: almond, Brazil, cashew, chestnut, coconut, hazelnut, macadamia, pecan, pine, pistachio, and walnut.

Generally speaking, nuts are a very good source of complete protein; all the essential life-supporting amino acids are generously supplied by the nut kingdom (refer to page 92). Nuts can easily replace all other foods for protein value and requirements.

We are fortunate these days to have a variety of nuts from around the world to choose from; however, many people consider nuts to be an expensive food item and may unfortunately avoid them for that reason. Economically speaking, nut protein is often comparable in price to meat or poultry (refer to the chart below). In addition, nuts provide an abundance of minerals and vitamins compared to meat and poultry, they don't contain any cholesterol, and they need no cooking, which saves on fuel bills. Nuts provide numerous other benefits due to their good supplies of fiber, trace minerals, and antioxidants. Nuts provide pure value per ounce. Furthermore, when nuts are eaten raw, their valuable unsaturated oil content is an excellent source of energy and other health benefits.

By contrast, the fat content of animal-protein foods such as meat is mostly composed of saturated fats. Once meat is cooked, protein value decreases and free radicals increase, which are really detrimental to health.

Nuts supply generous amounts of easily assimilated complete protein, minerals, vitamins—and no free radicals when eaten raw. For a simple protein snack, try a handful of almonds with a ripe peach or crisp apple.

Nuts supply all the essential nutrients for the utilization of their fat content, and because most of the fats are unsaturated, they can be readily used by the body. Over half the food value in nuts is composed of unsaturated fats, which provide a very satisfying effect on the appetite with no health risks. Research studies have shown that the unsaturated fats in nuts can actually reduce body weight when they replace the saturated fats of animal-based foods and meals. Nuts are the answer to the big appetite and the demand for calories and energy.

One 150 g serving (5.25 oz, or a little over 1 cup) of mixed nuts provides an average of 900 calories—which is one-third of the daily calorie allowance for men ages 20–50—and *all* the daily protein requirements.

Nuts also provide an abundance of the minerals calcium, phosphorus, iron, potassium, copper, selenium, and magnesium.

Read on to discover more about the enormous health benefits that are provided by the mighty nut kingdom.

Protein Food Comparison	Price/ 100 g* (3.5 oz)	Daily Req. for 70 kg Male	Cholesterol (mg)	Iron (mg)
Almonds	$1.75	180 g	0	4.6
Brazil	$2.19	210 g	0	3.4
Cashew	$2.19	200 g	0	3.7
A, B, C nut mix	$1.97	150 g	0	3.9
Pumpkin seeds	$1.31	130 g	0	11.3
Soybeans (roasted)	$0.65	150 g	0	5.1
Beef steak	$1.50–2.64	180 g	81	1.9
Cheddar	$1.32	120 g	107	0.6
Chicken	$0.72	140 g	90	0.7
Lamb	$1.10–2.64	160 g	75	1.0
Tuna	$1.16	100 g	38	1.5

* as of March 2013

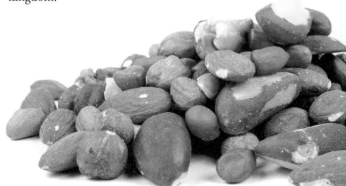

ALMOND – *Prunus dulcis, P. amygdalus*

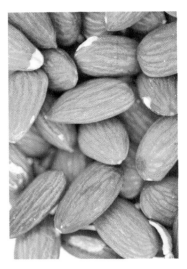

Almonds are alkaline and for this reason alone the almond nut in its raw state is a great food, ideal for obtaining the 75% alkaline daily food balance. All foods except fruits, vegetables, and rice are acid forming; the almond is a great exception. An alkaline balance in the body promotes natural healing.

Almonds are also a great provider of healthful lipids, especially monounsaturated fats (32 g); the content of polyunsaturated fat is 12 g and saturated is 4 g. In one study comparing two weight-loss diets, the "almond diet" proved to reduce weight and blood pressure 30% better than the standard low-calorie, low-fat diet. It was found that not all the fat in almonds is absorbed, as the cell walls of the nut act as a partial barrier to fat absorption. Furthermore, the abundance of monounsaturated fats in almonds is ideal for energy requirements and is readily used by the body; plus it reduces cholesterol levels in the blood.

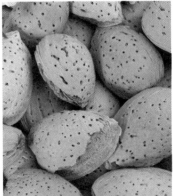

Almonds provide only a trace amount of omega-3 fatty acids, but they supply 10 g of omega-6, the other essential fatty acid. Almonds are an excellent source of vitamin E (26 mg), providing more than 100% of the daily value (DV) requirement. Vitamin E is a major antioxidant; it reduces the risk of heart disease by protecting against oxidation of LDL cholesterol, the bad cholesterol that leads to heart disease. Vitamin E also promotes blood circulation, heart muscle function, and the life of cells. One study showed a 45% decrease in the risk of heart disease by substituting the fats in almonds for the saturated fats in meat. In summary, lipids in almonds are safe and beneficial. For more information on almond oil, refer to page 140.

Raw almonds provide complete protein, as they supply the eight essential amino acids (refer to the table on page 89). Almonds consist of 20% protein, with 21 g or nearly 40% of the DV requirement for the average adult, but with only 20% of daily calories—that's a very impressive figure! Almonds are an excellent source of magnesium (275 mg, or close to 100% DV), which promotes blood flow and reduced risk of heart attacks. It is also essential for the health of the nervous system and brain because it nourishes the white nerve fibers and helps the nerves to relax. In addition, almonds' excellent phosphorus content (474 mg) is vital for repair of the nervous system, improved blood circulation, memory, and concentration. Don't forget almonds when you're working hard at a mental task! Almonds promote creativity, plus the good manganese content (3 mg) promotes memory abilities.

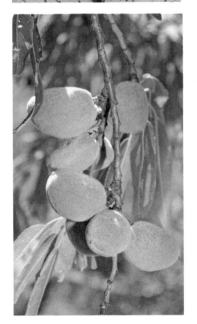

The calcium content in almonds is excellent (248 mg), making almonds ideal for those who are dairy intolerant. They are the best nut source of calcium. Apart from tahini and tofu, only dairy is higher, but it supplies considerable saturated fat and cholesterol. Almonds provide safe calcium. Almonds are a great source of dietary fiber (12 g), and when eaten as a snack with apples, their protein digestion is enhanced. Almonds are also full of copper (56% DV), iron (24% DV), zinc (22% DV), potassium (21% DV), B2 (48% DV), B3 (20% DV), and biotin (100% DV), which is essential for fat metabolism.

Besides being eaten in nut form, almonds can be ground and added to cereal. They merit a whole book devoted to them. They're the perfect alkaline protein.

ALMOND

NOTE: DV amounts listed refer to the daily value for women 25–50 years; refer to DRI tables on pages 95–96 for adult male and child values.

GLYCEMIC INDEX: VERY LOW	TOTAL CALORIES PER 100 G: 656	CALORIES FROM		
		CARB: 50 7%	PROTEIN: 50 8%	FAT: 556 85%

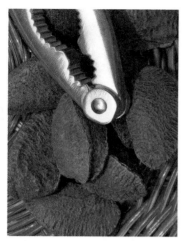

BRAZIL NUT – *Bertholletia excelsa*

Brazil nuts are exceptionally rich in the mineral selenium (1,900–2,960 mcg). The daily RDA for adults is 55 mcg, with an upper level intake of 400 mcg from supplements. Brazil nuts are so rich in selenium that it would be a big waste of money to buy a selenium supplement. One Brazil nut a day will provide all your selenium requirements—unless you want to eat a 100 g serving of liver, or 500 g of wheat germ, or 600 g of sunflower seeds, or 1 kg of tuna!

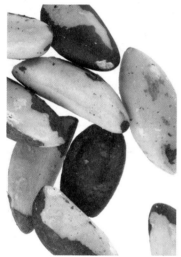

Brazil nuts really are an essential food item. A prolonged selenium deficiency can increase the risk of asthma, heart disease, HIV infections, arthritis, senility, Alzheimer's disease, epilepsy, mental fatigue, anxiety, and atherosclerosis. Selenium is vital for diabetics, as it stimulates glucose absorption. In a ten-year study, an optimum selenium intake decreased cancer mortality by 50%, especially cancers of the lung (46%), prostate (63%), and colon (38%). In combination with vitamin E, selenium acts as an antioxidant against free radicals, especially free radicals from cooked oils. The combo of selenium and vitamin E (6 mg) in Brazil nuts could be considered a life saver.

Another great benefit of Brazil nuts is their remarkable supply of the amino acid methionine (1,008 mg). Brazil nuts are the best natural source of this precious amino acid. Nearly all protein foods are deficient in methionine, which considerably lowers their real protein potential. Brazil nuts supply over 90% of required methionine. Most foods supply around 30%. A small sprinkle of ground Brazil nuts will add protein power to vegetable burgers or any other meal. Besides supplying complete protein (14 g), Brazil nuts are an excellent source of phosphorus (725 mg), potassium (650 mg), and magnesium (376 mg), and a good source of calcium (160 mg). Brazil nuts supply 66 g of lipids: 28 g monounsaturated, 21 g polyunsaturated, and 17 g saturated.

Most soils and foods are deficient in selenium. For the ultimate selenium antioxidant benefits, crack into the incredible Brazil nut.

GLYCEMIC INDEX: VERY LOW	TOTAL CALORIES PER 100 G: 155	CASHEWS (raw) CALORIES FROM		
		CARB: 35 22%	PROTEIN: 18 12%	FAT: 102 66%
GLYCEMIC INDEX: VERY LOW	TOTAL CALORIES PER 100 G: 748	CASHEWS (oil roasted) CALORIES FROM		
		CARB: 157 21%	PROTEIN: 75 10%	FAT: 516 69%

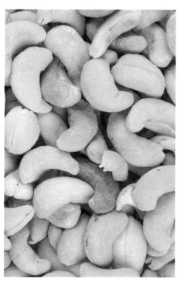

CASHEW – *Anacardium occidentale*

Cashews also originated from Brazil. Raw cashews have less fat than most nuts. Cashews supply 65% unsaturated fats, with 90% in the form of oleic acid, ideal for energy and reduced cholesterol. Cashews supply omega-6 fatty acids (8 g) and a trace of omega-3. Roasted cashews taste good, but the increase in free radicals is a problem; however, the rich supply of the trace mineral copper (2.2 mg) will help protect against such problems. One handful of cashews supplies a full daily dose of copper, essential for the heart muscles and for iron and fat metabolism. Cahsews also contain enzymes that provide flexibility to movable joints, blood vessels, and bones. Cashews are a complete protein food, but they're low in phenylalanine and methionine. To gain protein balance, add a few almonds and one Brazil nut, with an apple, for a perfect protein snack. Cashews are rich in magnesium (70% DV) and phosphorus (60% DV). Cashews are soft and great for children as well as adults. They are worth their weight in organic copper and brain minerals, and their pure energy value is wonderful.

GLYCEMIC INDEX:	TOTAL CALORIES PER 100 G:	CALORIES FROM		
		CARB: 200	PROTEIN: 15	FAT: 9
54	224	89%	7%	4%

CHESTNUT – *Castanea* spp.

Chestnuts grow on trees and in water. The sweet chestnut (*Castanea sativa*) grows on trees and belongs to the oak family. The water chestnuts include caltrops (*Trapa natans*) and the Chinese water chestnut (*Eleocharis tuberosa*).

Chestnuts have the lowest calorie and fat content (1 g) of any nut. Even when they're roasted in their shell, as is traditional in Switzerland and France, there are no problems with free radicals, as the chestnut is nearly pure carbohydrate (49 g). On a freezing cold day, a bag of roasted chestnuts is better than ice cream on a boiling hot day. Chestnuts have a soft texture when roasted or boiled and children love the experience of roasting them by the fireplace. Before roasting, it is best to slit the soft shell, to avoid explosions. Boys may think exploding chestnuts are a blast, but be careful!

Chestnuts supply good amounts of potassium (447 mg) and magnesium (21% DV); they're the second-best nut source of vitamin A (200 IU) and the best nut source of vitamin C (36 mg). Chestnuts need cooking to eliminate the *tannic acid*. In France the chestnut is a delicacy; in Italy it is a staple and is often ground into flour to make *farina dolce,* a specialty bread.

Chestnuts are a good source of folic acid (68 mcg, more than peas). They are also the least fattening of all nuts. Roasted chestnuts are the ideal food for anybody!

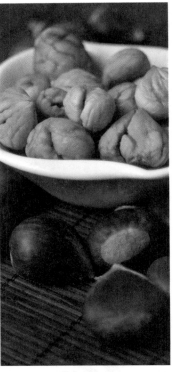

GLYCEMIC INDEX:	TOTAL CALORIES PER 100 G:	CALORIES FROM		
		CARB: 68	PROTEIN: 52	FAT: 508
VERY LOW	628	11%	8%	81%

COCONUT – *Cocos nucifera*

Coconuts are the biggest nut, and the coconut palm has been named the "tree that sustains life" from the Sanskrit *kalpha vrisha,* as it provides food, shelter, and a delicious milk that can be either drunk or used in numerous recipes. The flesh of the coconut, termed *copra,* available in shredded or desiccated form, is a great addition to many recipes. Coconut cream makes a dream dish come true.

Coconut is a very satisfying food; it would be nearly impossible to eat a whole one, primarily because of its rich supply of saturated fats. Coconut contains 32 g of fat, with 30 g as saturated fats, no polyunsaturated fats, and 2 g as monounsaturated fats. Ideally, saturated fats are best avoided as they raise blood cholesterol levels, The only saving grace is that coconut is eaten raw and therefore the free-radical problem is eliminated. If you were marooned on a tropical island for two weeks and coconut was your only food, you might actually consume fewer saturated fats than the average city dweller who relies on takeout foods. Coconut also provides a great supply of very beneficial fiber (9 g), much more than convenience foods. Coconut fiber can destroy tapeworms from infected meat, and it is an ideal snack for protection against constipation. Coconut milk is used in traditional medicine for relief from stomach ulcers and sore throats. Half the battle if you're a city dweller is to find a fresh coconut, one that has not been allowed to ferment, but is ripe. The taste of a quality coconut is incredible—but hard to eat in large quantities! Coconuts supply a fair amount of potassium (356 mg) and a good supply of beneficial organic sodium (20 mg).

Crack open a coconut next time you need a completely cool and super satisfying snack.

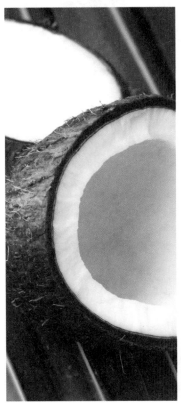

NOTE: DV amounts listed refer to the daily value for women 25–50 years; refer to DRI tables on pages 95–96 for adult male and child values.

GLYCEMIC INDEX: VERY LOW	TOTAL CALORIES PER 100 G: 628	CALORIES FROM		
		CARB: 68 11%	PROTEIN: 52 8%	FAT: 508 81%

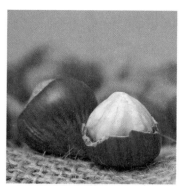

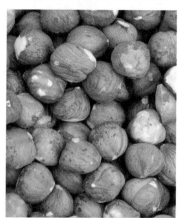

HAZELNUT – *Corylus avellana, C. americana*

Hazelnuts are a member of the *Corylus* family of trees, and depending on their country of cultivation hazelnuts may also be termed filberts or cob nuts. Hazelnuts are the second-best nut source of vitamin E (15–20 mg); the almond supplies 26 mg. A handful of hazelnuts is a most beneficial substitute for any vitamin E capsule. Hazelnuts are a fair source of omega-6 fatty acids (4 g), which in combination with vitamin E is vital for healthy arteries, regulation of cholesterol levels, and prevention of heart disease.

Hazelnuts are also a good source of zinc (2 mg), a mineral that is required for the breakdown of alcohol and is also a vital component of insulin. Hazelnuts supply fair amounts of calcium (110 mg), potassium (680 mg), and phosphorus (290 mg), and a very good supply of magnesium (160 mg). Hazelnuts' supply of copper is excellent (90% DV), which, in combination with their very good supply of iron (5 mg or 26% DV) and manganese (6 mg), makes them a complete blood builder, providing all the tools required. All of the basic B-group vitamins are supplied, especially B1 (43% DV) and B6 (28% DV). The protein value (21 g) of hazelnuts is complete in all the essential amino acids; in order to obtain very good protein value, combine hazelnuts with cashews and Brazil nuts and a few almonds. Hazelnuts are used in spreads: Try the pure spread, it's fantastic.

Hazelnuts are often roasted. They taste nice but may contain free radicals as a result of the cooking. By the time you buy them they may be of minimum nutrient value. For maximum benefits, raw hazelnuts can't be beaten!

GLYCEMIC INDEX: VERY LOW	TOTAL CALORIES PER 100 G: 718	CALORIES FROM		
		CARB: 56 8%	PROTEIN: 27 4%	FAT: 634 88%

MACADAMIA – *Macadamia integrifolia, M. tetraphylla*

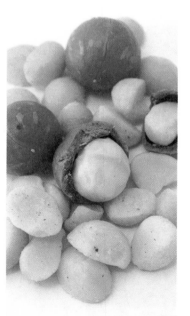

Macadamia nuts, also called the Queensland nut, are native to northeastern Australia. They are cultivated extensively in Hawaii. Macadamia nuts are the hardest nut to crack, but thanks to some inventors that problem has been solved. Breaking into them is well worth the effort. Macadamia nuts are soft inside, full of monounsaturated lipids (60 g), with polyunsaturated at 3 g and saturated at 13 g. But there's no cholesterol and no risk of free radicals—unless they are roasted.

Macadamia nuts, eaten raw, are the richest nut source of monounsaturated lipids. They are nearly a unique source of *palmitoleic acid,* a monounsaturated fatty acid that assists in fat metabolism. They help the body to use dietary fat efficiently as an energy source. Macadamia nuts supply 6% more oleic acid than olive oil. They contain vitamin E (1 mg) as well as flavonoids that provide antioxidant benefits. Their antioxidant power is increased by their good supply of copper (38% DV).

Macadamia nuts provide a fair supply of fiber (9 g, or 36% DV, 136% more than meat or fish). Macadamia nuts make a perfect addition to a fruit salad or a garden salad: no need for an oil dressing, unless it's a splash of delightful macadamia oil. Macadamias are a complete protein food (8 g, or 16% DV); when they're combined with a breakfast cereal their protein value increases to rival that of the common meat meal. A few macadamias go a long way toward satisfying the appetite. Unsalted are best nutritionally. When you need a big energy boost, macadamia nuts are cracked up for the job.

NOTE: Nutrient amounts are listed as milligrams (mg) per 100 grams (g), unless otherwise stated.

GLYCEMIC INDEX: VERY LOW	TOTAL CALORIES PER 100 G: 691	CALORIES FROM		
		CARB: 57 8%	PROTEIN: 32 5%	FAT: 602 87%

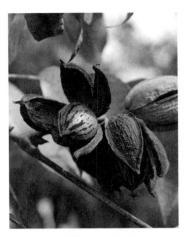

PECAN – *Carya illinoensis*

Pecans are similar to hickory nuts. They are the second-best nut source of lipids: 72 g to the macadamia's 76 g. But pecans have half the saturated fat (6 g) and ten times the polyunsaturated fat content (22 g) of the macadamia.

In a four-week study, when the pecan diet replaced a controlled low-fat diet, both with the same calorie content, the pecan diet lowered cholesterol by 6.7%, low density lipoproteins by 10%, and triglycerides by 11%. When pecans replace potato chips as a snack food, the benefits are undoubtedly even greater, as the number of free radicals from cooked chips is enormous. Try a handful of pecans with an apple, or a slice of pecan pie instead of chips.

Pecans are a good source of phosphorus (277 mg, or 28% DV), and their magnesium content (121 mg, or 30% DV) makes them a brain food. The magnesium content is four times that of perch (30 mg); however, pecans contain 11 grams less of protein (9 g) but 4% more potassium (410 mg).

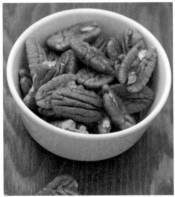

Pecans are a good source of dietary fiber (10 g, or 31% DV) and vitamin B1 (44% DV), an excellent source of copper (60% DV), and a small supplier of vitamin E (1 mg). All these factors provide antioxidant benefits. Pecans supply a fair portion of complete protein (9 g) and are great in recipes.

Pecans are a most popular nut. Try a piece of pecan pie with a scoop of ice cream, it's delightful!

GLYCEMIC INDEX: VERY LOW	TOTAL CALORIES PER 100 G: 673	CALORIES FROM		
		CARB: 53 8%	PROTEIN: 48 7%	FAT: 572 85%

PINE NUTS – *Pinus pinea*

Pine nuts, also known as pignoli, grow inside a large pine cone from a tree native to Italy. They are used in the famous basil pesto and are often included in stuffings and tossed into salads, including fruit salads. Pine nuts are best used in cooking, to reduce the turpentine flavor from the supply of lipids (68 g, or 105% DV). Half of their fat content (34 g) is in the form of polyunsaturated fats, including 1 g of omega-3 and 25 g of omega-6. The content of monounsaturated fat is 19 g and saturated fat 5 g. Pine nuts provide complete protein (14 g, or 27% DV), of which 50% is usable.

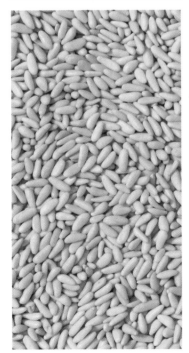

Pine nuts are full of phosphorus (575 mg, or 60% DV), which promotes utilization of the high calorie and fat content; it also benefits the nervous system, improves memory, and stimulates blood circulation. The magnesium content is excellent (250 mg, or 63% DV), more than that of almonds, and a real treat for the nervous system. Magnesium nourishes the white nerve fibers of the brain and spinal cord; 70% of the body's magnesium is contained in the bone structure. Pine nuts are a fair source of folate, for the nervous system and brain. If you think you're going nuts, pine nuts are tops in brain nutrition. Iron (6 mg), copper (1 mg), and manganese (4.3 mg) are all very well supplied by pine nuts, making them beneficial for the blood system, with three times the iron of beef, 4,000 times the manganese, and 150 times the copper.

Pine nuts will beef up your diet's blood-building and brain benefits.

NOTE: DV amounts listed refer to the daily value for women 25–50 years; refer to DRI tables on pages 95–96 for adult male and child values.

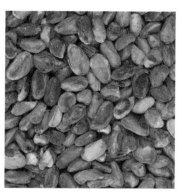

GLYCEMIC INDEX: VERY LOW	TOTAL CALORIES PER 100 G: 557	CALORIES FROM		
		CARB: 114 20%	PROTEIN: 72 13%	FAT: 372 67%

PISTACHIO – *Pistacia vera*

Pistachios are the best nut source of phytosterols, more specifically beta-sitosterol (198 mcg), which provides protection from some forms of cancer. It also assists in blood cholesterol reduction, especially in combination with pistachios' good supply of mono-unsaturated lipids (23 g). Pistachios have a low saturated fat content (5 g) and a fair polyunsaturated fat content (13 g).

Pistachios are the richest nut source of the mineral potassium (1,025 mg), making them beneficial for blood circulation (another benefit of the monounsaturated fat content), if they are not salted. Potassium is destroyed by excess coffee and alcohol consumption. A handful of pistachios after a "hard day's night" will really help. The good supply of B vitamins, especially B1 and B6, will boost the heart and calm the nerves. In addition, the magnesium content (125 mg, or 30% DV) will relax the nerves, replace the loss of the mineral from those extra drinks after work, and protect against heart attacks. Pistachio nuts are tiny in size but huge in potassium and heart-pumping benefits. They also contain calcium (107 mg), vitamin A (553 IU), lots of copper (65% DV), and vitamin E (2 mg), also of benefit for the heart muscles. The supply of zinc (2 mg) is vital, especially for people who drink alcohol regularly. Pistachio nuts will protect you!

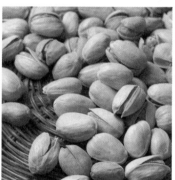

GLYCEMIC INDEX: VERY LOW	TOTAL CALORIES PER 100 G: 654	CALORIES FROM		
		CARB: 55 9%	PROTEIN: 53 8%	FAT: 546 83%

WALNUT – *Juglans regia, J. nigra*

Walnuts are a valuable food for many reasons. The excellent supply of omega-3 fatty acids (5.5 g) is nearly unique because most foods, including nuts, supply none or only a trace amount. Walnuts are the richest nut source of both of the essential fatty acids (see page 134). They are an omega-3 treat as they need no cooking and therefore the oils (see page 145) are at their maximum effectiveness, especially considering walnuts' good supply of biotin (1.3 mcg), which assists in fat metabolism.

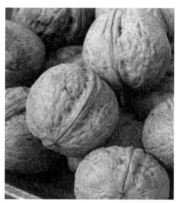

Walnuts are a good source of folate (98 mcg). They actually have more than spinach, and as folate is heat sensitive, the walnut wins the race, especially during pregnancy, since folate is essential to fetal development. In addition, walnuts' good iron content (3 mg) and protein supply (15 g, or 30% DV) all promote healthy fetal development.

The rich supply of polyunsaturated lipids (47 g) helps to lower cholesterol. Walnuts are a good source of phosphorus (346 mg, or 35% DV) and magnesium (158 mg, or 40% DV), both required for the brain. The great supply of omega-3 fatty acids, mentioned above, also help the brain, as brain cells or neurons need omega-3. They promote a flexible and fluid transfer of nutrients within brain cells and are also vital for the development of the infant's brain. Walnuts are the best "lookalike" brain food on the planet. The human brain is composed of 60% fat, and ideally, for maximum brain power, the diet's fat content is best made up of omega-3 fats. Give your brain a regular top up with walnut oil.

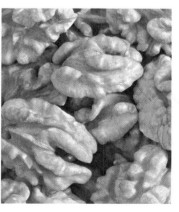

In addition, the combination of iron, manganese (3 mg), and copper (2 mg) is great for blood building, and the zinc (3 mg) is vital for hormone production and development of children's bones. Walnuts on toast with honey is simple, sweet, inexpensive, and full of omega-3, plus benefits for mother and baby. The best balanced nut, eating walnuts is one of the first steps you can take for your child. See page 220 for walnut recipes.

NOTE: Nutrient amounts are listed as milligrams (mg) per 100 grams (g), unless otherwise stated.

Nuts	Main Nutrients, Antioxidants, and Phytonutrients	Benefits Which Body Systems
Almond	vitamin E, protein, magnesium, phosphorus, manganese, calcium, biotin, lipids	skeletal, nervous, brain
Brazil	selenium, methionine, phosphorus, protein, potassium, magnesium, lipids	immune, growth, repair
Cashew	oleic acid, copper, protein, magnesium, phosphorus, lipids	brain, joint, circulatory
Chestnut	carbohydrate, potassium, magnesium, vitamin C, folate, lipids	muscular, blood, nervous
Coconut	fiber, sodium, potassium	elimination
Hazelnut	vitamin E, magnesium, copper, iron, manganese, B vitamins, protein, lipids	blood, nervous, circulatory
Macadamia	copper, fiber, lipids, protein	muscular
Pecan	copper, phosphorus, magnesium, potassium, fiber, protein, lipids	brain, blood
Pine	protein, phosphorus, magnesium, folate, iron, copper, manganese, lipids	nervous, brain, blood
Pistachio	phytosterols, potassium, magnesium, vitamin A, copper, zinc, lipids, protein	immune, circulatory, muscular
Walnut	omega-3, folate, iron, phosphorus, magnesium, manganese, copper, zinc, lipids	brain, growth, cellular, blood
Seeds		
Pumpkin	iron, protein, omega-3, phosphorus, magnesium, cucurbitacins, zinc, copper	blood, brain, nervous, repair
Sunflower	vitamin E, protein, magnesium, copper, phosphorus, silicon, potassium, selenium, zinc, iron, lipids, B vitamins	circulatory, growth, nervous, brain, joint, skin, muscular
Sesame	protein, methionine, calcium, fiber, copper, iron, magnesium, phosphorous, zinc, lecithin, phytosterols, manganese, folate	blood, nervous, brain, digestive, joint, skeletal, growth
Sprouts		
Alfalfa	phytoestrogens, iron, vitamin A, copper, selenium, cobalt, vitamin K, bioflavanoids	blood, urinary, immune
Buckwheat	rutin, magnesium, phosphorus, copper, zinc, iron	circulatory, brain
Wheatgrass	lycopene, chlorophyll, vitamin A, vitamin K, iron, cobalt, copper, manganese, potassium, selenium, sulfur, zinc, magnesium, vitamin C, vitamin E, fiber	immune, blood, repair, respiratory, circulatory, brain, skin, elimination

RECOMMENDATIONS FOR DAILY PROTEIN INTAKE FROM NUTS AND SEEDS		Adult Male	Adult Female	Teenager	Child
Total Daily Protein Intake (based on typical guidelines)		60 g	47 g	65 g	45 g
1. *UNH* recommendation:	25% of protein intake from nuts	15 g	12 g	16 g	11 g
	10% of protein intake from seeds	6 g	5 g	6.5 g	4.5 g
Note the average protein content in	100 g* (3–4 oz) nuts* or seeds* (on average)	approx. 23 g of carbohydrate on average			
2. U.S. MyPlate and DRIs (includes: meat, poultry, fish, legumes, eggs, nuts, and seeds)**		1–3 servings	1–2 servings	1–3 servings	1 serving
3. Australian Guide to Healthy Eating total protein food intake daily includes: meat, fish, poultry, eggs, and nuts. Does not include legumes.**		1 serving	1 serving	1 serving	1 serving

RECOMMENDATIONS FOR DAILY LIPID INTAKE FROM NUTS AND SEEDS		Adult Male	Adult Female	Teenager	Child
Total Daily Lipid Intake (based on typical guidelines)		58 g	50 g	60 g	44 g
1. *UNH* recommendation:	25% of lipid intake from nuts	14 g	12 g	15 g	11 g
	10% of lipid intake from seeds	6 g	5 g	6 g	4 g
Note the average lipid content in	100 g nuts: almonds, Brazil, and cashew mix*	approx. 78 g of lipids			
	100 g seeds: pumpkin, sesame, and sunflower*	approx. 48 g of lipids			
2. U.S. MyPlate guidelines include added lipids; do not include dairy or meat.		Use sparingly.			
3. Australian Guide to Healthy Eating (total lipid intake) includes added lipids; does not include dairy or meat.		Sometimes, or in small amounts.			

UNH = Ultimate Nutrition for Health; DRIs = Dietary Reference Intakes

* The average is calculated from a combination of: NUTS: almond, Brazil, and cashew; SEEDS: pumpkin, sesame, and sunflower

** 1 serving is equivalent to: ½ cup of almonds or peanuts, ¼ cup of sunflower seeds, 3–4 oz cooked fish fillets, 2 small eggs, or 3–4 oz cooked meat or chicken.

Seeds are the beginning of life. Seeds are the most compact form of life. Seeds are the universal code of nature. Seeds are latent life. Seeds are the force behind regeneration of new life. They are the most valuable asset of mankind.

From one seed we can assist nature and progressively create an infinite number of the same species. The seed you plant today will need care and attention, but when fully developed it will return the favor and supply you with an abundance of food for enjoyment and nutrition and energy requirements.

The following pages describe the main benefits associated with the most common edible seeds: pumpkin, sesame, and sunflower, as well as a section on sprouting seeds.

When seeds are eaten, they combine their life force. No other food group is more compact and generous. A handful of sesame seeds may contain nearly 500 individual life units; their capacity to promote your health and life are second to none. In contrast to animal products, seeds are a vital food: seeds contain no cholesterol, seeds are easy to digest, seeds are ready to sprout into life. There is no life without the seed kingdom.

A well-balanced diet must include seeds. They are full of complete protein, amino acids, and essential oils, and they provide a unique supply of essential nutrients and trace elements.

Seeds are also a source of the essential fatty acids. In particular, pepitas (or pumpkin seeds) are the second-richest natural source of omega-3 fatty acids.

Pumpkin, sesame, and sunflower seeds are compatible with various fruits, nearly all vegetables, whole grains, and some legume combinations. Refer to the chart on page 208 for food-combination ideas.

Seeds can be combined in numerous delicious ways, all depending on your imagination. If you have never tried any of the three basic edible seeds, know that you can greatly improve your health and range of recipes by experimenting.

Even though seeds may appear small and neglected in the packaged form, consider the colorful and abundant growth of their original source.

Numerous varieties of handy takeaway snacks now include seeds, and these are a very good alternative to chocolate bars. Sesame bars, pumpkin and honey crunch, and sunflower-coated energy bars are full of benefits. Pass me a pepita bar, please!

For a guide to ways to add seeds to your daily diet, refer to page 221. It is surprising how many basic meals can improve greatly with the addition of seeds, especially ground seeds sprinkled on top of breakfast cereal or pasta. Seeds can make a meal into a nutritional feast.

Seeds are unique providers of substances to protect against common ailments. Make the most of seeds; they will multiply your nutritional intake and provide abundant benefits.

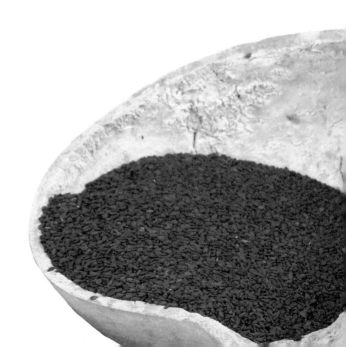

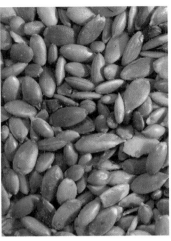

PUMPKIN SEEDS (PEPITAS) – *Cucurbita* spp.

One of the greatest natural foods is often forgotten when considering a highly nutritious diet. The seeds from the pumpkin are often referred to as *pepitas,* a name that is derived from the Greek word *pepon* and which translates as "cooked in the sun." Pepitas are available at most health stores and supermarkets. When purchasing pumpkin seeds, be sure to obtain only the inner kernel of the seed, usually a flat seed with a dark green/grey color, as the outer white shell is gritty.

Among the numerous benefits of pepitas, the organic iron content (11–14 mg) is second only to that of mussels (14.9 mg). The small amount of vitamin C (1.9 mg) will help with iron absorption. Pepitas have four times the iron value of lean beef (3.1 mg) and spinach (3.2 mg); a 100 g (3.5 oz) serving provides over 80% of daily iron values. For a big iron boost, in cases of anemia, after a surgical procedure, or following loss of blood due to menstruation, pepitas provide proper recovery. For an easy way to incorporate this tiny powerhouse into your daily diet, place a cupful of pumpkin seeds in a grinder or blender, process just long enough to produce a ground mixture or "pepi-mix," and add to soups or sprinkle over fresh garden salads. For the best Italian pasta recipe, add the mix to any pasta sauce, or sprinkle over pasta and cheese. It's incredibly nourishing, with a nutty texture.

Pepitas are an excellent protein food: a 100 g serving contains 24.5 g or 50% of the daily protein requirement—now that's potent protein! Pepitas have a low saturated fat content of 9 g, and a good supply of monounsaturated (14 g) and polyunsaturated lipids (21 g), with an excellent supply of precious omega-3 (7–10 g) and omega-6 (20 g). Compared to the omega-3 content of fish (0.1–2.2 g), pepitas are the champion omega-3 food. They need to take prime place in every pantry.

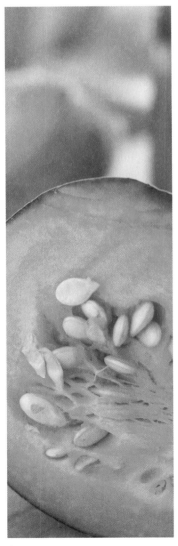

Pepitas provide numerous mineral benefits. The supplies of phosphorus (1,174 mg, or 167% DV) and magnesium (535 mg, or 134% DV) are exceptional. Pepitas get top marks as a brain food. They supply over five times the phosphorus and 17 times the magnesium of beef or fish. The excellent supply of phosphorus promotes healing of bone fractures, concentration, growth, blood circulation, and brain function.

Pepitas are a potent source of cucurbitacins, which are ideal for protection and relief from an enlarged prostate gland (prostatitis). The cucurbitacins retard the conversion of the male hormone testosterone into a more complex and potent hormone, *dihydrotestosterone,* which is used by the body to produce prostate cells. In addition, the excellent supply of zinc (7.5 mg, or almost 100% DV) assists to reduce prostate gland enlargement and is also essential for insulin conversion and protection from diabetes, ulcers, acne, dermatitis, and bone repair. The supply of the mineral copper (1.4 mg) is a bonus for iron absorption. Plus, pepitas supply manganese, also essential for iron absorption, as an antioxidant, and for brain function, memory, and regulating menstrual cycles.

Pepitas are a vital food for every man and woman, especially to counterbalance our era's highly processed foods, which have been stripped of most of their content of the minerals zinc, copper, magnesium, and phosphorus.

Pepitas also provide anti-inflammatory power against arthritis. For a life of bliss, strength, and good health, pumpkin seeds are a priority.

NOTE: DV amounts listed refer to the daily value for women 25–50 years; refer to DRI tables on pages 95–96 for adult male and child values.

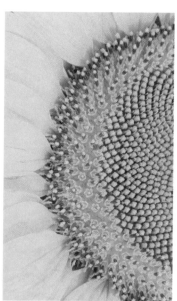

SUNFLOWER SEEDS – *Helianthus annuus*

Sunflower plants attract the sun's energy all day long with a happy golden face full of amazing nutritional benefits. The name "sunflower" is adapted from the botanical name and Greek words *helios* (sun) and *anthos* (flower). For thousands of years, originating in Mexico and Peru, the sunflower plant has provided nourishment and herbal benefits from its seeds, stems, and flowers. Hundreds of seeds develop within the enormous blossom. For edible purposes, only the inner kernel of the seed is used—unless you are a cockatoo and live for 100 years entirely on the whole sunflower seed.

Sunflower seeds are the richest natural food source of vitamin E (31–35 mg, or 200% DV). A regular intake of sunflower seeds will promote protection from aging, free radicals, and skin cell damage, as vitamin E is a powerful antioxidant. Delicious cookies or pancakes (refer to page 221) can be made with the sunflower kernels. Or you can grind them and sprinkle them over a fruit salad, or add them to your daily breakfast cereal; they have a soft nutty texture and are a soft gray in color. A sunflower butter spread is also delightful on breakfast toast.

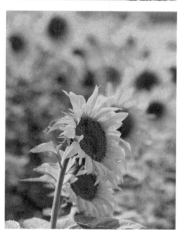

Sunflower kernels are low in saturated fat (5 g) and a good source of monounsaturated fat (9.5 g) and polyunsaturated fat (33 g), mainly in the form of omega-6 (30 g), with a trace of omega-3. The protein content of sunflower seeds is complete in all essential amino acids. They supply 23% protein and are the tenth-best protein food with 58% usable protein (NPU). The supply of minerals, especially magnesium (354 mg), is very good. Copper (1.8 mg, or 200% DV) is also abundant; it is vital for blood development, skin healing, nerve fiber protection, and cartilage repair. For a natural vitamin B1 boost, sunflower seeds provide (2.3 mg, or 200% DV) plus B2 (0.3 mg, or 27% DV) and B3 (4.5 mg, or 23% DV).

The supply of phosphorus (700 mg, or 100% DV) is most beneficial for the brain, nerves, and bones. This, in combination with the abundant supply of silicon (554 mg)—also essential for brain, nerves, and bones—will keep you thinking straight and walking strong. The supply of calcium (354 mg, or 35% DV) is good, and the supply of potassium (700–900 mg, or 20% DV) promotes strong muscular action and proper digestion. The price of sunflower kernels is really a big, bright bonus, considering the effort involved to make them edible. Add nutritional value to cookies with sunflower seeds or meal. Sunflower meal is available at most health stores; it is a rich source of protein (57%) with no fat content. Sunflower meal can be added to homemade bread or mixed with honey for a delicious spread.

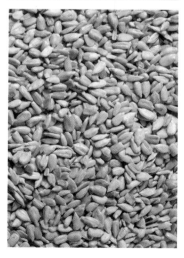

The selenium content of the kernels is very good at 59 mcg (55 mcg is the daily requirement). This combined with the exceptional vitamin E content makes the sunflower seed a potent antioxidant. Selenium works with vitamin E to protect against free radicals and promote DNA repair and also to induce *apoptosis,* or the self-destruction of cancerous cells.

Sunflower kernels are an excellent source of zinc (5 mg), essential for fighting infections and healing the body. Also, sunflower seeds are ideal for the reproductive system, in part due to their abundant vitamin E content. The seeds' content of manganese (2 mg) and iron (7 mg) are further proof that the sunflower is the brightest supplier of surprising sun-filled health benefits.

NOTE: Nutrient amounts are listed as milligrams (mg) per 100 grams (g), unless otherwise stated.

GLYCEMIC INDEX: VERY LOW	TOTAL CALORIES PER 100 G: 573	CALORIES FROM		
		CARB: 96 17%	PROTEIN: 61 11%	FAT: 416 72%

SESAME SEEDS – *Sesamum indicum*

Sesame seeds, from a plant native to Africa, Turkey, and Arabia, have been cultivated for thousands of years and are a staple food in China and India. The old saying "open sesame" originates from the fact that as soon as the sesame plant has ripened, the seeds pop out of the pods and scatter on the ground. The sesame seed is referred to as the "seed of immortality," and without a doubt some of its nutrient benefits promote long life. The seed can last for ages after harvesting, because the substance sesamol, unique to sesame seeds, prevents the oxidation and deterioration of the precious oils. Nearly half the seed weight is made up of oils (49 g). The seeds are low in saturated fat (7 g), and higher in monounsaturated (19 g) and polyunsaturated fats (23 g). Sesame seeds provide omega-6 fatty acids (25 g) and only a trace of omega-3.

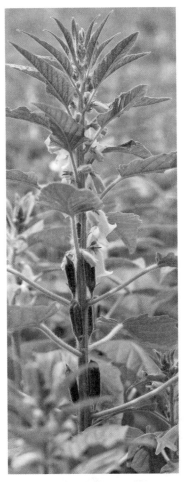

The protein value of sesame seeds is excellent (19 g whole and 18 g hulled). Their rich supply of the amino acid methionine (637 mg) promotes the metabolism of fats and offsets the low supply of methionine from numerous other foods—an important consideration when aiming for an intake of complete protein and a well-balanced supply of amino acids. A small amount of ground sesame seeds added to vegetable soup, bread, or legume dishes will greatly boost protein value. Sesame seeds are not easy to completely digest, unless they are ground into a paste, or eaten as tahini (sesame seed butter), halva (a sweet dish made of crushed sesame seeds in a binder of honey), or sesame meal, which can be used in numerous recipes such as cakes or cookies, sprinkled over fruit salad, or mixed into vegetable burgers.

The calcium content of sesame seeds is excellent (900–1,100 mg, or around 100% DV). Ground sesame seeds are the ideal nondairy calcium food; they provide more calcium than cheddar cheese (775 mg) and no cholesterol. Tahini supplies 420 mg of calcium. In addition, sesame seeds provide special fibers, termed *lignans,* that actually lower blood cholesterol.

The supply of the trace mineral copper is abundant (4.1 mg, or 350% DV) in sesame seeds. Copper provides benefits in cases of rheumatoid arthritis, as it is part of the enzyme that reduces inflammation; it is also required for the production of elastin and collagen. Besides liver, sesame seeds are the best copper food. The supplies of vitamins B1, B2, B3, B5, and B6 are also very good. Sesame seeds provide an excellent supply of iron (10–14 mg, or 60–80% DV). The supply of magnesium (350 mg or 110% DV) assists sleep patterns, promotes steady nerves, and may reduce migraine attacks, as magnesium reduces the spasms in the *trigeminal-nerve* blood vessels that cause the pain. Sesame seeds are full of phosphorus (630 mg) and zinc (7.8 mg), both close to 100% daily value.

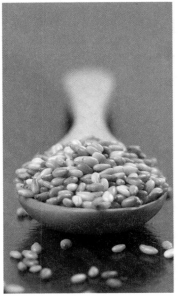

Sesame seeds are an excellent source of lecithin, which is required for the dissolving of fats and the reduction of cholesterol. Sesame seeds are a rich source of phytosterols (714 mg), plant sterols that inhibit the absorption of cholesterol. In addition, phytosterols can assist with the control of blood sugar levels for diabetics, reduce prostate enlargements, and decrease the inflammation of rheumatoid arthritis. Sesame seeds also supply manganese (2.5 mg), potassium (468 mg), selenium (5.7 mg), and folate (97 mcg).

Sesame seeds traditionally decorate rolls and buns, but let your imagination loose in the kitchen for the many other ways you can use this magical seed. Open the door to a new world of sesame sensations!

NOTE: DV amounts listed refer to the daily value for women 25–50 years; refer to DRI tables on pages 95–96 for adult male and child values.

Sprouting seeds, grains, and legumes is by no means a recent discovery. Over 3,000 years ago the Chinese discovered the potential of sprouted foods, and now, with modern methods of food analysis, the wisdom of their ways is revealed.

In this era, many people are still unaware of the potential of sprouted foods and are unaccustomed to preparing and combining sprouted foods with other meals. Throughout this section on sprouts, you will discover (if you don't already know) the methods of sprouting preparation, their associated benefits, and a few basic ways to include sprouted foods with other common foods.

Sprouting is a basic natural development: The original seed is transformed from a state of latent energy into a complete living form with the assistance of water, air, and sunlight.

Sprouting is also termed "seed germination." As the seed begins to sprout, elements contained in the seed are used to provide energy: the starches contained in the seed are slowly converted into natural sugars, the protein content of the seed is transformed into available amino acids, and the fat content is converted into essential fatty acids. All these changes improve the nutrient quality and digestibility of seeds, grains, and legumes. After a few days of seed development, the most substantial contribution is the "life-rate activity" within the seed, often termed the "enzyme activity."

The human body requires regular supplies of various enzymes for digestion, nutrient absorption, body development, and repair. Enzymes are the catalyst for all living development. Sprouted foods are one of the best sources of living enzymes. In fact, apart from fruits, vegetables, and sprouted foods, there are very few foods that contain living enzymes. Nearly all processed and refined foods are deficient in enzyme content. All cooked foods have very little enzyme content, and without enzymes a food cannot provide maximum nutritional benefits.

Sprouted foods provide a good source of vitamin C and various B-group vitamins, as well as a good supply of amino acids and such hard-to-get vitamins as P (another term for bioflavonoids), K, and U (antipeptic ulcer factor).

The mineral content of sprouted foods is based on the original source: whole grain, legume, or seed. Sprouts are a good source of trace minerals. You can start sprouting the seed of your choice today!

Sprouted foods are a most valuable addition to the regular diet, especially for overweight people. A large number of overweight people have developed their condition due to a decreasing rate of metabolism, often from a prolonged lack of essential living enzymes in the cooked foods they've eaten.

An overweight person can obtain excellent low-calorie, low-fat, regenerative energy from a regular supply of sprouted foods, fresh fruits, and fresh vegetables. Sprouted foods are also very economical. Just a tablespoon of seeds, when fully developed, will provide enough sprouts to fill a large salad bowl. So sprout off those excess pounds! If you're too busy to grow them yourself, visit the produce section of your local supermarket—or should that be sproutmarket?—and then start experimenting with the many great recipes available for sprouts.

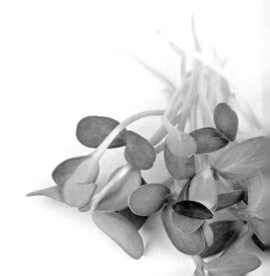

GLYCEMIC INDEX: VERY LOW	TOTAL CALORIES PER 100 G: 29	CALORIES FROM		
		CARB: 13 46%	PROTEIN: 10 34%	FAT: 6 20%

ALFALFA SPROUTS – *Medicago sativa*

Alfalfa sprouts are one of the most popular sprouts, available at nearly every supermarket and health food store. From the tiny alfalfa seed, great health benefits can be obtained. In fact, when considered in their *dry weight*, as 90% of the sprouts weight is water, the alfalfa sprout provides an enormous amount of nutrients.

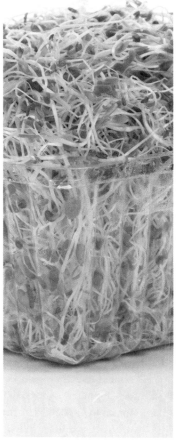

The calcium content of alfalfa sprouts (1,750 mg) is better than that of any cheese (parmesan, for example, has 1,100 mg). The iron (35 mg) and vitamin A (44,000 IU) content are also enormous. In comparison to lettuce and spinach, alfalfa sprouts provide over three times the value of calcium, iron, and magnesium, and for a super salad, alfalfa sprouts combined with tahini provides complete protein. On their own, alfalfa sprouts are not a complete-protein food as they lack four amino acids. Ensure that your alfalfa sprouts are fresh and rinsed properly, to obtain all the benefits and tasty flavor.

In their fresh state, alfalfa sprouts provide trace minerals such as zinc (0.9 mg), copper (0.2 mg), selenium (0.6 mcg), and manganese (0.2 mg), as well as cobalt. In the dry weight, values for molybdenum (2.6 ppm) have been recorded. A regular serving of alfalfa sprouts can promote blood building and elimination of excess body acids via the urinary system.

Alfalfa sprouts provide good supplies of vitamin K (30 mcg) and vitamin P, and in their dry weight, a measure of vitamin B12 (0.3 mg) has been recorded. The vitamin C content is low (8 mg), but a slice of red bell pepper will easily increase the supply. Alfalfa sprouts provide all the basic B vitamins in small amounts. A note of *caution* for persons with inflammatory or autoimmune conditions: high levels of the amino acid *canavanine* in alfalfa sprouts may irritate such conditions.

On a positive note, alfalfa sprouts have proven very beneficial in preventing the bacterium that causes stomach ulcers (*Helicobacter pylori*).

Alfalfa sprouts are a very good source of phytoestrogens, which are used by the body as antioxidants and for prevention of menopausal symptoms, osteoporosis, heart disease, and cancer. Let the freshly prepared alfalfa sprout add life and a beneficial bounce to your daily bread.

GLYCEMIC INDEX: VERY LOW	TOTAL CALORIES PER 100 G: 343	CALORIES FROM		
		CARB: 270 79%	PROTEIN: 45 13%	FAT: 28 8%

BUCKWHEAT SPROUTS – *Fagopyrum esculentum*

Buckwheat sprouts are hard to get but fairly easy to grow. The benefits from this relative of rhubarb are remarkable. Buckwheat and sprouts are the best natural food sources of rutin, a bioflavonoid and a component of vitamin P that is vital for healing varicose veins, poor blood circulation, and hardened arteries. Buckwheat sprouts promote the health of your circulatory system, plus the good supply of potassium (350–460 mg) will enhance the functions of rutin. Buckwheat in the form of groats can be eaten as a breakfast cereal or cooked like rice. The magnesium content (231 mg, or 58% DV) is very good for the nervous system and when combined with the phosphorus (347 mg) also benefits the brain. The supply of copper (1.1 mg, or over 100% DV) and zinc (2.4 mg) promotes healing and blood development, especially in combination with the iron content (2.2 mg). Buckwheat sprouts will help you to circulate all over!

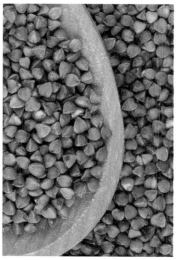

NOTE: DV amounts listed refer to the daily value for women 25–50 years; refer to DRI tables on pages 95–96 for adult male and child values.

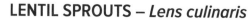

GLYCEMIC INDEX: VERY LOW	TOTAL CALORIES PER 100 G: 106	CALORIES FROM		
		CARB: 80 75%	PROTEIN: 22 21%	FAT: 4 4%

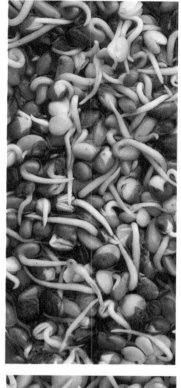

LENTIL SPROUTS – *Lens culinaris*

Lentil sprouts provide more iron (3.1 mg) than any other sprout, and more than milk, cheese, egg, lettuce, or spinach. Lentil sprouts are the ideal way to obtain the maximum benefits from this legume; they have a very low calorie content, a fair but complete protein supply (9 g), and a very low fat content (0.5 g).

Very few foods compare to the weight-watching power of lentil sprouts. During the sprouting stage, various changes in the protein and carbohydrate content (22 g) occur to improve the digestion of the compact lentil. There are numerous recipes for lentils but they often do not include sprouted lentils; plus, they may contain poor combinations. Ideally, lentil sprouts combine best with leafy vegetables and cottage cheese for a simple waist saver, or add the lentil sprouts last and make a great lentil vegetable soup, with carrots, spinach, broccoli, and parmesan cheese. For the cheapest meal in town, try lentil sprouts with rice and increase the protein value by 30%. Fresh lentil sprouts are a good source of vitamin C (17 mg or 23% DV), plus they provide all the basic B vitamins, especially folate (100 mcg or 25% DV). Keep a supply of lentils in your pantry for when times get tough; they can sprout new life into the kitchen and provide an abundance of energy. Lentils have been referred to as the poor man's meat, but they have none of the problems associated with meat: no saturated fat, no cholesterol, and no free radicals. Combine lentil sprouts with various spices and herbs for a lean lunch and a big boost to the blood system.

GLYCEMIC INDEX: VERY LOW	TOTAL CALORIES PER 100 G: 31	CALORIES FROM		
		CARB: 22 71%	PROTEIN: 7 23%	FAT: 2 6%

MUNG BEAN SPROUTS – *Vigna radiata*

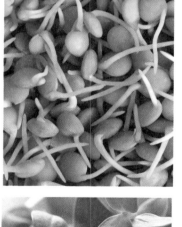

The Chinese discovered the method of sprouting the mung bean over 3,000 years ago; today, people from around the world utilize an important part of Chinese culture and cuisine when they enjoy bean sprouts. Mung beans in their sprouted form provide extra benefits, such as an increase in protein availability, from 23 g to 37 g per 100 g portion, complete in all the essential amino acids. The supply of B-group vitamins is also improved during the sprouting process, especially that of vitamin B1. Mung bean sprouts are a very good source of organic iron (refer to page 38 for more details). Take part in a little Chinese kitchen wisdom today. Mung bean sprouts will enhance any Chinese meal or Asian dish.

GLYCEMIC INDEX: VERY LOW	TOTAL CALORIES PER 100 G: 52	CALORIES FROM		
		CARB: 26 50%	PROTEIN: 13 25%	FAT: 13 25%

SUNFLOWER SPROUTS – *Helianthus annuus*

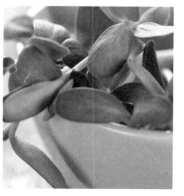

Sunflower sprouts are one of the tastiest and most delightful sprouts available. The minerals calcium, phosphorus, iron, potassium, and magnesium are well supplied, as are vitamins E and some B-group vitamins. Sunflower sprouts make an ideal addition to a tossed garden salad or a sandwich. They are easy to grow, and they are so cheap to buy that you can really save on your shopping bill while gaining a great increase in active enzymes, vitamins, and chlorophyll. If you are too busy to sprout, buy a handy pack of sunflower sprouts on your next shopping trip, and surprise yourself with the variety of meals that are enhanced by sunflower power. Sunflower sprouts will help you shine!

NOTE: Nutrient amounts are listed as milligrams (mg) per 100 grams (g), unless otherwise stated.

GLYCEMIC INDEX: VERY LOW	TOTAL CALORIES PER 100 G: 198	CALORIES FROM		
		CARB: 160 80%	PROTEIN: 27 13%	FAT: 11 7%

WHEATGRASS JUICE AND SPROUTS – *Triticum aestivum*

Wheat is the most dominant and versatile grain in the world; however, the greatest benefits of wheat are not obtained from products such as bread and cereals. In fact, numerous health problems can be attributed to the excess consumption of refined wheat products. The ultimate value from the humble wheat grain is obtained from sprouted wheat and wheatgrass shoots that are pressed into a juice, termed wheatgrass juice. Most juice bars prepare and applaud its health and healing benefits. Dr. G.H. Earp Thomas, a soil expert, calculated that 1 kg of wheatgrass is equivalent to 12 kg of the choicest vegetables. For those who are brave enough to sip or gulp a dose of wheatgrass juice, it is obvious from the taste and the headrush that it certainly is a potent tonic. The chlorophyll content is the major contributor of benefits, primarily because it is obtained so fresh and alive with enzymes and living nutrients. People typcially consume just a small quantity of wheatgrass juice (a "shot" of about 35 g, or 1.67 fluid oz) Surprisingly, the nutrients from such a small amount are enormous (refer to the chart below). In addition to supplying over 12 minerals and 13 vitamins, wheatgrass juice provides 830 mcg of lycopene—that's one-third the lycopene content of tomatoes, but that amount still provides proven protection from breast, lung, and prostate cancer. It's a powerful antioxidant and antitumor factor, able to fight against diseases caused by oxidative stress. The vitamin C content is four times that of oranges, and the vitamin A (beta-carotene) value is 47,700 IU per 100 g, or 16,600 IU per 35 g (1.67 oz) serving— that's potent! Both vitamin A and C protect against cancer.

Back to chlorophyll, the ultimate promoter of health and healing due to its oxygen content: Wheatgrass juice provides 185 mg per 35 g serving. According to Nobel prize winner Dr. Otto Warburg, oxygen deprivation is a major contributor to cancer. Obviously, exercise is the ideal way to oxygenate the blood, but for people with chronic illnesses, wheatgrass juice can provide a renewed supply of oxygen, directly into the bloodstream, within 15 minutes. Smoking, alcohol, pollution, drugs, fatty foods, and high-protein cooked foods all deplete oxygen in the bloodstream. The chemical composition of chlorophyll is nearly identical to that of human blood, except chlorophyll is based on a magnesium atom instead of an iron atom. This unique structure of chlorophyll was described by Dr. Birscher, a research scientist, as "concentrated sun power." He stated that it increases the functions of the circulatory system and the lungs, neutralizes toxins, and cleanses and rebuilds the body. Wheatgrass juice assists the body in manufacturing healthy new red blood cells, hemoglobin.

Wheatgrass juice also assists in the elimination of toxins such as fatty deposits, calcifications, hardened mucus, fecal matter, and crystallized acids; it purifies the liver, cleanses the skin, and can remove heavy metals from the body. One "shot" per day will promote renewed energy, healing of various ailments, and a positive outlook, due to its remarkable supply of nutrients, such as the rich iron content (8.7 mg). In this era of depleted, processed, and snack foods, a "shot a day" may be the simple answer to the hectic pace of city living. Make it at home, get it from shops, buy it at a juice bar—whatever. Just remember, wheatgrass juice is tops for healing!

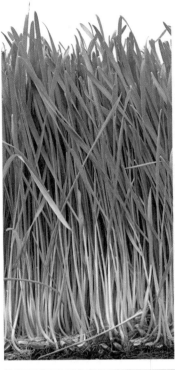

WHEATGRASS JUICE

Nutrients	3.5 g	"shot" 35 g	100 g
Calories	13	130	371
Carbohydrate	1.6 g	16 g	45.7 g
Protein	860 mg	8.6 g	24 g
Fiber	1 g	10 g	28 g
Chlorophyll	18.5 mg	185 mg	529 mg
Calcium	15 mg	150 mg	429 mg
Cobalt	1.7 mcg	17 mcg	48 mg
Copper	17 mcg	170 mcg	485 mcg
Iodine	8 mcg	80 mcg	228 mcg
Iron	870 mcg	8.7 mg	24 mg
Magnesium	3.9 mg	39 mg	111 mg
Manganese	240 mcg	2.4 mg	6.8 mg
Phosphorus	14 mg	140 mg	400 mg
Potassium	137 mg	1,300 mg	3,918 mg
Selenium	3.5 mcg	35 mcg	100 mcg
Sodium	1 mg	10 mg	28.6 mg
Sulfur	10.5 mg	105 mg	300 mg
Zinc	62 mcg	620 mcg	1.7 mg
Vitamin A	1,668 IU	16,668 IU	47,704 IU
Vitamin C	7.5 mg	75 mg	214 mg
Vitamin E	320 mcg	3.2 mg	9.15 mg
Vitamin K	35 mcg	350 mcg	1 mg

NOTE: DV amounts listed refer to the daily value for women 25–50 years; refer to DRI tables on pages 95–96 for adult male and child values.

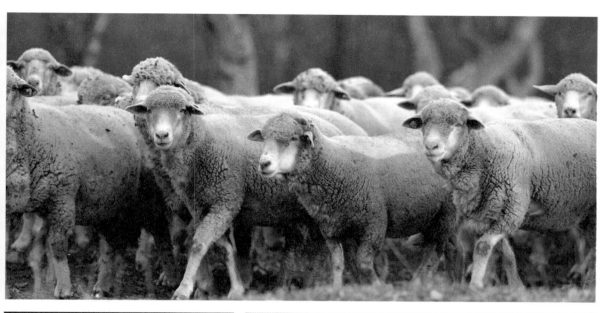

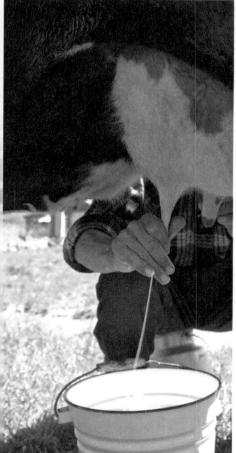

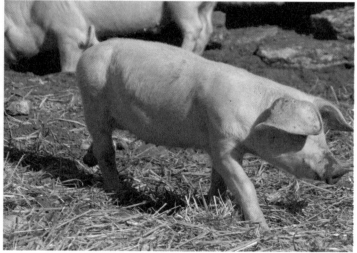

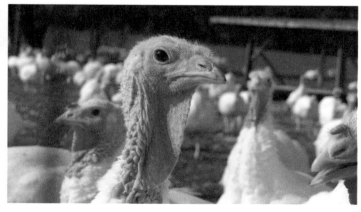

ANIMAL PRODUCTS – SECONDARY PROTEIN

CHEESE

Cheese has been made for thousands of years. The origin of cheese is thought to have occurred accidentally when nomads and tribespeople carried milk in containers that were made from the stomach of a milk-producing animal: cow, goat, sheep, camel, or buffalo. The contact between the milk and the container produced the earliest method of milk storage: cheesemaking. The special active ingredient obtained from the animal stomach is called rennet, a digestive enzyme that assists the calf to digest milk from the cow. The human child, up to the age of around seven, also produces a milk-digesting enzyme. The majority of traditional and modern methods of cheesemaking are based on the curdling effect produced by the enzyme rennet. But some cheese is curdled by the effects of lemon juice, and, more recently, a vegetable rennet has been developed. It is less expensive and is greatly increasing in popularity as a large variety of aged cheese and cottage cheese can be produced from vegetable rennet.

Today, there are over four hundred individual types of cheese, each with a different taste, texture, and appearance. From Switzerland the famous Swiss cheese has unique characteristics nutritionally as well as visually (by virtue of its large holes). From Italy comes the famous mozzarella and parmesan; from France, camembert; and from England and the United States, cheddar cheese. All over the world different types of cheese are produced and available in urban areas from the delicatessen or supermarket.

POSSIBLE BENEFICIAL FACTORS

1. low lactose content
2. high protein content
3. high calcium content
4. meal maker

Natural cheese made from raw milk contains the active enzymes lipase, for fat digestion, and lactase, for lactose conversion. During the natural cheesemaking process, rennet and "natural bacteria" are added; these promote lactose conversion and digestion of the concentrated milk product. Natural cheese may cost more, but it provides true value and easier digestion.

Cheese is an excellent source of *complete protein,* and it boosts the protein value of many recipes. The simple "peasant's lunch" of cheese on bread provides the protein, energy, and other nutrients to continue a hard day's work. Because cheese is a good supplier of the common limiting amino acid methionine, it improves the overall (net) protein value (NPU) of many meals. A small amount of cheese, 50 g, when combined with kidney beans or rice or a veggie sandwich, can provide over half the daily protein requirements. However, depending on other foods in the daily diet, over 100 g of cheese per day is excessive. Refer to the table on page 92 for details on cheese protein.

The *calcium content* of cheese is excellent, making cheese a far better choice than milk, especially because it is easier to digest. Cheese supplies on average 700 mg of calcium per 100 g, and it easily supplies over half the daily calcium in one serving: in the form of a cheese and veggie sandwich, or grated parmesan on pasta. Up to one-quarter of the weekly calcium supply can be obtained from natural cheese.

Cheese is a *meal maker.* It adds flavor to numerous recipes due to its rich saturated fat content and the individual cheese's culture. Grilled cheese, however, is not recommended for good health as it contains free radicals. Enjoy cheese's natural "meal-making" benefits at work or play.

CALCIUM CONTENT PER 100 G (3.5 OZ) OF CHEESES	
Cheddar	728 mg
Edam	738 mg
Feta	500 mg
Mozzarella	653 mg
Parmesan	1,200 mg
Ricotta	208 mg
Swiss	971 mg

RECOMMENDED DAILY CALCIUM INTAKE			
Child 4–8	Child 9–18	Male 19–50	Male 51–70
1,000 mg	1,300 mg	1,000 mg	1,000 mg
female 9–18	female 19–30	female 31–50	female 51–70
1,300 mg	1,000 mg	1,000 mg	1,200 mg
pregnant, under 18 years 1,300 mg		pregnant, 19–50 years 1,000 mg	
lactating, under 18 years 1,300 mg		lactating, 19–50 years 1,000 mg	

There are two main groups of cheese: soft cheese and hard cheese. There are also two main types of cheese: natural cheese and processed cheese.

Processed cheese is available in numerous varieties and flavors with any number of additives. Processed cheese was invented by Mr. J. L. Kraft in 1917; since then, it has taken over the diet of many people. Check labels for bleaching agents, preservatives, and colors. Ideally, avoid *processed cheese.* The packaging of individual slices in plastic adds to the price, and the cheese spoils fairly quickly compared to true natural cheese, which can last for months and just gets better with age.

Most "natural" supermarket cheese provides the benefits mentioned but may only last a week, refrigerated.

All cheese may promote the following problems, if consumed in excess. Natural cheese, however, has the long-lasting benefits and rich, full flavor.

POSSIBLE DETRIMENTAL FACTORS

1. excess saturated fats/cholesterol
2. processed cheese additives
3. high in calories
4. high salt content

Cheese is full of fats, especially *saturated fats,* and it also contains a fair amount of cholesterol. It is easy to obtain both excess fats and cholesterol from cheese. On average, hard cheese is 30% fat and also contains 100 mg of cholesterol.

Cheese is full of *salt,* and it also provides abundant *calories,* which is ideal for energetic kids and athletes. For the not-so-active, cheese is best in small amounts. The charts on this page compare the supply of nutrients to the recommended daily allowance (RDA). Cheese easily supplies the daily protein, calcium, sodium, and lipids, but it is best to keep cheese intake to about one-quarter of total daily calories, as 200 g (7 oz) of cheddar cheese alone, with 66 g of total fat, will start to tilt the scales on daily lipids (87 g is the adult RDA).

Two cheese sandwiches contain about 200 g of cheese. Add as much lettuce and other veggies as you can to obtain balance without so much cheese.

Keep your cheese intake to a bare minimum, and enjoy it to the maximum.

RECOMMENDED DAILY ALLOWANCES FOR LIPIDS / SODIUM / IRON / PROTEIN

Age Group	Lipids* (Fats and Oils)	Sodium (approx.)	Iron	Protein	Calories* (kcal)
Children 6–12 months	31 g	0.12 g	0.27 mg	9.1 g	650
Children 1–3 years	38 g	1.0 g	7 mg	13 g	1,300
Children 4–6 years	58 g	1.2 g	10 mg	19 g	1,800
Children 7–14 years	80 g	1.5 g	8–10 mg	19–34 g	2,000
Teenagers 15–22**	80 g	1.5 g	11–15 mg	46–52 g	2,500
Females 11–23**	78 g	1.5 g	15–18 mg	46 g	2,200
Men 23 and over**	87 g	1.3–1.5 g	8 mg	56 g	2,900
Women 23–50**	66 g	1.5 g	18 mg	46 g	2,200
Men and women* 51 and over	59 g	1.2–1.3 g	8 mg	46–56 g	1,900–2,300

*In the U.S., no RDAs are established for total lipid intake (above age 12 months) or calorie intake. What's listed here are Australian recommendations, from the original edition of this book.
**Cholesterol maximum daily intake 300 mg (adult)

CHEESE SUPPLY OF LIPIDS AND CHOLESTEROL

Per 100 g (3.5 oz)	Total Fat	Choles-terol	Saturated	Poly	Mono
Cheddar	33 g	107 mg	22 g	1 g	9.5 g
Edam	27 g	89 mg	18 g	0.7 g	8.2 g
Feta	21 g	89 mg	15 g	0.6 g	4.6 g
Mozzarella	21 g	78 mg	13.5 g	0.8 g	6.7 g
Parmesan	26 g	67 mg	17 g	0.6 g	7.2 g
Ricotta	13 g	50 mg	8.3 g	0.4 g	3.7 g
Swiss	28 g	92 mg	18 g	1 g	7.5 g

CHEESE NUTRIENT COMPARISON CHART

Per 100 g (3.5 oz)	Sodium	Iron	Protein	Calories
Cheddar	628 mg	0.67 mg	25 g	406
Edam	978 mg	0.42 mg	25 g	360
Feta	1,128 mg	0.64 mg	14 g	267
Mozzarella	387 mg	0.17 mg	19.6 g	285
Parmesan	1,620 mg	0.82 mg	35 g	397
Ricotta	84 mg	0.36 mg	11.3 g	175
Swiss	264 mg	0.17 mg	29 g	382

NOTE: Nutrient amounts are listed as milligrams (mg) per 100 grams (g), unless otherwise stated.

MILK – INFANTS AND CHILDREN

Milk is the first natural food. Mother's milk is the perfect food for development of content, healthy infants. Depending on the duration of breastfeeding and the health of the mother, a child will obtain from breast milk all the essential nutrients to assist in the early vital stages of growth and development.

Because mother's milk is the best food for babies, special care should be taken by the mother to ensure that she also obtains the best foods, including natural foods to promote milk production, such as carrot juice.

There are a few other, very important elements supplied by mother's milk, such as colostrum and *Bacillus bifidus*, a natural bacterium that protects the child from other harmful bacteria and also assists in digestion of milk sugar (lactose).

As the child is weaned off of its mother's milk, formula, cow's milk, and other milks may be given as the next main food. For children who obtain a supply of both mother's milk and other milk, the natural bacteria provided by the mother's milk will assist in digestion of the other milk, until such time that no more mother's milk is available. From that time onward, the "new" milk will supply its own bacteria. The addition of acidophilus yogurt is the best way to supply the "friendly bacteria" needed to help protect and promote the infant's/child's digestive system. It will also promote the digestion of milk and the breakdown of lactic acid. The addition of mashed foods, especially carrots, pumpkin, and broccoli, will soon provide the child with nutrients not supplied by cow's milk or goat's milk.

Within the developing digestive system of children, a very important temporary digestive enzyme is produced, called rennin. On average, this digestive enzyme will remain within the child's digestive system until the first full set of permanent teeth commence to develop, usually around the age of seven.

Slowly, from that time onward, the ability of a child to digest milk depends greatly on their health and their body's ability to adapt to a new system of milk digestion. The enzyme rennin is required to convert the caseinogen content of milk into casein. Rennin curdles milk by converting the soluble protein caseinogen into insoluble casein, which combines with calcium to form calcium caseinate, the curd that is digested by the hydrochloric

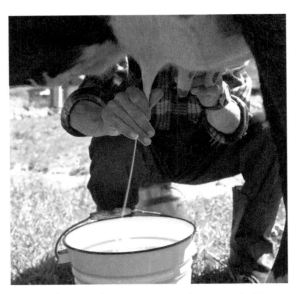

acid and pepsin (pepsinogen) in the stomach. Human "mother's milk" protein comprises 40% casein and 60% whey. Cow's milk protein comprises 80% casein and 20% whey. Cow's milk contains 200% more caseinogen than human milk. Cow's milk contains so much caseinogen because it is designed for calves, which have a growth rate four times that of human children. The function of caseinogen is mainly to assist in the production of the hormone thyroxine, used by the thyroid gland to control general metabolism, nervous system, glandular system, mental development, and growth rate.

Physical and mental imbalances may occur in some children and teenagers from excessive consumption of cow's milk, more than 1 liter (1 quart) per day for teenagers, or 500 ml (half a quart) for children ages 7–12. For most adults, cow's milk is not recommended as a regular food source. In addition, for babies and children, the thymus gland provides lymphocytes to protect against disease and infection. Up to the age of seven, the thymus gland continues to grow and protect the body, and by the time of puberty, it ceases to function. The thymus gland functions as a "junior" immune system and needs more than milk to maintain its functions.

Finally, it is the fat content of milk that promotes rapid growth in babies. Mother's milk contains 4.5 g of fat per 100 g, and whole cow's milk contains 3.3 g of fat, with both having a similar saturated fat and cholesterol value.

NOTE: DV refers to the daily value for women 25–50 years, refer to RDI tables on pages 95–96 for adult male and child values.

MILK – LACTOSE INTOLERANCE

Milk is a popular drink among the general public, possibly due to powerful marketing campaigns that claim benefits such as protection from osteoporosis; however, there are more factors than meet the eye when evaluating milk, especially for adults. One survey of Australian adults showed that water was the most popular drink, with 215 liters (l) consumed per year, followed by soft drinks (150 l), coffee (106 l), beer (94 l), milk (82 l), tea (28 l), juices (23 l), and wine and spirits (14 l). The *total* of all these drinks equals about two liters per person per day. Because 2.1 liters of *pure water* alone is required by the body for proper functioning (kidneys, evaporation, food oxidation, during sleep) in a cold climate, it is clear that insufficient water is obtained, on average, per day, per person.

The average milk consumption is about 220 ml (a little over one cup) per day, per adult, or the equivalent of the milk added to five cups of tea or coffee. This amount of milk is not considered excessive, but the kidneys may suffer from a poor supply of pure water, as tea, coffee, milk, soft drinks, beer, etc., require filtration by the kidneys.

POSSIBLE DETRIMENTAL FACTORS

1. overconsumption
2. lactose intolerance
3. teenage acne
4. homogenization/pasteurization
5. calcium content/iron content
6. respiratory disorders

Overconsumption of cow's milk may easily occur in teenagers and the elderly due to the advertising campaigns that promote milk. Teenagers may consume over a quart of milk per day, thinking it is necessary for their growth. Milk often takes the place of other important foods that are necessary for growth. Milk satisfies the appetite quickly and is available at every corner store. For the elderly, milk is promoted for prevention of osteoporosis and brittle bones, but other factors are important for strong bones: moderate regular sunlight (for vitamin D) and exercise, plus the minerals magnesium, phosphorus, and zinc, which are undersupplied by milk. Only humans drink milk after the infancy stage; animals survive on other foods.

Lactose intolerance is a very common problem with milk consumption. Lactose is the sugar portion of milk; it is a disaccharide, made of glucose and galactose. No other food contains lactose. It is the perfect food for infants: mother's milk contains approximately 75 g of lactose per liter; cow's milk supplies 45 g per liter.

The enzyme lactase in the small intestine is usually active in children up to the age of about five years; after that production of lactase progressively slows down. Without the enzyme lactase, milk is not digested properly, possibly leading to the development of lactose intolerance. One survey showed that 15% of white Americans and 70% of African Americans in the United States had lactose intolerance. Over 80% of all people from Japan, Taiwan, the Philippines, Thailand, and many Arab countries are lactose intolerant or lactase deficient. About 5% of people from Switzerland and Denmark have lactose intolerance.

Undigested lactose ferments in the colon by bacterial action, causing carbon dioxide gas and lactic acid, possibly resulting in flatulence, cramps, and diarrhea. Everybody has a different lactose tolerance. Decide for your own health whether it's worth all that gas to drink milk from a cow.

Teenage acne may result from excess milk protein (casein), which may overstimulate the thyroid gland, general metabolism, and secretion of hormones. Furthermore, milk may contain traces of hormones as residue from the cow's diet. The fat content of milk after pasteurization is not beneficial as it does not contain the essential fatty acids; plus, it contains saturated fats, which can enter the bloodstream before filtration by the lymphatic system. Another common problem comes from the hormone progesterone contained in the milk of pregnant cows. About 80% of all cow's milk is derived from pregnant cows. Progesterone is broken down into androgens, which promote premature sexual development and hormone production. Research has shown that teenage acne was reduced remarkably when milk drinking was stopped. The bacteria produced from milk digestion is also a problem. Avoid milk if you have a teenage skin problem. Instead, try a freshly made carrot juice every three days for the best skin-cleansing and anti-acne drink. Three cheers for the carrot!

NOTE: Nutrient amounts are listed as milligrams (mg) per 100 grams (g), unless otherwise stated.

MILK – PROCESSING

Homogenization is the process that unifies the milk and cream content; it saves you the effort of shaking the milk but places great effort on the body later. During homogenization, the fats in the cream and milk get pulverized and fragmented. These minute fats are able to "hide" from the lymphatic system, which is designed to initially process and filter all digested fats. The milk fats thus enter the bloodstream directly, where they may accumulate to cause problems with the heart and circulatory system. More fat enters the bloodstream from homogenized milk than from unprocessed cheese, cream, or butter.

Pasteurization is the process in which raw milk is heated to 62°C (144°F) for 30 minutes or 161°C (322°F) for 15 seconds. Pasteurization was implemented to protect the community against possibly harmful bacteria in batches of spoiled milk from the dairy farm. It is recognized that the pasteurization process does not eliminate all bacteria and microorganisms. In addition, pasteurization may alter the protein structure of milk, as heating ruptures and "tangles" the protein molecules, making them difficult to digest or break down. For better digestion, pasteurized milk can be reboiled quickly to help dismantle the "tangled" protein molecules. For many centuries, the practice of boiling raw milk quickly has resulted in a sterile product, and according to modern research, it does not destroy the nutritional value.

The calcium content of milk is possibly the main marketing factor, especially for the prevention of osteoporosis. Calcium is required to promote strong bones. Milk does supply calcium, but considering the fact that many people are lactose intolerant, it cannot be classified as the ideal calcium food. Foods such as natural cheese, yogurt, carob, tahini, tofu, almonds, green vegetables, and salmon are full of calcium (refer to the table on this page for a few examples).

Other factors associated with osteoporosis are just as vital to address as one's calcium intake: lack of sunlight, lack of weight-bearing activities, menopause and hormone action, lack of other minerals, and an unstable supply of calcium.

The efficiency of calcium absorption can vary considerably. Ideally, maintain a regular intake of calcium foods rather than ingesting large amounts in one day. The body adapts to a pattern of calcium absorption. Ideally, a good serving of yogurt an hour before bedtime provides maximum value; during sleep the body requires calcium for various processes, and when it is not available bone demineralization may occur. Vitamin D from sunlight promotes calcium absorption. Rest easy with a regular intake of yogurt: the calcium promotes a good night's sleep, and yogurt does not trigger the lactose problem.

The iron content of milk is really overestimated; it is best not to rely on milk for iron. The RDA for iron for children ages one to ten is 7–10 mg. To achieve that would require drinking approximately 20 cups of milk! Also, most other minerals, vitamin A, and the B vitamins are undersupplied in milk.

Milk provides a basic supply of a few nutrients but has a range of possible adverse factors. In some children, excess milk intake has lead to anemia and leukemia.

NUTRIENT COMPARISON CHART				
Per 100 g (3.5 oz)	Milk	Almonds	Kidney Beans	Pumpkin Seeds
Calcium (mg)	119	232	28	51
Iron (mg)	0.04	4.6	3	11.3
Potassium (mg)	151	768	358	801
Magnesium (mg)	13	270	45	531
Phosphorus (mg)	93	502	147	1166
Manganese (mg)	0.004	1.9	0.47	2.9
Zinc (mg)	0.38	2.9	1.1	7.4
Vitamin A (IU)	126	9.8	0	72

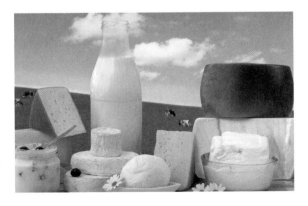

NOTE: *DV refers to the daily value for women 25–50 years, refer to RDI tables on pages 95–96 for adult male and child values.*

GOAT'S MILK/CHEESE

The benefits of goat's milk when compared to cow's milk are numerous. The composition of the fat globules in goat's milk is finer than in cow's milk, thereby allowing better digestion. Goat's milk is composed of more medium-chain triglycerides (MCTs), or fatty acids, than cow's milk. These MCTs are absorbed more easily into the digestive and lymphatic systems. In addition, the MCTs have lower cholesterol and provide a special form of energy that is easy to metabolize. Goat's milk supplies about 20% more calcium and phosphorus than cow's milk. One cup of goat's milk supplies approximately 33% of the daily calcium for adult females and 27% of phosphorus.

Goat's milk and cheese are used throughout the world. Goat's milk is often preferred to cow's milk as it is less allergenic. (Obviously, soy milk or rice milk is the best choice for those with high lactose intolerance or milk allergies.) The protein in goat's milk and cheese is easier to digest. It contains fewer beta-lactoglobulins than cow's milk; these are the most complex milk proteins to digest. The beta-lactoglobulins in goat's milk are digested more efficiently, leaving less protein residue in the digestive system after ingestion and thereby protecting against bacterial problems and mucus development that clogs the respiratory system.

Goat's milk does not need to be homogenized. Because the fat globules are smaller than in cow's milk, they remain evenly suspended in the milk. When considering whether to feed infants goat's milk, once breastfeeding has ceased, it is best to obtain advice. Due to the low folate content (0.40 mcg) compared to human milk (5.2 mcg) or cow's milk (4.9 mcg), it is best not to give infants only goat's milk. Add foods such as mashed broccoli (64 mcg of folate) and foods with vitamins C and E. Goat's milk provides 3.6 g of complete protein; human milk only supplies 1 g, and cow's milk supplies 3.2 g. The casein in goat's milk (alpha-s3 casein) is softer and more flexible than the alpha-s1 casein in cow's milk. Goat's milk contains only small amounts of alpha-s1, compared to cow's milk, making it easier to digest. Goat's milk is sweet and sometimes salty due to a very good source of organic sodium. Over half the milk consumed in the world is from the goat.

YOGURT

Yogurt has a health history dating back thousands of years, possibly to just after the domestication of farm animals. From the early 1900s to the present day, research into the nutritional qualities of yogurt has provided very encouraging results that are backed up by generations of people throughout the world, especially in Turkey, the Balkans region, Greece, Egypt, Arabia, Algeria, India, and China. Today, many people all over the planet obtain the benefits that only yogurt can provide. Yogurt can be prepared from cow's milk, goat's milk, buffalo milk, sheep's milk, and soy milk.

During the process of making yogurt, the raw milk is boiled to kill any "wild" bacteria that could interfere with the added culture. The culture used is a natural bacterium, the two most common of which are *Lactobacillus acidophilus* and *Lactobacillus bulgaricus*. Both are closely related; however, the acidophilus has proven to be more effective in maintaining a correct and prolonged supply of natural bacteria within the digestive system—for up to 48 hours.

The word "bacteria" may concern some people, so it must be pointed out that various types of bacteria are obtained from other food products: meat, cheese, milk, eggs, poultry, fish, and seafood, as well as processed and carry-out foods. The bacteria that is formed from those foods can produce harmful effects if allowed to accumulate in the lower digestive system.

Natural yogurt destroys harmful bacteria within the lower digestive system and colon and replaces it with "friendly bacteria" containing valuable antibiotic qualities, which provide a natural balance and cleansing for the lower digestive system. An estimated 450 different types of bacteria can live in the human digestive system. Ideally, you should choose yogurt made from nonpasteurized milk.

BENEFICIAL FACTORS OF YOGURT

1. acidophilus bacteria
2. easy digestion
3. high calcium content
4. B vitamins and other benefits
5. high protein value

NOTE: Nutrient amounts are listed as milligrams (mg) per 100 grams (g), unless otherwise stated.

The *Lactobacillus acidophilus* bacterium is considered the most powerful yogurt culture. Other strains of bacteria used in yogurt making, and often combined with acidophilus, are *Lactobacillus bifidus, Lactobacillus bulgaricus,* and *Lactobacillus thermophilus.* As a group they are termed probiotics. It is possibly better not to obtain a yogurt that has more than one culture as they may interfere with each other's function.

The term "dysbiosis" is used to describe the condition in which the balance of "bad" or pathogenic bacteria are prevalent in the intestines, as opposed to "friendly" bacteria. Such factors as antibiotics, analgesics, the contraceptive pill, and steroids can cause dysbiosis. In addition, a diet low in fresh fruits, vegetables, legumes, and fiber, and high in animal protein, animal fats, and processed foods promotes dysbiosis. Acidophilus yogurt taken regularly will balance the bacteria and avoid the problems associated with dysbiosis, such as flatulence, constipation, diarrhea, bloating, chronic fatigue, skin problems, and irritable bowel syndrome. Acidophilus bacteria also secrete antibacterial and antifungal substances termed "bacteriocins," which stop the growth of pathogens. Acidophilus is available in *tablet form* for anyone who is unable to digest yogurt. However, the calcium content is missing from tablets.

Yogurt is a *simple food to digest.* The common ingredient in all types of milk products is lactose, or milk sugar. Most adults are unable to digest lactose properly. Lactose is converted by the digestive system into the energy-providing sugar glucose via the enzyme lactase. As mentioned in the section on milk, there are two main considerations regarding lactose. First, most children have the digestive enzymes lactase and rennin, which are necessary to assist in the conversion of lactose. After the age of 7 to 14, these enzymes are no longer active in the human body. During the yogurt-making process, lactose is converted into simple sugars, glucose and galactose, by the bacterial action of fermentation. For adults, yogurt is the best way to obtain the benefits of dairy products.

The *calcium content* of yogurt is ideal and one of the best natural ways to obtain the daily calcium requirement. One cup (227 g) of plain, nonfat yogurt supplies 450 mg of calcium. That is nearly half the daily requirement for men and women ages 19 to 50. For the elderly, yogurt is an excellent food as it requires no chewing and is simple

to digest. Ideally, 1 cup of natural acidophilus low-fat yogurt midmorning or 1 cup before bedtime will ensure a very regular intake of calcium. That's exactly what the body needs—in combination with the vitamin D provided by moderate, regular sunlight—to protect against osteoporosis.

For growing children, yogurt is really an essential food, especially between ages nine and 18, as the digestive system needs help to process the milk and cheese in their diet; plus they no longer have the enzymes to assist in lactose conversion. They also need 1,300 mg of calcium a day. Meat supplies hardly any calcium, and it promotes toxins in the lower digestive system.

The *protein content* of whole-milk yogurt by weight is only 3.5%; the average woman would require approximately 1,600 g of yogurt to satisfy her protein RDA. Low-fat yogurt provides about 5.2 g of protein. The Net Protein Utilization (NPU) of yogurt is very good, the same as milk at 80%, so the protein value is used effectively. Yogurt contains high-quality protein, meaning it does not require other foods to increase the amino acid balance. Because yogurt is about 60% water content by weight, it may not appear to supply good protein, but a cup of yogurt a day supplies about one-fifth the protein requirement for women. Yogurt has so many other benefits; the protein is just a bonus.

CALCIUM CONTENT IN YOGURT AND DAIRY			RECOMMENDED DAILY CALCIUM INTAKE	
	Calcium in 1 cup	Calcium in 100 g	child 4—8	male 9—18
Plain low-fat yogurt	415 mg	182 mg	1,000 mg	1,300 mg
Plain nonfat yogurt	452 mg	198 mg	female 9—18	female 19—30
Fruit low-fat yogurt	314 mg	138 mg	1,300 mg	1,000 mg
Plain whole-milk yogurt	227 mg	100 mg	male 19—50	male 51—70
Whole milk (3.25% fat)	291 mg	119 mg	1,000 mg	1,000 mg
Low-fat milk (2% fat)	297 mg	121 mg	female 31—50	female 51—70
Low-fat milk (1% fat)	300 mg	123 mg	1,000 mg	1,200 mg

NOTE: DV refers to the daily value for women 25–50 years, refer to RDI tables on pages 95–96 for adult male and child values.

EGGS

Eggs are a symbol of life. The chicken comes before the egg alphabetically, but the egg is first in protein availability with the highest net protein utilization (NPU) of any food at 93%; chicken has an NPU of 65%. One large egg contains approximately 6 g of protein, 93% of which is usable by the body.

To obtain all your daily protein from eggs would be more than difficult; it would be harmful, mainly due to eggs' cholesterol content. The average adult requires 45–55 g of protein per day—which is supplid by about eight eggs. But hold on: Eight eggs also supply nearly 1,700 mg of cholesterol. The recommended daily maximum of cholesterol per adult is 300 mg. *One large egg contains approximately 200 mg of cholesterol,* or two-thirds the daily limit. People cannot live on eggs alone. Enjoy your free-range eggs, but carefully manage your intake.

CHOLESTEROL AND EGG FACTS

1. Only the egg yolk contains cholesterol.
2. Cholesterol is also made by the liver for the absorption of fats and the utilization of fat-soluble vitamins.
3. Obese people produce more cholesterol than average-weight people. Weight-loss diets can decrease the body's manufacture of cholesterol.
4. One survey showed that the average dietary intake of cholesterol was about 330 mg per day for men, 212 mg per day for women.
5. The liver can increase and decrease cholesterol manufacture according to dietary intake.

The choline (a B vitamin) content of eggs is abundant, with 215 mg per large egg. Choline contains a phospholipid known as lecithin that can lower blood cholesterol and remove cholesterol from tissues. A lack of choline can contribute to high blood-cholesterol levels. The high cholesterol content of eggs may be reduced by the rich choline content, but to be really sure add some *lecithin granules* as a supplement to your next dish of scrambled eggs, or add them to soup and be confident about your cholesterol.

The supply of other nutrients from eggs is fairly basic. The iron content is 2.8 mg per 100 g. For comparison purposes, kidney beans supply 3 mg, almonds 4.6 mg, beef 1.9 mg, pumpkin seeds 11.3 mg, and parsley 6 mg. The vitamin A content is fair at 520 IU per 100 g, but carrots supply 16,705 IU—no comparison there!

The vitamin D content is fairly good. For people stuck indoors in the hospital, or unable to tolerate any sunlight, or who live in a region with long dark winters, the egg may provide a small but valuable dose (but the best food source is fish oils). Dairy products also provide a fair source of vitamin D.

Eggs are not a calcium food, and neither is meat, so if your diet has few other foods, add some almonds or cheese. The biotin (a B vitamin) content of eggs is good, but raw egg white contains avidin, which can prevent biotin from reaching the blood. The raw egg white in eggnog, etc., also contains albumen protein, which can pass into the blood undigested, causing allergies.

The great benefit of eggs is their versatility in recipes: They are featured in omelets, cakes, pastries, and pasta, to name just a few. Eggs are best kept refrigerated to prevent bacterial growth. Proper cooking of eggs is essential to avoid bacteria and salmonella poisoning. Hard-boiled eggs are simple and free of added fats. Bring eggs to room temperature before boiling. Fried eggs are full of saturated fats and free radicals if butter is used; ideally, use cold-pressed olive oil or canola oil, or poach eggs, scramble them, or mix them into an omelet with leafy green vegetables. Children enjoy dipping toast into soft-boiled eggs, a meal that provides them with high-density protein.

Nutrient Content (1 large egg)	Whole Egg	Egg Yolk	Egg White
Protein (grams)	6.25	2.78	3.47
Calories (kcal)	75	59	17
Total lipids (g)	5.12	5.11	0.01
Saturated fat (g)	1.55	1.55	0
Polyunsaturated fat (g)	0.68	0.68	0
Monounsaturated (g)	1.91	1.91	0
Cholesterol (mg)	213	213	0
Calcium (mg)	25	23	2
Iron (mg)	0.9	0.9	0
Vitamin D (IU)	24.5	24.5	0
Biotin (mcg)	9.98	7.58	2.34
Choline (mg)	215	214	1
Vitamin A (IU)	317	317	0

NOTE: Nutrient amounts are listed as milligrams (mg) per 100 grams (g), unless otherwise stated.

POULTRY

The term "poultry" includes chicken, as well as duck, goose, turkey, pheasant, and quail. Poultry varies in its supply of nutrients, as can be seen from the chart below. In regards to protein, chicken and turkey are on par at about 21 g per 100 g with an NPU of 65%. Three hundred grams (10.5 oz) of chicken will supply all the daily protein for an adult male, but no fiber and no carbohydrate. Without the addition of fiber-rich foods, chicken is "lost" in the digestive system, which may lead to toxins in the colon. Chicken is classed as a nutrient-dense food, implying that it supplies protein, iron, and zinc, but the iron content is fairly low at 0.7 mg per 100 g, and the zinc content is 0.8 mg—neither are big in value, but the protein makes up the balance, enabling it to be classed as a nutrient-dense food.

Poultry are very low in calcium at 11 mg, a content even lower than that of eggs (25 mg) or beef (25 mg). With many people relying on these three foods for a majority of their daily protein and food supply, a calcium deficiency is likely to develop, especially considering that the average RDA for adults is about 1,000 mg. Regular intakes of natural yogurt, cheese, tahini, and almonds are required to balance the calcium deficiency. In addition, acidophilus yogurt will help reduce harmful bacteria in the lower digestive system (colon) that often result from diets high in chicken and meat. Ideally, obtain free-range chicken, and serve it roasted, alongside generous amounts of fiber-rich vegetables or a large serving of coleslaw.

With regard to total fat content, chicken (containing about 9 g) is similar to lean beef (9.6 g)—depending on the part of the chicken used and whether the skin is consumed. With regard to saturated fat, lean beef (4.2 g) has more than chicken (2.6 g). Duck is very rich in saturated fats, with 23 g. All poultry contain similar amounts of cholesterol. Chicken supplies 63 mg and beef 78 mg—again, depending on the cut of meat. Unless cholesterol-containing fats are added during cooking, the cholesterol levels are fairly safe in one serving of either per day. Fried chicken is more of a concern than roasted chicken due to the excess fats, free radicals, and cholesterol absorbed into the outer layer, especially if the cooking oil is used several times. A home-roasted chicken is the safest way to ensure quality control of the oils. Most fast-food outlets have chicken as their number-one seller, and undoubtedly it is one of the most overconsumed carry-out foods. Limit your craving for chicken by indulging in other meals—such as bean tacos, fish, nuts, and baked vegetables—before the hunger rush starts!

The topic of free-range poultry has been discussed for years, but mass-produced eggs and poultry still find their way onto dinner plates. The nutritional value of eggs is said to be the same between factory and farm eggs. The color of the yolk is determined by the feed type: Wheat-based feed produces a pale yellow yolk, corn-based produces a golden yolk. Mass-produced hens are given a well-controlled diet of mainly soy and corn, plus added antioxidants, mold inhibitors, and scraps from beef or chicken production. Hormones are not used, generally speaking, but antibiotics are required to protect against disease outbreaks—some flocks number over one million. The cage system is preferred for sanitation, the air is force ventilated, there's no sunlight, and automatic feeders activated by a time clock move food mash into troughs. Hens produce eggs for about 19 months and then molt (shed feathers) and rest for about six weeks; then they produce again for about eight weeks until molting. That is usually the end of their life. A free-range bird gets sunlight, fresh green feed and insects, and can exercise and relax when the sun goes down. The price is often more for free-range poultry and eggs, especially in the city, but the cost is worth its weight if the hens are given a decent outdoor life and not treated like machines.

Poultry per 100 g serving (3.5 oz)	Chicken	Duck	Goose	Turkey
Protein (g)	20.8	11.4	16	21
Calories (kcal)	172	403	370	158
Total lipids (g)	9.2	48	33	7.3
Carbohydrate	0	0	0	0
Fiber	0	0	0	0
Saturated fat (g)	2.6	23	8	2
Polyunsaturated (g)	1.9	5	3.8	1.6
Monounsaturated (g)	3.8	19	18	2.7
Cholesterol (mg)	63	75	80	65
Calcium (mg)	11	10	12	13
Iron (mg)	0.7	2.4	2.5	1.2
Sodium (mg)	62	1.3	73	58

NOTE: *DV refers to the daily value for women 25–50 years, refer to RDI tables on pages 95–96 for adult male and child values.*

FISH

Humans have eaten fish for thousands of years. In the early days primitive hooks and nets were used to catch fish, a tradition that continues in some parts of the world today.

Freshly caught, fire-roasted fish is well worth the effort of a few hours' fishing. *Fresh fish,* kept on ice, is fish that has been caught less than one day ago. Ask any fisherman about the taste of fresh fish compared to canned, deep-fried, or previously frozen fish, and enjoy fresh fish yourself at least once a week.

POSSIBLE BENEFICIAL FACTORS

Fish is an excellent source of *complete protein;* on average the protein content is 24% by weight. The NPU of fish is 80%, whereas beef contains only about 67% usable protein. Therefore, fish is considered a higher-quality protein than meat and most other foods.

The table below lists the individual amino acid values for a variety of fish. Refer to the table on page 92 to see how these amounts compare to the amino acid content of other foods. Most commonly eaten fish supply similar protein. Sardines have a lower NPU of 69%. Tuna is the best supplier of protein with an NPU of 80% and 28% complete protein. Refer to the table on page 89 for information about the NPU of various foods.

Refer to the tables on pages 93 and 94 to see the daily amino acid requirements for individuals of various body weights. You can see that a 100 g (3.5 oz) serving of tuna (and most other fish) easily provides the daily requirements of all of the essential amino acids except phenylalanine.

Note that children *need more protein per pound of body weight than adults.* For some amino acids, children weighing over 75 lbs (35 kg) have a requirement more than twice that of adults. Fish is the *ideal food* at least twice a week *for growing children;* it provides *compact protein while satisfying their hearty appetites.* A 140 g (5 oz) serving of fish (or 120 g of tuna) will supply the total daily protein for a child of 35 kg. For beef, it would take about 180 g (6.5 oz).

Adults, male and female, require approximately 180 g (6.5 oz) of fish (or 140 g of tuna) to supply their *total daily protein requirements.* For beef, it would take about 220 g (7.75 oz). It is recommended that adults consume fish twice a week. And whenever the *choice between meat or fish* is available, catch the fish for its protein and other benefits.

For *absolutely amazing protein,* try fish coated with a mixture of wheat germ, two ground Brazil nuts, and a beaten egg. Fish is the complete protein dish.

FISH—PROTEIN (AMINO ACID) COMPARISON CHART (CONTENT PER 100 G PORTION)										
	NPU	**HIS**	**ISL**	**LEU**	**LYS**	**MET**	**PHA**	**THR**	**TRY**	**VAL**
Bass	80%	523	818	1451	1628	526	658	778	199	916
Cod	80%	525	823	1451	1640	528	697	783	199	919
Mackerel	80%	549	859	1510	1711	552	728	817	208	960
Perch	80%	549	860	1522	1711	552	729	818	210	962
Salmon	80%	585	916	1616	1829	588	777	873	223	1025
Sardines	69%	730	1142	2016	2276	735	970	1087	277	1276
Tuna	80%	880	1481	2198	2556	842	1074	1249	290	1554

NOTE: Nutrient amounts are listed as milligrams (mg) per 100 grams (g), unless otherwise stated.

FISH – OMEGA-3 FATTY ACIDS

Fish—especially tuna, salmon, mackerel, lake trout, mullet, sardines, herring, and anchovies—is a good provider of the essential fatty acid *omega-3*, as can be seen in the table below. Omega-3 is valuable for control of cholesterol and for the brain, nervous system, skin, eyes, and growth (refer to page 167). The saturated fat content of fish on average is low compared to other animal-protein foods.

Fish supplies approximately 50–70 mg of cholesterol per 100 g serving, but the content of omega-3 and the tracec mineral vanadium will help utilize the cholesterol. Use a cold-pressed olive or canola oil to bake the fish, or, ideally, steam fish with rice and a sprinkle of cold-pressed olive oil, and serve with green beans, potatoes, and carrots for a complete "catch" of benefits.

You can also see from the chart below that meat does not supply omega-3 fatty acids. Meat does, however, supply omega-6 fatty acids (not shown on the chart). Both omega-3 and omega-6 are essential in the diet. Fish does not supply omega-6, but it is available from all nuts and seeds, dairy foods, margarine, and all oils.

There are two types of fish: oily fish and low-fat fish. Mackerel, mullet, and sardines are the "oiliest" fish, with salmon, trout, and tuna also supplying a fair amount. It is these fats that supply all the omega-3. And don't be concerned about total fat content. When compared to meat, fish is always lower in fat, especially saturated fat. For a complete low-fat, high-protein meal, baked perch, snapper, or cod is an excellent choice. The low-fat fish contain only about 10% fat—compare this to meat. Over the course of a year, by replacing two meat meals per week with baked fish you can obtain 90% less fat and over 120% less saturated fat. That can potentially produce a big savings in body weight, cholesterol, and saturated fat. Fish will reduce your weight on the scales!

Long before nutrition became a common term, fish oils from cod and halibut liver provided a unique food source of vitamin D, especially for people in Arctic and low-sunlight areas. Vitamin D is easily obtained via sunlight, but if it happens to be dark for many months, or you have to live indoors or work indoors during daylight hours, or if you work in a mine, get your supply of vitamins D and A from fish oil supplements. Also, if you are in the hospital for months, or playing computer games all day instead of out on the playground, your supply of vita-min D will be inadequate, especially for growing children and people with bone problems.

Fish, especially tuna, is a good source of the trace mineral selenium. Fish supplies all the main minerals in fair amounts, plus vitamins A, E, and most of the B complex, including B12. Ocean fish also supply iodine. Fish is often termed a "brain food"; the minerals magnesium, phosphorus, iodine, zinc, manganese, and the trace mineral vanadium are all brain nutrients available from fish. These nutrients combined with the high protein content really does make fish a brain food. Fish and seafood are the best reliable source of vanadium. Vanadium is required for cholesterol control and prevention of cholesterol formation within arteries. Fish, on average, supplies similar cholesterol compared to meat; however, nearly all "land foods" are deficient in vanadium. Fish also supply the omega-3s to protect against cholesterol accumulation.

Hook into the great benefits of fish!

FISH AND SEAFOOD—PROTEIN/FAT CONTENT

Fish and Other Animal Products (100 g cooked)	Total Protein (g)	Total Fat (g)	Sat. Fat (mg)	Omega-3 (mg)	Cholesterol (mg)
Bass	13	1.6	0.5	0.74	80
Cod	18	0.67	0.67	0.23	44
Crab	18	2	0.08	0.12	41
Crayfish/lobster	18	2	0.17	0.15	96
Mackerel	19	13.8	3.2	3.3	71
Oysters	6	2.5	0.62	0.94	54
Perch	19	1.6	0.24	0.42	42
Prawns/shrimps	20	2	0.32	0.65	153
Salmon	20	6.3	0.98	2.5	55
Sardines	25	11.4	1.5	1.4	142
Scallops	17	0.75	0.07	0.25	30
Shark	21	4.5	0.92	1.1	50
Snapper	20	1.3	0.28	0.46	36
Trout	21	6.5	1.1	1.5	58
Tuna	24	4.9	1.2	1.4	38
Frankfurter	11	29	12	0	50
Lamb chops	15	17	8	0	58
Round steak	19	17	7	0	66
T-bone steak	17	25	11	0	71
Veal breast	14	14	6	0	56

NOTE: DV refers to the daily value for women 25–50 years, refer to RDI tables on pages 95–96 for adult male and child values.

SEAFOOD/SHELLFISH/CRUSTACEANS

The term "seafood" includes an incredible range of products affording a wide variety of benefits. Clams, eel (technically a fish), mussels, octopus, oysters, scallops, snails, and squid are the main seafoods. Crustaceans include crabs, crayfish, lobster, and shrimp or prawns. Kelp (seaweed) and spirulina (a type of blue-green algae) can be considered seafood, even though they're algae rather than animal products.

Clams are an excellent source of the mineral iron with 13.8 mg per 100 g (meat supplies only 1.9 mg, pumpkin seeds supply 11.3 mg). Clams also provide the other essential blood-building minerals, manganese and copper. If you feel weary and get sick often, iron may be lacking in your diet. Clams are low in fat and have only 73 calories per 100 g.

Crab meat is a good source of the mineral zinc, with 6.4 mg per 100 g, and is low in fat. Compared to other crustaceans, the cholesterol content is low. The protein content of 18% is complete with all essential amino acids. Crab meat is also low in calories (83 per 100 g) and has no carbohydrate, so it is advised to enjoy your crab feast with plenty of salad and rice. Crayfish and lobster are full of selenium for antioxidant benefits and to promote vitamin E effectiveness. But cholesterol is abundant in these crustaceans; so even if you can afford to eat them in terms of economics, can you afford the added cholesterol problems?

Eel has a similar fat content to mackerel and sardines with 12% fat, over 60% in the form of monounsaturated fats. The cholesterol content is fairly high, but fortunately the monunsaturated fats reduce blood cholesterol. In some countries the eel is a delicacy, but some people find them too fatty. I've heard it said about a person that they were "as slippery as a bag of eels!"

Kelp is generally obtained from the botanical species *Macrocystis pyrifera* or *Fucus vesiculosus*. It is considered the "first crop" in ancient Roman, Greek, and Chinese history. Kelp is the richest source of natural iodine; for people living inland or whose ancestors lived by the sea and are now inland, iodine deficiencies are likely unless regular seafood is obtained. Kelp is known to contain nearly all the trace minerals, as well as the main ones, and many vitamins. A kelp shaker is the best way to obtain the trace nutrients regularly, or try kelp crackers to balance your body. That is actually the most formidable function of kelp: It restores a natural balance to the glands and entire body. Don't be weary, give kelp the chance to help! The ocean is full of minerals washed from the earth which form sediment on the ocean floor, where kelp grows. Kelp is food for the future; it may become the "new penicillin"!

Oysters are the richest food source of zinc. If you need to boost your reproductive life, zinc is essential; plus, it promotes healing of numerous disorders. The RDA of zinc is 8–11 mg; one medium oyster supplies approximately 13 mg. Zinc promotes the functions of the immune system, but excess amounts depress the immune system. One dozen oysters is definitely excessive at 156 mg of zinc. Instead, split half a dozen (for 39 mg of zinc per person) with your sweetie, and share the fun and benefits once a fortnight—or every anniversary!

Prawns (shrimp) are an overconsumed seafood. They may get thrown on every barbecue, but they are also the seafood richest in cholesterol. They are a good source of protein, but the risk of high blood cholesterol needs to be noted, especially if you eat a few sausages on the same day, or eggs, ham, or especially kidneys or liver.

Scallops are a safe seafood in regard to nutrients and cholesterol but, as with all seafood, the risk of toxins from polluted water can be a concern. The same applies to land products, of course: Chemicals grouped as dioxins are more prevalent in meat (81 picograms/gram), dairy (24 pg/g), and fish (7.8 pg/g). Dioxins accumulate in fat tissues of animals (including humans), posing a cancer hazard and reproductive problems. Keep our oceans clean!

Spirulina is a supplement. It is full of organic iron and may boost the blood and immune system. Take it in moderation under supervision from a naturopath.

SEAFOOD—NUTRIENT COMPARISON CHART									
100 g serving	Protein %	Fat %	Choles-terol	Iron (mg)	Sele-nium (mcg)	Zinc (mg)	Vit. A (IU)	Vit. B12 (mcg)	Vit. E (IU)
Clams	13	0.97	71	13.8	24	1.3	300	49	1.5
Crab	18	0.60	41	0.59	36	6.4	23	11	—
Eel	18	12	126	0.50	6.5	1.6	3485	3	6
Kelp	17	0.56	0	2.8	0.7	1.2	120	0	—
Lobster	19	0.89	95	0.63	41	3	70	0.92	2.1
Oysters	7	2.5	54	6.6	52	90	332	19	1.2
Prawns	20	1.7	153	2.4	37	1.1	10	1.2	1.1
Scallops	17	0.7	33	0.3	22	0.95	51	1.5	1.5
Snails	23	0.4	65	5	—	1.6	84	9	—
Spirulina	57	7.7	0	29	7.3	2	570	0	7.5
Almonds	18	54	0	4.7	7.8	2.9	10	0	39
Cheese	25	33	107	0.67	14	3.1	1071	0.83	0.53

NOTE: Nutrient amounts are listed as milligrams (mg) per 100 grams (g), unless otherwise stated.

MEAT

Possibly the greatest nutritional debate centers on the question of meat. No other natural food causes such heated controversy. The general public is often pushed into meat consumption because it is always on the menu or carry-out display.

The overconsumption of meat can cause problems. This section on meat first lists the problems associated with a regular meat diet and then outlines the possible benefits of meat consumption.

POSSIBLE DETRIMENTAL FACTORS

1. excess consumption of meat
2. excess saturated fat intake
3. low carbohydrate content
4. excess cholesterol intake
5. uric acid, nitrates, adrenaline
6. antibiotics, hormones, drugs
7. low calcium content
9. excess body acids
10. obesity
11. processed meats
12. bacteria, long digestion time
13. free radicals
14. lacking omega-3
15. low in numerous nutrients
16. other factors

POSSIBLE BENEFICIAL FACTORS

1. moderate protein content
2. supply of vitamin B12
3. long lasting, "full stomach" feeling

As is true of nearly all foods, consuming meat in excess is not beneficial. The serving of meat often takes up 70% of the dinner plate, and the small quantity of "side dishes" barely provides sufficient nutrition for a proper balanced diet. The balanced diet requires a calorie distribution of 50% carbohydrate, 35% protein, and 15% lipids. On average, meat (steak) supplies a ratio of 0% carbohydrates, 28% protein, and 72% lipids. Unless the diet supplies a balance of carbohydrate foods without added fats, the typical meat meal, when consumed on a regular basis, can become a big problem!

The fat from two lamb chops or two sausages or two slices of bacon easily exceeds the daily lipid limit. The average beef steak supplies 45 g saturated fat, 1 g polyunsaturated fat, and 9 g monounsaturated fat. The essential fatty acid omega-3 is not supplied by meat. Saturated fats can be used for energy, but carbohydrate foods are the best energy foods as they require less digestive effort and, generally speaking, they supply the associated nutrients to support energy production. Excess saturated fat intake can lead to heart disease. You risk an excess consumption of saturated fats if you eat more than one meat meal per day, or over 100 g of cheese, or one meal of bacon and eggs.

Saturated fats do provide a "full stomach" feeling for many hours, which can be considered both a bonus and a detriment. Once meat is consumed, the digestive system attempts to process the protein content of meat within the stomach. Saturated fats slow down the protein conversion and can cause problems later in the small intestine and colon. Saturated fats are not processed in the stomach; they are converted into fatty acids and glycerol in the upper part of the small intestine (duodenum). This delay factor can make it seem like you've had a satisfying meal, but it overworks the digestive system. Saturated fats increase blood cholesterol levels—and this is in addition to the dietary cholesterol supplied by meat.

As mentioned previously, meat supplies hardly any carbohydrate content—or, more to the point, no roughage or fiber content. Both of these factors can become a problem for the regular meat eater, especially if the diet also includes refined foods—white bread, chips, etc.—as there will be insufficient natural movement in the lower digestive system. This can lead to constipation and, over the long term, possibly to colon cancer, which may develop due to the bacteria caused by the buildup of toxins within the large intestine. Nearly all animal-protein foods are very low in fiber and carbohydrate.

It is essential to regularly obtain such foods as pears, apples, rice bran, figs, coconut, legumes, bananas, and other fruits and vegetables in order to protect against the meat getting "stuck in a rut"!

NOTE: DV refers to the daily value for women 25–50 years, refer to RDI tables on pages 95–96 for adult male and child values.

MEAT — CHOLESTEROL/SATURATED FATS

Meat supplies both dietary cholesterol (beef: 81 mg) and saturated fat. The risk of an excess blood cholesterol level (BCL) is common for people who consume meat-based meals plus other cholesterol-rich foods every day and who have other risk factors. Foods that are vital for lowering blood cholesterol are those that are rich in omega-3 fatty acids: for example, walnuts, hazelnuts, pecans, cold-pressed flaxseed oil, and oily fish. Apart from lowering the BCL, the omega-3s can also lower blood triglycerides, or blood fat levels. Omega-6 fatty acids also help to lower blood cholesterol. Both omega-3 and omega-6 are poly-unsaturated fatty acids. Monounsaturated lipids also lower blood cholesterol, and in addition they moderately reduce the bad low density lipoproteins (LDL) and maintain the good high density lipoproteins (HDL). Olive oil is a rich source of monounsaturated lipids and is recommended for its ability to reduce "bad" cholesterol. Other risk factors that increase BCL for regular meat eaters are smoking, obesity, lack of exercise, refined foods, takeout foods, chocolate, milk, cream, cheese, eggs, and especially prawns, crabs, crayfish, brains, kidney, liver, and sausages. Adding fats during cooking can easily top the scales.

The maximum recommended daily cholesterol intake for an adult is 300 mg. One meal of two sausages and one egg will easily exceed this. Many common meat-based meals exceed not just the maximum daily cholesterol but also the maximum saturated fat. To be sure your cholesterol is not increasing, get a medical checkup, especially if you have a regular meat diet and other associated risk factors.

Cholesterol is produced by the liver at about 1,000 mg per day. It is required for hormone production, cell structure, vitamin D synthesis, and the metabolism of fats. Excess cholesterol intake from foods can lead to the narrowing of arteries, which directly affects blood flow and blood pressure because the cholesterol particles, especially the LDL, can attach to the arterial walls.

In addition, refined carbohydrates—those contained in white bread, sugar, etc.—increase both LDL and total blood cholesterol levels. Finally, research has shown that dietary cholesterol inhibits the anticancer action of the large white blood cells.

RECOMMENDED LIPIDS INTAKE PER DAY

	Minimum	Maximum
Child (5–12)	30 g	60 g
Teenager	40 g	80 g
Man, sedentary	30 g	40 g
Man, physically active	40 g	80 g
Woman, sedentary	30 g	40 g
Woman, physically active	40 g	60 g
Athlete, very physically active	80 g	120 g

MEAT—CHOLESTEROL/FAT CONTENT

100 g Cooked	Total Fat (g)	Sat. Fat (g)	Cholesterol (mg)
Beef steak, lean	22	9	81
Chicken, lean	5	4.5	90
Crab	2	0.5	70
Crayfish/lobster	2	0.5	150
Ham	10	4	100
Kidney	3	1.5	550
Lamb chop	14	7	75
Liver	12	5.5	400
Oysters	2.5	1.5	53
Pork	27	11	100
Prawns	2	1	110
Rabbit	4	2	65
Salami	38	13	99
Sausages (2 med.)	20	10	200
Veal roast	1	0.5	100
Milk chocolate	30	19	100
Eggs (2 average)	12	4	420
Pâté	30	13	150

BLOOD CHOLESTEROL LEVELS
Measured in Milligrams per Deciliter (mg/dl)

Very high	240 and above
Borderline high	200–239
Desirable	Below 200

NOTE: Nutrient amounts are listed as milligrams (mg) per 100 grams (g), unless otherwise stated.

MEAT — SUBSTANCES/LOW CALCIUM

Uric acid, a compound formed from the breakdown of purine, is a problem because it builds up in the bloodstream, forming sharp crystals. No foods contain uric acid itself, but foods high in purine, such as animal foods, break down to yield higher levels of uric acid in the body. White blood cells attempt to rid the blood of the uric acid; however, they are unable to digest the uric acid crystals and unfortunately are destroyed in the process. The resulting dead white cells release a corrosive digestive liquid which is known to attack the delicate lining of joints, possibly one major cause of arthritis and certainly of gout. Uric acid also causes kidney stones. Coffee, chocolate, and tea also contain high levels of purine.

Some meats such as sausages, frankfurters, and some processed lunch meats contain nitrites, which can be linked to cancer-causing nitrosamines in the stomach.

Adrenaline is produced in animals and humans during conditions of fear, excitement, and other states of heightened awareness. At the abattoir animals are penned in for a few days, without food, until finally they are lined up for slaughter. During this latter stage the animals sense fear. Adrenaline is pushed through their system into the blood and tissues. Adrenaline can be transferred to humans from the eating of meat and it can cause overstimulation of the thyroid gland and the general metabolism. In some cases it can promote aggressive tendencies. For thousands of years in India warriors were allowed meat; the rest of society was forbidden meat. The elephant is generally a placid plant-eating animal; however, the tiger is a pure carnivore and becomes aggressive quickly. It is the adrenaline that triggers the action.

CALCIUM COMPARISON (per 100 g)	
Beef steak	25 mg
Almonds	235 mg
Cheddar cheese	734 mg
Tahini	422 mg
Adult RDA	1,000–1,200 mg

Antibiotics, hormones, and other drugs are often contained in meat and meat products. The use of antibiotics in humans is already at peak levels. As any farmer will tell you, antibiotics, hormones, and drugs are used to maintain the health of the herd and to promote growth, and these may transfer to the person who eats the meat. Even though DDT has been banned for over 40 years, animals can still show trace amounts, which transfer to the human via meat. Other chemicals that are used in meat production include tranquilizers, toxaphene, chlordane, stilbestrol, methoxychlor, dieldrin, lindane, and aureomycin. Be scrupulous about purchasing only organic meat, to avoid these added chemicals. Research also shows that fresh fruits and vegetables can help to remove some toxic chemicals from the body.

The low calcium content of meat is a concern as calcium is the body's main mineral. Conditions such as osteoporosis, brittle bones, and low-density bones are certainly not helped by eating meat. For women after menopause, bone loss increases and calcium-rich foods are essential. Excess meat reduces the appetite for other foods and possibly increases bone leaching due to its low calcium supply. Muscle cramps and high blood pressure may also result from a calcium deficiency. Meat makes weak bones, so balance your diet with calcium-rich foods!

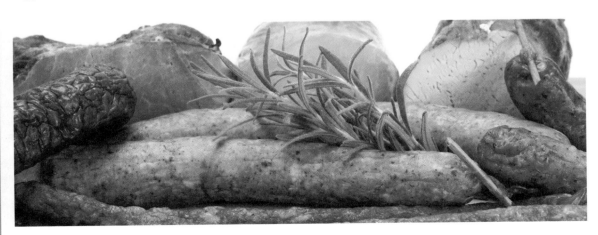

NOTE: DV refers to the daily value for women 25–50 years, refer to RDI tables on pages 95–96 for adult male and child values.

MEAT — OBESITY/BACTERIA/FREE RADICALS

The ideal balanced diet requires 75% raw foods and 25% cooked foods. Nearly all cooked foods are acid forming. Meat is one of the most acid-forming foods. When the blood is in an acid state it can lower the immune system's ability to protect and heal the body. Excess acidic foods cause the body to produce more mucus in an attempt to protect against the acids. Alkalinity in the blood is vital for the process of reproduction. For maximum healing, the blood needs an alkaline balance. Minerals are the main provider of both acid and alkaline elements. The pituitary gland controls the body's acid–alkaline balance. Nearly all fruits and vegetables, almonds, and rice are alkaline foods. Most other foods, especially crustaceans, meat, poultry, fish, and eggs, are acid forming. A constant acid diet can cause a person to experience considerable discomfort. Conditions such as headaches, sluggish liver, poor circulation, and constipation can all be attributed to excess body acids. Coffee, alcohol, soft drinks, and tannin tea are also acid forming. The best advice for the regular meat eater is to ensure that adequate servings of fruit and vegetables are obtained regularly and to choose legume meals whenever possible.

Obesity is a "growing" problem in some countries, and there are a few connections between eating meat and obesity. Calories do add up in the diet, and with meat, over 50% of the calories are from fats (lean ham 75% fat, sirloin steak 76%, and trimmed sirloin steak 35% fat). Most of the fat is saturated and often extra fats or oils are added to the meat when cooking; these are 100% lipid content. Overeating is a major cause of obesity, and with meat it is common to see large portions on the plate that are eaten completely and followed by extra servings later. To encourage the appetite and make the meal full of flavor, some people often add rich sauces, because the saturated fats satisfy the appetite. Over the years, a person can consume more as their stomach and intestines stretch, and if there is no reason to stop eating, obesity increases. Obesity is often related to a slow metabolism and the excess intake of processed and convenience foods, soft drinks, alcohol, chocolate, and those "traditional" family meals.

The digestion time for meat is longer than for any other food group, especially if fats are added. Meat requires five to six hours of digestion in the stomach, poultry four to six hours, cheese three to four hours. The problem really occurs later, in the small intestine, and particularly in the large intestine, the colon. The adult human digestive system is approximately 30 feet long; most carnivorous animals' digestive system is only six feet long. Because meat putrefies easily in a warm environment, the digestive system of humans is an ideal breeding ground for bacteria as it can take 18 hours or more for the meat chyme to pass out of the body. Meat provides no fiber, and unless the diet includes fiber-rich foods the meat can hang around the colon for days. This is a major cause of colon cancer in that it allows for the absorption of numerous toxins, leading the way to poor health due to the strain on the immune system.

Free radicals are abundant in cooked, fried, and roasted meat. The barbecue is the greatest provider of free radicals, so make sure you also eat salads with flax or olive oil to protect against the damage. Free radicals are now recognized as cancer-causing elements within cooked fats and oils.

Omega-3 is an essential fatty acid that is required from the diet. Meat supplies omega-6 (another essential fatty acid) and large quantities of saturated fats, but few omega-3s. Refer to the table on page 134.

When meat is cooked all heat-sensitive nutrients are depleted. Meat is not a nutritious food, due to its low mineral and vitamin content (refer to the chart below), plus the numerous detrimental factors mentioned above.

NUTRIENT COMPARISON				
per 100 g	Beef	Almonds	Kidney Beans	Pumpkin Seeds
Calcium (mg)	5	232	28	51
Iron (mg)	1.9	4.6	3	11.3
Potassium (mg)	318	768	358	801
Magnesium (mg)	20	270	45	531
Phosphorus (mg)	188	502	147	1166
Manganese (mg)	0.013	1.9	0.47	2.9
Zinc (mg)	3	2.9	1.1	7.4
Vitamin A (IU)	0	1.0	0	380

NOTE: *Nutrient amounts are listed as milligrams (mg) per 100 grams (g), unless otherwise stated.*

MEAT — PROTEIN EVALUATION AND SUMMARY

Meat protein is often considered to be the only source of the essential amino acids, or what is commonly termed "complete protein."

This is certainly not true. In addition to seafood, poultry, and dairy foods, numerous other food groups such as nuts, seeds, grains, and legumes also provide the eight essential amino acids or complete protein. Refer to pages 89 and 92 for tables verifying that complete protein is available from numerous natural foods.

On pages 93–94 another table provides a guide to the average amino acid supply of the main food groups, plus the amount of each amino acid required per day for different body weights. It is obvious from these charts that meat/beef is not the best protein food. On page 88 the question "what are the best protein foods?" is answered in a complete evaluation of all protein factors.

Apart from the *numerous* possible detrimental factors detailed in the previous pages on meat, the protein from meat is complete, and it provides a fair supply of the essential amino acids. The protein value of meat, however, can be considerably less than the "ideal lean beef" value given on the charts.

Excess cooking of meat is common, which reduces the protein (amino acid) value and increases the risk factors. Furthermore, many of the nutrients are leached out during cooking, via the juices. Any added fats greatly decrease the protein value of meat by retarding and reducing proper protein digestion in the stomach, resulting in poorly prepared proteoses and peptides. Animal protein foods, especially meat, require considerable digestive energy to convert the food into usable protein. Primary proteins—nuts, seeds, grains, and legumes—require half the digestive time and energy of meat. Primary proteins do not have a list of possible detrimental factors.

Vitamin B12 is often a bone of contention when the requirement for meat is discussed. Meat is not the only source of vitamin B12 (see page 171).

The countryside is *cleared* for meat production and in some places has become desolate due to overgrazing. Consequently, the major problem of soil salination occurs with a huge expense (in the form of reforestation) required to rectify the problem.

Meat takes the place of numerous other meals as people become less able to cook. The typical meal of meat and three veggies *every night* is overkill! It takes just as much time to prepare any of the hundreds of meatless meals. The habit of eating meat can be so compelling that people say they can't live without it. That is because it has been the major food in their diet for years and without meat their plate would be empty.

There are over 100 complete-protein meals that don't include meat, and many of them have supported civilizations for centuries. See if you can get a piece of the action from a properly prepared meatless meal and take a stab at discovering new recipes. Don't let the habit of daily meat eating take over your health, food budget, and life.

THE BEST PROTEIN FOODS			
Natural Protein Foods	Protein % of Food (by weight)	NPU Net Protein Utilization	Usable Protein per 100 g
1 Tuna	28%	80%	22
2 Soybeans	34%	61%	21
3 Cheese	26%	70%	18
4 Fish	22%	80%	17
5 Eggs	12%	94%	17
6 Wheat germ	25%	67%	17
7 Pumpkin seeds	29%	60%	17
8 Beef	24%	67%	16
9 Chicken	21%	65%	13
10 Sunflower seeds	23%	58%	13
11 Peanuts	26%	43%	11
12 Cashews	18%	58%	10
13 Sesame/tahini	19%	55%	10
14 Oats	14%	66%	9
15 Almonds	18%	50%	9
16 Brazil nuts	14%	50%	9
17 Walnuts	14%	50%	7
18 Chickpeas	20%	43%	7
19 Rice	7%	70%	5
20 Milk/yogurt	3%	80%	3

NOTE: DV refers to the daily value for women 25–50 years, refer to RDI tables on pages 95–96 for adult male and child values.

WHAT ARE LIPIDS?

"Lipids" is the term used to describe fats and oils.

WHAT ARE THE SIX PRIMARY TYPES OF FOODS THAT SUPPLY LIPIDS?

1. nuts, 2. seeds, 3. fish, 4. seafood, 5. meat, 6. dairy products

WHAT OTHER TYPES OF FOODS SUPPLY LIPIDS?

1. cooking oils from seeds, grains, legumes, and vegetables; 2. avocadoes, olives; 3. margarine;
4. fried foods; 5. convenience or takeout foods; 6. snack foods

ARE ALL LIPIDS BENEFICIAL?

No. Lipids that are heated or chemically altered are not beneficial.

WHAT EFFECT DOES COOKING HAVE ON LIPIDS?

Lipids that are heated undergo a chemical change in their molecular structure. Oxygen, which is naturally attached to the lipid structure, becomes *oxidated* during frying, cooking, or intense heat. These "oxidated molecules" are released from the lipid structure and become free radicals. These *free compounds,* in search of more oxygen and nourishment, attach to other nutrients within the blood, such as vitamins, causing them to become oxidized and to deteriorate. This process damages skin cells and other bodily cells. Refer to page 137 for more details on the problems with cooked oils.

HOW CAN YOU PROTECT AGAINST FREE RADICALS?

The simple answer is to restrict the intake of deep-fried foods and cooked oils and to use methods of cooking such as steaming, boiling, and shredding to prepare most meals. Other methods such as baking and roasting can reduce the need for added lipids. Ideally, the balanced diet contains 75% raw foods and 25% cooked foods.

Vegetables can be either steamed or baked without added fats, and once the meal is served add fresh, cold-pressed oils—olive, flaxseed, canola, sunflower, or walnut oil—or tahini or butter to provide the flavor-enhancing benefit without the free radical problem.

Chicken is an overconsumed food, and even though it is a low-fat food when roasted, deep-fried chicken contains lots of harmful fats within the crumb coating. Eggs can be boiled or poached.

NOTE: Nutrient amounts are listed as milligrams (mg) per 100 grams (g), unless otherwise stated.

Barbecuing is another common cooking method; barbecued sausages, when overconsumed, are especially a concern with their enormous supply of saturated fats and free radicals.

By choosing foods and preparing meals carefully, it is possible to avoid over 90% of common cooked lipids. Increasing one's intake of vitamin E foods like tahini, almonds, hazelnuts, or wheat germ oil, and selenium-rich foods like Brazil nuts can also provide protection from free radicals, as they promote cell life and protect against rapid oxidation. The ideal diet must also include foods that provide the essential fatty acids, which are vital for numerous body functions.

WHAT ARE THE ESSENTIAL FATTY ACIDS?

There are two essential lipids, meaning they must be obtained from the diet as they cannot be produced by the body and are required for numerous vital body functions: alpha linolenic acid, also referred to as omega-3 fatty acid; and linoleic acid, also referred to as omega-6 fatty acid. Omega-3 and omega-6 are collectively termed the "essential fatty acids" (sometimes referred to as vitamin F). These essential fatty acids belong to the group of *polyunsaturated lipids* (see below).

The word "omega" is the last letter in the Greek alphabet and it means "last of series" or "final development," but for those seeking the ultimate lipids, let the omegas be first!

WHAT ARE THE THREE MAIN GROUPS OF LIPIDS?

Monounsaturated lipids have one space in the chain of carbon atoms; this allows for two carbon atoms to share two bonds with each other.

Polyunsaturated lipids have four or more "free carbon atoms" forming two or more double bonds, which gives them the ability to transport many nutrients.

Saturated lipids have all their carbon atoms attached to hydrogen atoms; they are usually solid at room temperature and come mainly from animal fats.

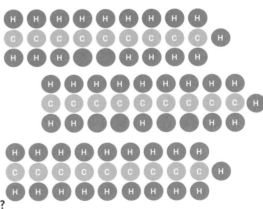

WHAT ARE THE MAIN FUNCTIONS OF THE THREE GROUPS OF LIPIDS?

Monounsaturated lipids, such as those contained in olive oil, hazelnuts, almonds, and macadamia nuts, are used by the body for energy and for the breakdown of cholesterol; they are also stored as body fat in the adipose tissues. Monounsaturated oils are the best to use in cooking, if you have to fry, but ideally they are consumed in the natural state, as a cold-pressed oil.

Polyunsaturated lipids, especially omega-3 and omega-6, are the great carriers of nutrients such as vitamins A, D, E, and K. They also transport and break down cholesterol, manufacture other fatty acids, regulate the transfer of oxygen, and aid in the protection of the nervous system and the cellular system and cell structure. They are vital for the blood-clotting process, they participate in the manufacture of hormones, regulate healing, and are required for development of the fetus and for mental

NOTE: DV refers to the daily value for women 25–50 years, refer to RDI tables on pages 95–96 for adult male and child values.

development, especially in infants. Polyunsaturated lipids oxidize quickly and are best consumed as cold-pressed oils with a fresh garden salad. Canola oil and walnut oil are rich sources of both omega-3 and 6. Flaxseed oil is the richest source of omega-3. When used for cooking, especially frying, oils oxidize into peroxides or free radicals. They cause damage to the arteries and skin cells and may eventually cause cancer. If you have to fry a food to enjoy a meal, restrict the quantity and make sure the oil you're using is fresh, not rancid. Don't toil over spoiled oil!

Saturated lipids are not essential for health or life. Most natural foods provide a portion of saturated fats in addition to mono- and polyunsaturated fats (see the table on page 135). Saturated fats are used mainly for energy. Animal foods are the primary source of saturated fats in the average diet. Saturated fats provide a "full stomach feeling" and easily satisfy the appetite for lengthy periods. These two benefits are often the reason for their common consumption; however, numerous problems are associated with a regular consumption of saturated fats from animal products (see pages 114–130). Saturated fats are the hardest to digest and are the most likely to be stored as body fat.

WHAT FOODS ARE THE BEST SOURCES OF OMEGA-3 AND OMEGA-6?

Omega-3 is the "hard to get" essential fatty acid. Flaxseed oil, nuts, seeds, and oily fish are the best sources of omega-3. Meat supplies only a trace of omega-3. Foods such as margarine and most cooking oils are rich sources of omega-6. The ideal dietary ratio of the essential fatty acids is three omega-6 to one omega-3. The average diet consists of 20 omega-6 to one omega-3. Due to this common imbalance, it is generally recommended to increase the intake of omega-3 foods.

WHAT ARE THE MAIN FUNCTIONS OF OMEGA-3?

The main function of the essential omega-3 is in the production of prostaglandins, compounds that regulate blood pressure, kidney function, blood clotting, inflammatory responses, and nerve transmission. They are also required for the production of hormones, cell maintenance, supple skin, and various digestive functions.

In addition, a regular balanced intake of omega-3 fatty acids may help prevent depression, obesity, asthma, diabetes, high blood pressure, cancer, attention deficit syndrome, rheumatoid arthritis, and heart disease. Omega-3 foods reduce the appetite by stabilizing blood sugar levels, and help to increase metabolism and thereby promote activity and weight loss. Omega-3 is vital during the early stages of a baby's development, especially for the brain. Numerous mental disorders can be traced to a prolonged omega-3 deficiency. See page 167 for more detail on the vital functions of omega-3.

Approximately 2–4 g of omega-3 per day is the recommended minimum. An excess of omega-6 foods and products, such as margarine, can reduce the activity of omega-3 and its numerous essential functions.

WHAT ARE THE MAIN FUNCTIONS OF OMEGA-6?

The main function of omega-6 is the transportation of nutrients, oxygen, and energy throughout the body. Omega-6 is also required for blood clotting, regulating healing, and the manufacture of hormones.

NOTE: Nutrient amounts are listed as milligrams (mg) per 100 grams (g), unless otherwise stated.

HOW DID OMEGA-6 AND OMEGA-3 GET THEIR NAMES?

As mentioned, both omega-6 and omega-3 belong to the group of polyunsaturated lipids. Omega-6 has three double bonds within the chain of carbon atoms, the first of which is located at the number-six carbon atom, hence the name omega-6. Omega-3 has two double bonds, the first of which is positioned at the number-three carbon atom. (Refer to page 133 for the polyunsaturated carbon chain diagram.)

WHAT FOODS PROVIDE MONOUNSATURATED AND SATURATED LIPIDS?

As can be seen from the table on page 135, the main foods containing monounsaturated lipids are almonds, cashews, hazelnuts, macadamia nuts, pecans, pistachios, and olive oil. Seventy-six percent of the lipids in olive oil are monounsaturated. See page 142 for details on the benefits of olive oil.

The main foods containing polyunsaturated lipids are walnuts, soybeans, and fish, with the oils—corn, safflower, and sunflower—all providing over 50% polyunsaturated lipid content.

The main sources of saturated fat are *coconut, butter, cheese, cream, chocolate, ice cream, milk, yogurt, beef, and lamb.*

Note that the figures in the chart add up to less than 100% as some of the values for the minor fatty acids in each group are not available.

In addition to the foods in the chart, there are numerous other foods that supply both unsaturated and saturated lipids.

IS MARGARINE A BENEFICIAL FOOD?

Margarine is often classed as polyunsaturated; however, most of the lipid content (45%) is in the form of monounsaturated fat. Margarine is processed via hydrogenation, which converts vegetable oils into a semi-saturated state. In addition, margarine usually contains additives such as coloring, food acid, antioxidants, preservatives, emulsifiers, added vitamins, and salt.

The oils used for margarine originate from a heat and chemical process. These oils are then hydrogenized, a process that mixes hydrogen into the oils, causing saturation of the fatty acids. This converts them into "trans fatty acids," which increase blood cholesterol levels, deplete skin cell life, and tax the immune system. So the question is: what do I spread on my bread, sandwich, or roll? Ideally, cold-pressed olive, flaxseed, or canola oil should be sprinkled on bread, or use avocado or tahini, all of which promote health. Trans fatty acids need to be avoided. They promote heart disease and hardened

OMEGA-3 & -6 CONTENT OF FOODS
(measured in g per 100 g)

Natural Foods/Oils	Omega-3	Omega-6
Almonds	trace	10
Brazil nuts	trace	23
Cashews	trace	8
Pine nuts	1	25
Walnuts	5.5	28
Linseed/flaxseed	20	6
Pumpkin seeds	9	20
Sunflower seeds	trace	30
Sesame seeds (tahini)	trace	25
Canola oil	7	20
Soy oil	7	51
Chicken	0.1	1
Fish (average)	2	0.1
Meat	trace	6

OMEGA-3 IN FISH AND SEAFOOD
(measured in g per 100 g)

Bass	0.74
Cod	0.23
Mackerel	3.3
Perch	0.42
Salmon	2.5
Sardines	1.4
Shark	1.1
Snapper	0.46
Trout	1.5
Tuna	1.4
Crab	0.12
Crayfish	0.15
Prawns/shrimps	0.45
Scallops	0.25

NOTE: DV refers to the daily value for women 25–50 years, refer to RDI tables on pages 95–96 for adult male and child values.

FOOD LIPID BALANCE CHART (%)			
	Mono.	Poly.	Sat.
Almonds	68	19	8
Brazil nuts	33	37	25
Cashews	58	16	20
Hazelnuts	77	10	7
Macadamia nuts	76	3	14
Pecans	60	25	8
Pistachios	68	13	14
Walnuts	18	68	8
Avocado	43	12	18
Chickpeas	42	42	trace
Peanuts	47	29	30
Millet	33	33	33
Margarine	45	32	19
Poultry	45	20	30
Olive oil	76	7	11
Sesame seeds	38	42	14
Soybeans	23	51	17
Wheat germ	27	46	18
Coconut	6	2	88
Butter	34	2	57
Eggs	40	12	30
Cheese	28	4	64
Cream	29	4	62
Chocolate	38	2	57
Ice cream	29	4	63
Milk	29	4	63
Yogurt	27	3	65
Fish (average)	20	50	25
Beef	35	2	60
Lamb	36	3	54
Veal	40	2	40
Pork	40	2	40
Corn oil	28	53	10
Safflower oil	15	72	8
Sunflower oil	19	63	13

arteries and may upset hormone function and the delicate balance in the glandular system.

Another problem with margarine is that an excess intake of omega-6, contained in high levels in margarine and in processed foods, upsets the important functions of omega-3. Keep a lid on things and balance your omegas. Choose margarine made from canola oil, mix in a tablespoon of flaxseed oil, and remember that margarine was invented for convenience, not for health.

WHAT IS CHOLESTEROL AND WHAT DOES IT DO?

Cholesterol is described as a waxy, fat-like substance. As an essential component of cell membranes, it is part of every living cell in the human body. It is required for functions such as the manufacture of hormones like estrogen, cortisone, and testosterone.

Cholesterol is produced by the liver—about 1,000 mg per day. The bodies of animals also produce cholesterol, which is present in their cells, too. When humans consume animal foods such as meat, chicken, seafood, and dairy, they obtain dietary cholesterol. Such foods as organ meats and crustacea are especially rich in dietary cholesterol.

Many people experience a great increase in blood cholesterol levels not only from an excess intake of animal foods, but also from processed foods and other foods with a high glycemic index, such as soft drinks, French fries, rice cakes, baked potatoes, white bread, and refined carbohydrates. The conversion of such foods into energy results in carbon fragments, which the body uses to make cholesterol. Saturated fats also supply carbon fragments after digestion and conversion into fatty acids, thereby promoting an increase in blood cholesterol.

Cholesterol is vital for cell construction, but excess cholesterol is lethal and can cause obstruction.

HOW DO I REDUCE BLOOD CHOLESTEROL NATURALLY?

To reduce blood cholesterol naturally, it is advised that you:
1. Restrict the intake of foods that are high in cholesterol.
2. Restrict the intake of foods rich in saturated fats (butter, cheese, chocolate, meat, sausages, etc.).

NOTE: Nutrient amounts are listed as milligrams (mg) per 100 grams (g), unless otherwise stated.

3. Reduce the intake of foods that have a moderately high glycemic index, high glycemic index, or very high glycemic index.

4. Ensure that the diet includes legume meals regularly—e.g., kidney bean tacos, hummus, lentil soup.

5. Obtain a regular intake of rolled oats or barley.

6. Obtain foods rich in natural lecithin such as sweet corn and soy in the form of soy grits.

7. Consider taking a natural lecithin supplement, available at health stores; it is a concentrated source and may be helpful for promoting a reduction in blood cholesterol.

8. Limit total cholesterol intake to less than 300 mg per day.

9. Limit intake of pastries, cakes, and cookies.

10. O0p8.5040p8.504btain regular moderate exercise.

NOTE: The ideal blood cholesterol level is less than 200 mg/dL (milligrams per deciliter). Borderline high cholesterol is 200–239. High cholesterol is 240 or above.

CHOLESTEROL LEVELS (measured in mg per 100 g)	
Beef steak	70 mg
Brains	1800 mg
Butter	250 mg
Cheddar cheese	100 mg
Chocolate	100 mg
Cream cheese	120 mg
Swiss cheese	85 mg
Chicken (cooked, lean)	100 mg
Egg (whole, raw)	550 mg
Egg yolk	1500 mg
Fish (average)	50 mg
Hamburger meat	80 mg
Kidney	550 mg
Lamb chops	70 mg
Lard	95 mg
Liver	400 mg
Lobster	150 mg
Milk (cow, full fat)	11 mg
Oysters	250 mg
Pâté (average)	150 mg
Prawns	110 mg
Salmon (canned)	50 mg
Sardines	140 mg
Sausage (cooked)	200 mg
Tuna	40 mg
Turkey (no skin)	60 mg
Veal chops	90 mg

IS LECITHIN REALLY THAT IMPORTANT?

Lecithin is a part of every living cell in the body, especially those in the brain and liver. Lecithin is also part of the glandular system and is required in the tissues and muscles of the heart and kidneys.

Lecithin is made from a mixture of substances that are collectively known as phospholipids. They consist of the essential fatty acids, phosphorus, and the B-complex vitamins choline and inositol. Research has shown that mentally impaired people often have a brain lecithin content as low as 19%. For mentally stable people, the brain lecithin content is 28%.

Lecithin, in combination with the B-complex vitamins and magnesium, is vital for mental health. It is termed "nature's tranquilizer." During times of stress, the body uses lecithin rapidly. If it is not replaced through diet, fatigue, irritation, and mental confusion may develop. The majority of processed, refined, and convenience foods have no lecithin content, are loaded with cholesterol or trans fatty acids, and often have a high glycemic index. Protect your body, nervous system, and brain with a little lecithin. Lecithin granules are available at most supermarkets and health stores. They can be added to soups, gravy, bread, muffins, omelets, or scrambled eggs. Try a "pinch" every few days. Your brain will regain, your blood cholesterol will naturally level, your nerves will not be disturbed, and your health will be better than wealth.

Some margarines have added lecithin—that's one positive thing—but they still contain those nasty trans fatty acids.

NOTE: DV refers to the daily value for women 25–50 years, refer to RDI tables on pages 95–96 for adult male and child values.

IS BUTTER BETTER THAN MARGARINE?

Butter is a natural food, and as such it contains no trans fatty acids. Margarine does contain trans fatty acids. Once heated, however, butter is no better than margarine because the fats are converted into free radicals.

BUTTER/MARGARINE/SPREADS (all measured in 1 teaspoon or 5 g portions)			
Food Type	Cholesterol (mg)	Total Fat (g)	Saturated Fat (g)
Butter	10	4	2.5
Margarine	0	4	1
Margarine, reduced fat	0	3	0.5
Margarine with olive oil	0	3	0.5
Avocado	0	0.7	0
Tahini	0	3	0.2
Hummus	0	0.8	0
Cream cheese	6	1.6	0.9
Olive oil	0	5	0.5

Butter is made from cream and milk, a rich source of saturated fats, which the body can use only in moderation. If your diet is well balanced, with ample fruits and vegetables, legumes, and oats, the addition of a small amount of butter to bread or toast, corn on the cob, rice, or potatoes will be of no concern. Choose unsalted butter to avoid adding to your sodium intake. If your diet is rich in animal products, especially bacon, sausages, meat, and cheese, the extra butter will add up quickly to a cholesterol and weight concern.

If you want a "better butter," add cold-pressed oil to soft butter. Using the food processor, mix approximately one-fourth cup cold-pressed canola oil with three-fourths cup softened unsalted butter. Add 1 teaspoon of wheat germ oil, 2 teaspoons flaxseed oil, 1 teaspoon of lecithin granules, and a dash of kelp salt. More healthful ingredients and more flavor!

WHY ARE COOKED OILS HARMFUL?

Eating cooked oils is possibly the most common health risk, especially for people who regularly consume takeout foods, deep-fried foods, and chips cooked in oils. Nearly half the fat that people eat is termed "hidden fat"; you can be sure it's there because the food is so tasty.

Any oil or fat that has been heated will go through a process wherein the oxygen attached to the lipid structure becomes "oxidized," so it tries to attach to other compounds, such as nutrients, within the bloodstream. As mentioned earlier, these oxidized particles are termed "free radicals," and as the name implies they are free to roam around causing trouble. They destroy skin cells, and the result is premature aging. They destroy cellular structures, resulting in damage to the internal linings of arteries. They break down DNA, resulting in possible birth defects. They attack the immune system when it's compromised, so they are truly nasty. Why do we enjoy them? Because they taste good for a few seconds and provide long-lasting satiety.

Instead, learn to enjoy the abundance of flavor from pure, cold-pressed oils: canola, flaxseed, sunflower, soy, safflower, olive, and walnut oil. In addition, fresh nuts are really underestimated as a delicious source of healthy fats and are often rejected due to their cost. As they say, you get what you pay for.

Rescue yourself from the menace of "radicals" in your diet!

NOTE: Nutrient amounts are listed as milligrams (mg) per 100 grams (g), unless otherwise stated.

DO LIPIDS REALLY ADD CALORIES AND INCREASE BODY WEIGHT?

Lipids supply nine calories per gram; carbohydrates and proteins each supply only four calories per gram. The balanced diet requires a caloric ratio of about 45–65% carbohydrates, 10–35% proteins, and 20–35% lipids.

If the carbohydrate intake comes mostly from refined foods, that can lead to an increased need for insulin, and excess insulin causes an increased storage of body fats.

Protein foods on their own are less likely to increase body weight, unless they are consumed with added fats and oils. Excess protein can be stored as fat or used for energy, but it is not a clean-burning energy fuel, as it produces harmful ammonia during conversion into energy.

The 20–35% daily intake of lipids includes added fats and oils from cooking, fats added to processed foods, and the actual fat content of the foods consumed. It is very easy to obtain excess fats and associated calories from the diet, especially if the diet does not follow the recommended formula of 75% fresh foods and 25% cooked foods. Furthermore, added fats make a meal or snack food more tasty, which can easily result in overconsumption. Also, cooked foods lack numerous nutrients that control fat metabolism.

Don't let cooked foods take over your diet, keep in ship shape naturally! Regular exercise is also key to natural weight control.

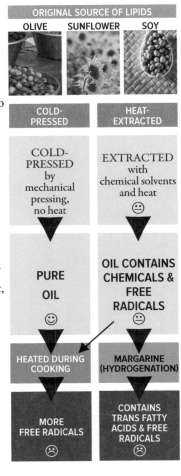

ORIGINAL SOURCE OF LIPIDS
OLIVE · SUNFLOWER · SOY

COLD-PRESSED | **HEAT-EXTRACTED**

COLD-PRESSED by mechanical pressing, no heat | EXTRACTED with chemical solvents and heat ☺

PURE OIL ☺ | OIL CONTAINS CHEMICALS & FREE RADICALS ☺

HEATED DURING COOKING | MARGARINE (HYDROGENATION)

MORE FREE RADICALS ☹ | CONTAINS TRANS FATTY ACIDS & FREE RADICALS ☹

NOTE: DV refers to the daily value for women 25–50 years, refer to RDI tables on pages 95–96 for adult male and child values.

Oils can be extracted by various methods. The best method for human consumption is when the oil has been "cold-drawn" or "cold-pressed." The cold-pressed method, usually achieved with hydraulic equipment, does not change the chemical structure of the lipid, thereby preserving the correct balance for human digestion, absorption, and metabolism. Cold-pressed or "virgin" oil is obtained with one pressing.

The majority of oils that are available from the supermarket are extracted with chemical solvents and heat processes, as this is the most economical way to produce oils. In addition, further processing and bleaching techniques are used to make the oil clean-tasting, odorless, and light-colored.

All those extra processing techniques are designed to get every drop of oil from the original source; however, the amount of chemical residue that remains in the oils is something to be avoided. The only way to be sure of obtaining top-quality oil is to see the phrase "cold-pressed" on the label.

Heat and chemical processes destroy an oil's vital vitamin E content. One of the most noticeable effects from regular use of chemically extracted oils is poor skin condition, due to a deficiency of vitamin E in particular. Very few processed foods and natural foods supply a good amount of vitamin E. A deficiency of vitamin E may be a major factor contributing to skin cancer, as vitamin E protects against ultraviolet radiation. Whole-grain bread is meant to supply a daily serving of vitamin E; white bread supplies no vitamin E. Almonds are rich in vitamin E. It is important to know that the more polyunsaturated oils and margarine one consumes, the greater the need for vitamin E in order to prevent cellular deterioration and arterial damage.

Another vital factor is the supply of the essential fatty acids, in particular omega-3. Very few oils and foods supply the hard-to-get omega-3.

Canola oil and walnut oil are well balanced with both the essential fatty acids. Flaxseed oil is exceptionally rich in omega-3, with nearly four times the omega-3 content compared to omega-6. Add flaxseed oil to other oils or margarine.

Margarine and most seed oils supply abundant omega-6, but most oils supply either no omega-3 or only a trace of omega-3. Refer to pages 134–135 for details on the unique functions of omega-3 and the problems with margarine and excess omega-6 intake.

The following pages provide details about several types of cold-pressed oils. Due to the ability of oils to enhance a food's flavor, most processed foods, takeout foods, and restaurant meals include considerable amounts of added fats and oils, but it is hard to know what types of oil they use. Ideally, when at home, make up for the restaurant meals by adding cold-pressed oils to salads, especially well-balanced oils such as flaxseed, canola, and walnut oil.

NOTE: The following chemical additives and preservatives may be found in oils that have not been extracted with the cold-pressed method: propyl gallate, methyl silicone, BHT, BHA, polyglycerides, polysorbate 80, oxystearin. A common solvent used to extract some oils is hexane, a derivative of crude petroleum oil refinement.

AVOCADO OIL

Avocado oil is second best to olive oil for the rich supply of monounsaturated fats, with 70% of all lipids in the form of oleic acid. The benefits of using avocado oil on a fresh salad or as a replacement for butter or margarine are well worth discovering. Oleic acid is known to reduce low density lipoproteins and also to protect against the accumulation of arterial plaque, thereby reducing high blood pressure. The avocado fruit supplies 77% lipid content, and with 70% in the form of oleic acid, avocado butter is without doubt a great way to obtain a nourishing spread that can be consumed regularly as it contains no cholesterol; plus, it has the potential to reduce blood cholesterol levels. Avocado oil supplies a trace amount of omega-3 (0.1 g) and a fair supply of omega-6 (1.9 g). The avocado fruit is an excellent source of glutathione, a potent antioxidant with the power to inhibit numerous carcinogens. The consumption of deep-fried foods and cooked oils is the main source of dietary carcinogens. Foods such as potato chips, French fries, and barbecued meats are full of cooked oils; they contain the free radicals that lead to cell destruction and the onset of cancerous tissues. The avocado and avocado oil are ready for the rescue. Mix two teaspoons of flaxseed oil and 1 teaspoon of wheat germ oil to a cup of avocado oil. The power of vitamin E and omega-3 will provide the force to knock out those dangerous radicals.

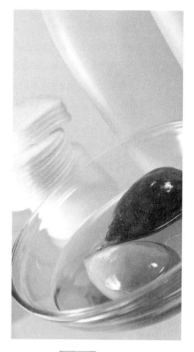

VITAMIN E: **CALORIES** – total: 884 kcal per 100 grams
39.2 mg   Saturated: 8.2 g Poly: 17.4 g Mono: 69.9 g

ALMOND OIL

Almond oil has been used for thousands of years as a facial cosmetic. Roman women cherished its rejuvenating benefits, and today you can, too, with little expense. A small bottle of pure almond oil will go a long way to providing essential nourishment for the skin. A rich supply of vitamin E (39 mg) is the main factor. Almond oil comprises 87% unsaturated lipids, mainly in the form of monounsaturated (70%), of which nearly 60% is in the form of oleic acid. The oleic acid content of almond oil is completely digestible and has the ability to improve the transfer and absorption of the fat-soluble vitamins: A, D, E, and K. Almond oil is a good source of omega-6 (10 g) but it supplies only a trace of omega-3. When added to a salad dressing, the rich oleic acid content in almond oil will enhance the effectiveness of vitamin E and promote skin cells' life, as vitamin E protects against oxidation. Excess use of margarine is a major cause of poor skin condition as it increases the rate of vitamin E oxidation. Almond oil is ready to liven your life internally and externally with beautiful benefits.

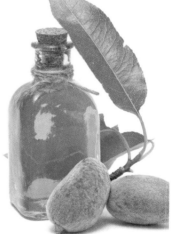

VITAMIN E: **CALORIES** – total: 884 kcal per 100 grams
8.7 mg   Saturated: 7 g Poly: 31 g Mono: 62 g

APRICOT KERNEL OIL

Apricot kernel oil is a rare beauty, a rich source of oleic acid (62%) and a fair source of vitamin E, both of which contribute to healthy skin when used externally. Apricot oil provides an excellent supply of phytosterols (580 mg; for more on phytosterols, refer to corn oil on the next page). Apricot oil is ideal for sensitive skin, prematurely aging skin, and baby's skin. It provides a softening effect and easily penetrates the skin; it is odorless and does not feel oily. Apricot kernel oil can also be added to a fruit salad. Appreciate the benefits of apricot kernel oil.

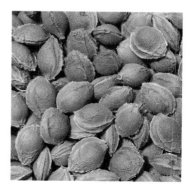

NOTE: DV amounts listed refer to the daily value for women 25–50 years; refer to DRI tables on pages 95–96 for adult male and child values.

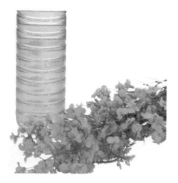

VITAMIN E:	CALORIES – total: 884 kcal per 100 grams
17 mg	Saturated: 7 g Poly: 31 g Mono: 62 g

CANOLA OIL

Canola oil has become a common cooking oil, but cooked oils are of no health benefit. Canola oil is a good source of both omega-3 (7 g) and omega-6 (20 g), and a good source of vitamin E. The balance between omega-3 and omega-6 is in the ideal proportion (one omega-3 to three omega-6). Canola oil is nearly 70% monounsaturated. Canola oil also provides a good supply of vitamin K (122 mcg). Canola oil is a great choice for daily use and for a balanced supply of the essential fatty acids. Cold-pressed canola is the best.

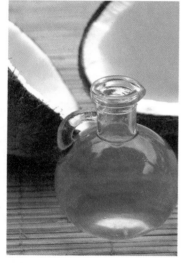

VITAMIN E:	CALORIES – total: 862 kcal per 100 grams
0.1 mg	Saturated: 86.5 g Poly: 1.8 g Mono: 5.8 g

COCONUT OIL

Coconut oil is 86% saturated fat, the richest source from any food, and its minute supply of polyunsaturates means it provides none of the essential fatty acids omega-3 or omega-6. The small amount of monounsaturates (6 g) may just be sufficient to help offset the increase in blood cholesterol from the saturated fat content of the coconut. Fortunately, neither the coconut nor its oil contains any dietary cholesterol, so it seems that on its own the oil is safe, but preferably used externally only. Numerous suntan lotions contain coconut oil; it is a rich oil and can provide a unique "beachy" glow and scent when applied liberally. In these days of increasing ultraviolet radiation, the use of coconut oil has decreased due to the risk of skin cancer from excess sunlight. Coconut oil is extracted from the white fleshy part of the nut; termed "copra," it is also used for desiccated coconut, as livestock feed, and as a fertilizer. Nearly all calories from the coconut are derived directly from its concentrated saturated lipid content.

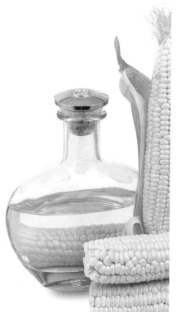

VITAMIN E:	CALORIES – total: 884 kcal per 100 grams
14.3 mg	Saturated: 12.7 g Poly: 58.7 g Mono: 24.2 g

CORN OIL

Corn oil has been used in Peru for thousands of years. It is easily extracted from the corn kernels and is a good general-purpose cooking oil. Corn oil is a good source of vitamin E and provides a small amount of vitamin K (1.9 mcg). It is a rich source of omega-6 (50 mg) but it does not supply omega-3. A combination of half corn oil with half flaxseed oil provides a balance of the essential fatty acids, as flaxseed oil provides 15 g omega-6 and 58 g omega-3. The corn–flax oil combo would be as good as oil gets if both are cold-pressed.

Corn oil is exceptionally rich in phytosterols (968 mg), containing more than wheat germ oil (553 mg) and olive oil (221 mg). Most other oils supply either no phytosterols or only a small amount. Phytosterols are recognized to block cholesterol from entering the bloodstream, and they have been shown in clinical research to reduce symptoms of an enlarged prostate, reduce inflammation in cases of rheumatoid arthritis, and help control blood sugar levels in diabetics. Ideally, make a salad dressing from cold-pressed corn oil, add a dash each of vinegar and flaxseed oil, and reap the benefits, including the good supply of vitamin E and omega-6. Corn oil on its own is too rich in omega-6. An excess of omega-6 can interfere with the functions of omega-3, as they both compete for enzymes to manufacture other essential fatty acids. Corn oil is ready to combine for numerous benefits; cob onto them!

NOTE: Nutrient amounts are listed as milligrams (mg) per 100 grams (g), unless otherwise stated.

VITAMIN E: 17.5 mg	CALORIES – total: 884 kcal per 100 gram Saturated: 10 g Poly: 68 g Mono: 22 g

LINSEED/FLAXSEED OIL

Linseed oil is obtained from the *Linaceae* family, or the common flax plant. The early Romans and Greeks used linseed oil as a food, and it is common in some European countries. Edible linseed/flaxseed oil is available; it is deodorized and refined and can also be used externally as a poultice for boils. It makes an excellent addition to other common oils, especially to increase their omega-3 content.

Linseed oil is the richest source of the vital omega-3s (58 g) and a good source of omega-6 (15 g). No other oil or natural food, apart from fish, has such an abundance of omega-3 compared to omega-6. An increased use of polyunsaturated margarine in the average diet has led to an excessive intake of omega-6; furthermore, the trans fatty acids can lead to increased cholesterol, damage to cell membranes, and compromised hormone production.

The excellent supply of omega-3 in linseed oil is vital for the nervous system, brain function, fetal development, and for protection from depression, autism, and learning difficulties. Adding just a drop of edible linseed oil to margarine can make a bright difference, or add it to salad dressing. Add some ground flaxseeds to bread or breakfast cereals. Flaxseeds are full of O-3s!

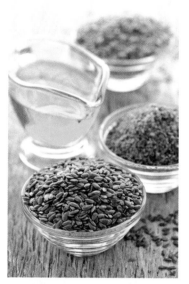

VITAMIN E: 1 mg	CALORIES – total: 718 kcal per 100 grams Saturated: 12 g Poly: 2 g Mono: 59 g

MACADAMIA OIL

Macadamia oil is obtained from the nut tree native to the north coast region of New South Wales, Australia, where the trees flourish amidst the rolling hills. Macadamia oil is nearly 60% monounsaturated, which is helpful for lowering cholesterol and reducing low-density lipoproteins. Macadamia oil is mainly oleic acid with a nearly unique source of palmitoleic acid. It is low in the essential fatty acids omega-3 and 6. Macadamia oil makes a marvelous addition to a salad dressing with a taste that's hard to crack!

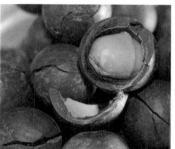

VITAMIN E: 1 mg	CALORIES – total: 884 kcal per 100 grams Saturated: 13.5 g Poly: 10 g Mono: 73.9 g

OLIVE OIL

Olive oil has become a popular addition to the Western diet; after thousands of years, the nutritional benefits of olive oil are being researched and acclaimed the world over. The exceptionally rich monounsaturated content (74%) is ideal for lowering blood cholesterol levels and especially for protection from the low-density lipoproteins, as olive oil is less likely to oxidize and form into arterial plaque. The substance oleuropein in olives inhibits the sticking of monocyte cells to the arterial walls.

When olive oil replaces saturated animal fats in the diet, a great improvement in arterial health and cholesterol levels occurs. The polyunsaturated content of olive oil supplies a small amount of both omega-3 (0.7 g) and omega-6 (8 g), plus a good supply of vitamin E (14 mg) and vitamin K (60 mcg). Olive oil can be used as a replacement for butter; in Italy, bread is dipped into olive oil and served with lunch salads and pasta. The oleic acid content of olive oil is helpful for reducing inflammation in cases of rheumatoid arthritis and may also help in cases of asthma. Olive oil has proved beneficial in reducing the risk of colon cancer and also for reduction of high triglyceride levels in some diabetics. Virgin olive oil mixed with walnut oil in salad dressings is wonderful.

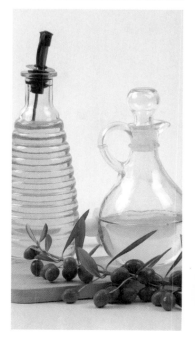

NOTE: DV amounts listed refer to the daily value for women 25–50 years; refer to DRI tables on pages 95–96 for adult male and child values

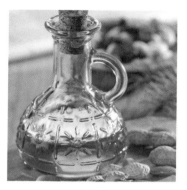

| VITAMIN E: | CALORIES – total: 884 kcal per 100 grams |
| 15.7 mg | Saturated: 16.9 g Poly: 32 g Mono: 46.2 g |

PEANUT OIL

Peanut oil, sometimes referred to as arachis oil, is obtained from the *Arachis hypogaea* plant. The peanut is actually a legume. Cold-pressed peanut oil is composed of 80% unsaturated lipids and 20% saturated. The valuable supply of essential unsaturated fatty acids is mainly in the form of oleic acid (70%) and polyunsaturated linoleic acid, or omega-6 (20%). The method of oil extraction is most important to the quality of peanut oil. Cold-pressed oil is the best choice. Peanut oil helps transport adrenaline throughout the body. It is a good cooking oil as it can be used several times without breaking down. The fair supply of vitamin E with cold-pressed peanut oil is a bonus for the circulatory system.

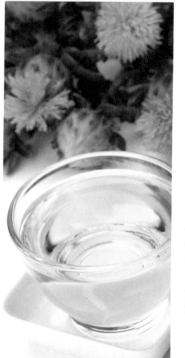

| VITAMIN E: | CALORIES – total: 884 kcal per 100 grams |
| 34.1 mg | Saturated: 6.2 g Poly: 74.6 g Mono: 14.4 g |

SAFFLOWER OIL

Safflower oil is obtained from the safflower seed, which is a member of the *Compositae* family of plants and one that ancient civilizations cultivated near the banks of the river Nile. Safflower oil is the richest source of unsaturated lipids, with linoleic acid being the dominant essential fatty acid. Nearly 90% of safflower oil is unsaturated—over 70% (74 g) in the form of linoleic acid (omega-6) and 20% oleic acid. Safflower oil supplies 10 g of linoleic acid per tablespoon. A most common result of a linoleic acid deficiency is dermatitis, a condition also prompted by excess emotional stress and physical exhaustion. Its high proportion of unsaturated lipids gives safflower oil the ability to protect your body against high cholesterol levels caused from excess consumption of animal fats and a lack of natural whole foods such as fruits, vegetables, whole grains, legumes, nuts, and seeds. A high blood cholesterol level can be most detrimental to the heart muscles and the circulatory system. Such symptoms as arteriosclerosis, heart disease, chilblains, and cramps may all be due to excess blood cholesterol levels. As safflower oil does not provide omega-3 (linolenic acid), it is best to ensure that the diet also includes such foods as salmon, fish, walnuts, pepitas, and flax oil, as there may be a link between excess intake of omega-6 and heart disease. Margarine is a common source of omega-6, so spread lightly.

Add a tablespoon of flaxseed oil to your bottle of safflower oil for a balanced oil.

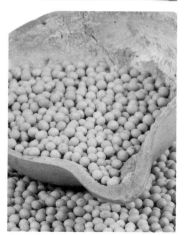

| VITAMIN E: | CALORIES – total: 884 kcal per 100 grams |
| 9.2 mg | Saturated: 14.4 g Poly: 57.9 g Mono: 23.3 g |

SOY OIL

Soy oil is a reliable source of the two essential unsaturated fatty acids; however, the balance of omega-6 is high compared to omega-3. Over 85% of soy oil is made up from unsaturated lipids with omega-6 at 51 g and omega-3 at 7 g.

Soy oil also supplies approximately 25% oleic acid, or monounsaturated lipids. To obtain a well-balanced oil and greatly increase the omega-3 value, mix 2 teaspoons (about 30 g) of edible flaxseed oil to 5 teaspoons (about 70 g) of soy oil. The combined oil provides approximately 22 g of omega-3 and 40 g of omega-6. A teaspoon a day provides 3 g of omega-3 and 5 g of omega-6.

NOTE: Nutrient amounts are listed as milligrams (mg) per 100 grams (g), unless otherwise stated.

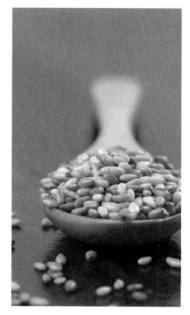

SESAME OIL

The sesame seed has been called the "queen of the oil-bearing seeds." Sesame seeds comprise 45% protein and mineral content and over 50% lipid content. From every 500 g of sesame seeds you can obtain over 1 cup of top-quality oil. Sesame oil is an excellent source of unsaturated lipids; over 80% are unsaturated and 14% are saturated. The extraction of sesame oil is a simple process that requires no chemical solvents or additives as there are no husks to be removed. A top-quality oil can be obtained with one cold pressing. Sesame seeds are grown throughout many parts of the world, especially in Turkey, China, Africa, South and Central America, India, and the southwestern United States. In some of these places, sesame oil is referred to as gingelly oil or benne oil.

The sesame plant produces a special substance known as sesamol, an excellent natural preservative that retards sesame oil from turning rancid. In places that have very hot weather, such as Turkey, from where the sesame paste tahini originated, sesame oil lasts longer than other cold-pressed oils. Sesame oil supplies an abundance of phytosterols (865 mg), which reduce blood cholesterol and retard the absorption of dietary cholesterol. Sesame oil has a rich and distinct flavor; for an authentic Middle East recipe, use sesame oil.

| VITAMIN E: | CALORIES – total: 570 kcal per 100 grams |
| 40 mg | Saturated: 6.7 g Poly: 21 g Mono: 18.1 g |

SESAME SEED PASTE (TAHINI)

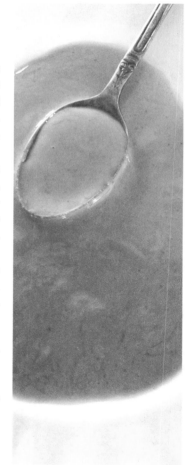

Tahini is made from ground sesame seeds and has a consistency similar to that of thick honey. One of the main benefits of tahini is that it is easily digested; within half an hour after digestion, the valuable nurients from tahini begin entering the bloodstream. Tahini is an excellent source of vitamin E (40 mg), which provides numerous health benefits. Vitamin E promotes the functioning of linoleic acid, which retards aging of body cells, thereby helping to preserve that youthful look and the ability of the eyes to focus.

Tahini is one of the most versatile foods—as a great spread for bread or toast, as an alternative to butter, as an ingredient in salad dressings, as a dip, in hummus or halva, mixed into a fruit salad, or poured over a fresh garden salad. It is a most nourishing complete-protein food. It is also an excellent source of calcium (420 mg); if you are allergic to dairy, tahini is the best alternative. The phosphorus content (750 mg) is excellent, making it ideal for the nervous system and brain, and it is also a top source of the substance torulitine (sometimes referred to as vitamin T, or the sesame vitamin), which affords another boost to the brain and memory. Tahini has an abundant content of magnesium (96 mg), copper (1.6 mg), and zinc (4.6 mg)—all vital for the nerves, skin, bones, blood vessels, healing, and immune system. The content of vitamins B1, 2, and 3 is very good; these vitamins are essential for the nerves, skin, and digestion.

There are two types of tahini: made from hulled and unhulled sesame seeds. They have similar nutrient benefits, but the tahini from hulled seeds is more palatable and lighter in color. No kitchen or breakfast or lunch is complete without tahini; it is one of the greatest natural foods for strength, growth, repair, and health. Add a teaspoon of flaxseed oil to your tahini for a complete supply of the essential fatty acids. Tahini also contains lecithin, choline, and inositol. Regular servings of tahini will ensure that your body has all it needs to heal, regenerate, and think!

NOTE: DV amounts listed refer to the daily value for women 25–50 years; refer to DRI tables on pages 95–96 for adult male and child values

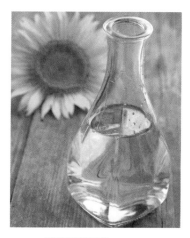

VITAMIN E:	CALORIES – total: 884 kcal per 100 grams
41.4 mg	Saturated: 9.7 g Poly: 3.8 g Mono: 83.6 g

SUNFLOWER OIL

Sunflower oil is composed of approximately 90% unsaturated lipids and 10% saturated lipids. The dominant unsaturated lipids are linoleic acid (60%) and oleic acid (30%). By using cold-pressed sunflower oil on your salads, you will obtain a very good supply of vitamin E (41 mg) and omega-6 (63 g) but only a trace of omega-3, so add a teaspoon of linseed/flaxseed oil to your sunflower oil bottle for greater benefits and balance. Sunflower oil is available at all supermarkets. It is produced via a chemical extraction process; such oil is best used for baking or frying, but keep the cold-pressed oil on hand for salad dressings. The vitamin E content of sunflower oil will help preserve the quality of the oil, as vitamin E retards oxidation and the formation of free radicals. Sunflower oil has hardly any taste, making it suitable for cooking pancakes, scones, and other delicately flavored recipes. Let the sunshine in with sunflower oil.

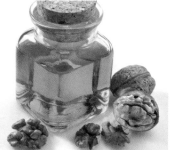

VITAMIN E:	CALORIES – total: 884 kcal per 100 grams
0.4 mg	Saturated: 9.1 g Poly: 63.3 g Mono: 22.8 g

WALNUT OIL

Walnut oil was once used exclusively for timber finishing, but today its very good supply of omega-3 (11.5 g) makes it a beneficial edible oil, ideal for those special salad dressings. Keep the guests guessing: Add a teaspoon of walnut oil to the Waldorf salad and get the best of both worlds, or add a drop to the pancake mix, the guacamole, or other dips. Walnut oil provides an abundance of omega-6 (58 g) and a fair supply of phytosterols (176 mg), for cholesterol reduction. Walnut oil is nearly 90% unsaturated with over 20% in the form of monounsaturated (oleic acid). Walnut oil is a well-balanced oil for daily use. Serve up the Waldorf, waiter!

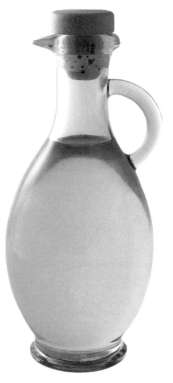

VITAMIN E:	CALORIES – total: 884 kcal per 100 grams
149 mg	Saturated: 18.8 g Poly: 61.7 g Mono: 15.1 g

WHEAT GERM OIL

Wheat germ oil is the most potent source of vitamin E (149 mg); in fact, it was the original source from which vitamin E was discovered. The whole wheat grain is an excellent food for your daily vitamin E requirements; however, very few people have tasted whole wheat and have a diet that is generally deficient in vitamin E foods. A small (200 ml) bottle of cold-pressed wheat germ oil should be an essential addition to the fridge, especially if you eat refined bread and other refined foods, smoke, and want to protect yourself from polluted air. By taking half a teaspoon per day, twice a week, of cold-pressed wheat germ oil you can be assured that your arteries and heart muscles will be given assistance for protection from pollution.

Wheat germ oil should also be part of every first aid kit; use it for skin irritations, to heal scar tissue, and to help prevent wrinkles. People with heart problems, blood clots, and other ailments should check with their medical practitioner before taking wheat germ oil. Wheat germ oil is a fair source of omega-3 (5 g); over 60% is unsaturated with 15% monounsaturated. Wheat germ oil provides an abundance of phytosterols (553 mg), which protect against low-density lipoproteins. It oil is very rich in texture and is best used as a supplement. Wheat germ oil is ready, willing, and waiting to heal.

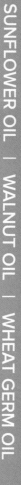

NOTE: Nutrient amounts are listed as milligrams (mg) per 100 grams (g), unless otherwise stated.

LIPID RECOMMENDATION: 20–35% OF DAILY CALORIC INTAKE

(Examples show 30% of calories coming from various sources of lipids)

		Calories
Male 18–50 years (example) approx. 870 calories daily		
Dairy foods	20%	174
Nuts	30%	261
Seeds	10%	87
Avocado	10%	87
Pure oil	10%	87
Margarine	5%	44
Cooking oil	5%	44
Other foods	10%	87
Total	**100%**	**871**
Female 18–50 years (example) approx. 600 calories daily		
Dairy foods	20%	120
Nuts	30%	180
Seeds	10%	60
Avocado	10%	60
Pure oil	10%	60
Margarine	5%	30
Cooking oil 5% 44	5%	30
Other foods 10% 87	10%	60
Total	**100%**	**600**
Teenager 13–17 years (example) approx. 660 calories daily		
Dairy foods	20%	132
Nuts	30%	198
Seeds	10%	66
Avocado	10%	66
Pure oil	10%	66
Margarine	5%	33
Cooking oil 5% 44	5%	33
Other foods 10% 87	10%	66
Total	**100%**	**660**

The table below provides a guide to the approximate amount of calories from lipids (fats and oils) required per day, based on the U.S. DRI guidelines. It is not necessary to consume all the foods listed in the chart each day. The chart is designed to provide an indication of the total quantity of foods required per day to satisfy the "nutritional appetite" for lipids. Some lipids are very beneficial and preferably are eaten daily.

TOTAL DAILY INTAKE OF LIPIDS—APPROX. FOOD QUANTITY/SERVING SIZE

	Proportion of Maconutrients		
	Carb.	Protein	Lipid
7 oz whole milk or 6 oz yogurt or 1 oz cheddar cheese	0	30	70
1 oz almonds (25–30) or 1 oz Brazil nuts (7–8) or 1 oz raw cashews (30)	0	40	60
¾ oz pumpkin seeds or ¾ oz sesame seeds or 3–4 oz sunflower seeds	0	60	40
½ small avocado	30	0	70
½ teaspoon of any cold-pressed oil (canola or walnut are best)	0	0	100
1 teaspoon of canola-based margarine	0	0	100
1 teaspoon of peanut, olive, or canola oil	0	0	100
a small snack or ⅔ oz chocolate or ½ oz potato chips	30	0	70

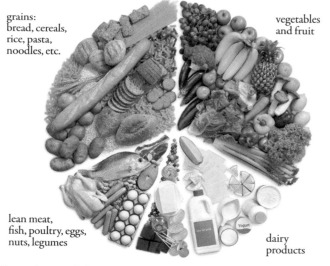

grains: bread, cereals, rice, pasta, noodles, etc.

vegetables and fruit

lean meat, fish, poultry, eggs, nuts, legumes

dairy products

Choose these snack foods only occasionally and in small amounts: potato chips, tortilla chips, ice cream, chocolate, candy, soft drinks, takeout foods.

The illustrated pie chart shows recommended proportions of the major food groups. As you can see, no specific mention of lipids is made. This is because lipids are automatically included with dairy and snack foods, and are typically added when cooking meat, fish, poultry, and other foods. For cooking, use cold-pressed oils and moderate their use. Obtain a variety of the lipid groups every week. Consume the pure oils with salads or bread, and combine dairy products with grains, legumes, or vegetables.

NOTE: DV refers to the daily value for women 25–50 years, refer to RDI tables on pages 95–96 for adult male and child values.

Minerals perform a multitude of vital functions throughout the body. They are required for the construction of cells. Every day the body builds new cells—blood, bone, connective, epithelium, muscular, nerve, skin, and skeletal cells. Minerals, along with amino acids and fatty acids, are the major building blocks for cells.

There are 14 essential main minerals and five essential trace minerals. Minerals are converted into organic salts via digestion. These organic salts are dissolved in bodily fluids such as water and blood. The following pages list the individual minerals and outline over 200 functions they accomplish.

Besides building new cells, minerals convey electrical stimuli along nerves to activate the body. Minerals have either positive or negative ions. Similarly charged ions repel and oppositely charged ions attract. This action, triggered by stimuli from the brain and nervous system, is involved in all bodily movements, such as relaxation and contraction of muscles.

Minerals are also involved in maintaining the acid–alkaline balance of the blood and body. Ideally, the diet should provide 75% alkaline-forming foods and 25% acid-forming foods. The main alkaline-forming foods are fruits, vegetables, almonds, millet, and brown rice. Most other foods are acid-forming. Every food has both acid and alkaline minerals. A food is termed "acid" when the end product, after digestion, provides an acid ash or residue.

Various common ailments can be attributed to a prolonged deficiency of a particular mineral. Processed foods are often depleted in their supply of minerals, especially the trace minerals. Balance your system with the foods that give; avoid the foods that take away!

A list of best food sources for the various minerals is provided on pages 156–158. Check the list to make sure you are regularly obtaining at least a few of the foods from each mineral group. Also refer to the individual foods throughout this book to obtain more details on the quantity of the minerals supplied, and refer to the Dietary Reference Intake (DRI) table on page 95.

The chart below lists the approximate proportion that minerals and other essential nutrients make up of the human body.

ELEMENTS AND MINERALS: PROPORTION OF BODY WEIGHT		
Carbon	18%	
Nitrogen	3%	
Hydrogen	10%	
Oxygen	65%	
Water H_2O	55%	96%
Calcium	2%	
Phosphorus	1%	
Potassium	0.4%	
Sulfur	0.25%	
Chlorine	0.25%	
Sodium	0.25%	
Fluoride	0.20%	
Magnesium	0.05%	
Iron	0.008%	
Manganese	0.003%	
Silicon	0.002%	
Copper	0.002%	
Iodine	0.00004%	4%
		100%

NUTRIENT COMPOSITION OF THE HUMAN BODY	
Carbo-hydrates	2%
Protein	20%
Lipids	15%
Water	55%
Minerals	7%
Vitamins	1%
	100%

NOTE: Nutrient amounts are listed as milligrams (mg) per 100 grams (g), unless otherwise stated.

CALCIUM (CA) – ALKALINE MINERAL

1. CIRCULATORY SYSTEM

Calcium regulates the heartbeat and, in combination with the mineral magnesium, is vital for the nourishment of the cardiovascular system: heart, arteries, veins, and capillaries.

2. DIGESTIVE SYSTEM

Calcium is essential for the involuntary muscular movements of the digestive system (peristaltic action), thereby protecting against constipation.

3. GLANDULAR SYSTEM

The parathyroid glands regulate the storage of calcium throughout the body, a process that requires vitamin D, available through sunlight. Obtaining moderate sunlight on a regular basis is vital for healthy glands and for calcium metabolism.

5. MUSCULAR SYSTEM

Muscles need calcium to contract and relax. Cramps are often due to a calcium deficiency as muscle fibers cannot contract or slide and mesh properly without a steady flow of calcium ions. Eating yogurt the night before a big race can prevent cramps.

6. NERVOUS SYSTEM

Calcium combined with magnesium is required for the transmission of nerve impulses to muscles.

20. REPAIR SYSTEM

Calcium is essential for the repair of bone fractures, in combination with a regular daily supply of vitamin D (available from sunlight) and the minerals phosphorus, magnesium, zinc, silicon, fluorine, copper, and the vitamins A and C. Foods such as almonds, tahini, and fresh vegetables are good sources of these nutrients. For a great bone-repair lunch, enjoy a veggie sandwich with cheddar cheese and a spread of tahini on rye bread, while sitting outside in the sunlight.

8. SKELETAL SYSTEM

Calcium is the most important bone mineral, and with two hundred bones in the adult skeleton it is vital to ensure a regular supply of calcium. This is especially important for growing children, for women during pregnancy and lactation, and for the elderly.

Various factors are important for a strong skeletal system. 1. Bones become weak without weight-bearing exercise or daily activities. 2. Vitamin D (sunlight) is vital for proper calcium absorption and strong bones. 3. Ideally the body needs a regular supply of calcium from the diet to maintain strong bones. 4. Over 95% of the body's calcium is contained in the bones, teeth, and skeletal system. 5. The total calcium content of the body is entirely renewed over a six-year period.

12. GROWTH SYSTEM

Calcium is the dominant mineral for the growth system. Milk and dairy products are the most common source of calcium, and they are very good sources; however, it is important that children obtain a good supply of fruits and vegetables to help cleanse the body of excess mucus produced from the digestion of dairy foods.

13. IMMUNE SYSTEM

Calcium is required to increase the body's general resistance to infections. Only when the calcium levels are low can a viral infection occur.

14. JOINT SYSTEM

Calcium obtained from refined foods such as white bread, cookies, etc., is converted from organic to inorganic by heat and processing. Inorganic calcium can cause deposits within the joint system, eventually leading to conditions such as arthritis.

CALCIUM

NOTE: DV refers to the daily value for women 25–50 years, refer to RDI tables on pages 95–96 for adult male and child values.

CHLORINE (CL) – ACID MINERAL

2. DIGESTIVE SYSTEM

Chlorine stimulates the production of hydrochloric acid in the stomach, which is vital for the initial stage of protein digestion: converting protein into smaller units known as proteoses and peptones.

Chlorine also assists in the digestion of fats and cleanses the body of excess fats. Tomatoes are an excellent source of organic chlorine, but cooking destroys the chlorine content.

Chlorine assists with the function of the liver, protects against digestive problems, and assists with the distribution of hormones. It helps regulate the acid–alkaline balance of the blood.

A deficiency of organic chlorine in the diet can lead to a sluggish liver, general body congestion, and even heart disease.

3. GLANDULAR SYSTEM

Chlorine is vital for the glandular system because it assists the functioning of the pancreas, spleen, and gallbladder. It also helps to cleanse the bloodstream and glands.

4. LYMPHATIC SYSTEM

Chlorine cleanses the lymph glands and blood, promoting the production of antibodies to fight infections.

9. BLOOD SYSTEM

Chlorine purifies the blood and regulates blood pressure. The liver needs a regular flow of blood to maintain the functioning of the adrenal glands, the balance of salt levels, and correct fluid retention. Otherwise, conditions such as swelling in the legs, excess water retention, obesity, and heart problems may develop.

COPPER (CU) – ALKALINE MINERAL

2. DIGESTIVE SYSTEM

The vital trace mineral copper is an ingredient of many digestive enzymes. The copper content from natural foods is stored in the liver, kidneys, heart, brain, bones, and muscles. Over half the body's copper stores are located in the bones. Copper is required for the metabolism of fats.

9. BLOOD SYSTEM

Copper, together with the mineral manganese, is required for the proper assimilation of iron. Copper and iron are required for the development of hemoglobin.

Copper is required for the conversion of ascorbic acid into vitamin C and for protection from infection, especially in the lungs, as it promotes tissue respiration.

Copper is a very important blood mineral. It is vital for the prevention of blood vessel ruptures and may prevent the degeneration of heart muscles.

A balance between the minerals zinc and copper is crucial; if an excess of either occurs, which can happen from supplementation, levels of the other mineral will be lowered. Natural copper foods such as tahini and most nuts provide an excellent—and naturally balanced—supply of both minerals.

19. BRAIN SYSTEM

A copper–zinc imbalance may be the problem in some cases of schizophrenia and various other mental problems; the mineral zinc may be depleted in such patients, causing an excess of copper. Natural foods supply balance. When an excess of vitamin C is taken regularly, copper metabolism may be reduced.

Copper is also required for the central nervous system and glandular system.

FLUORIDE (F) – ACID MINERAL

8. SKELETAL SYSTEM

Fluoride from natural foods is termed calcium fluoride, whereas fluoridated water contains sodium fluoride. It is deposited into some cities' drinking water as an inorganic element. The synthetic fluoride in drinking water can inhibit the functions of vitamin C, which promotes hardening of the bones and tooth enamel. Excess intake of fluoridated water can also retard calcium absorption. Teflon-based cookware increases synthetic fluoride intake; in contrast, aluminum cookware destroys the fluoride from city water but also from foods. Organic fluoride is essential for the strength and growth of bones. A prolonged fluoride deficiency can lead to curvature of the spine and decalcification of bones.

9. BLOOD SYSTEM

Fluoride from natural foods helps to increase the number of red blood cells: 90% of fluoride is contained in the bloodstream. Beets are tops on the list for building blood as they provide natural fluoride as well as iron, manganese, copper, sodium, potassium, calcium, magnesium, chlorine, and iodine—the full range of blood minerals. A juice of fresh carrots and beets is one sure way to give your blood a boost.

15. OPTIC SYSTEM

Fluoride promotes the optic system functions, especially for the delicate iris of the eye. Lettuce with asparagus, mayonnaise, and finely grated carrot will bring a sparkle to the iris of the eye!

17. SKIN SYSTEM

Fluoride foods promote a youthful skin and complexion. Rolled oats soaked in milk overnight and served with grated apple is the ideal breakfast for anyone.

IODINE (I) – ACID MINERAL

2. DIGESTIVE SYSTEM

Iodine is required to maintain a proper rate of digestion and for the utilization of fats. It is necessary for the oxidation of both fats and proteins, thereby promoting proper digestion. It also assists in regulating cholesterol levels. A prolonged deficiency may lead to obesity.

For people who live near the ocean and eat fish and seafood regularly, a deficiency of iodine is less likely to occur.

Kelp is the richest source of iodine. Try crisp kelp crackers once a week with tahini or grated cheese for an iodine boost.

3. GLANDULAR SYSTEM

Iodine is the major mineral for the thyroid gland. Approximately 30% of all iodine is required by the thyroid glands for effective internal functions and control of general body metabolism, digestion, and rate of hormone secretion. The thyroid gland produces the hormone thyroxine, which is composed of 65% iodine. Its functions include energy production, conversion of carotene into vitamin A, growth, healthy mental condition, and healthy skin, hair, and nervous system.

Iodine is vital for the development of infants' mental and physical structure.

The condition known as goiter, an enlargement of the thyroid gland, is often caused by an iodine deficiency.

Kelp is the ideal natural food to create a proper iodine body balance.

12. GROWTH SYSTEM

Iodine is vital for the growth system because the hormone thyroxine is required for bodily growth. Iodine is also required by the thyroid gland to keep the skin and hair in good condition, for maintenance of the nervous system, and for normal cellular growth.

NOTE: DV refers to the daily value for women 25–50 years, refer to RDI tables on pages 95–96 for adult male and child values.

IRON (FE) – ALKALINE MINERAL

9. BLOOD SYSTEM

Iron is the main blood mineral; it is essential in the formation of rich red blood cells and is vital for supplying oxygen to the body. About two-thirds of the iron content in the body is stored in the bloodstream; the remainder is located in organs such as the liver and spleen, in the muscles (a small amount), and in the bone marrow, where it is stored until it is required in the formation of hemoglobin, a protein that transports oxygen throughout the body. Hemoglobin transports oxygen from the lungs via the bloodstream to bodily tissues, where oxygen separates from hemoglobin and attaches to myoglobin, a protein that stores oxygen in the muscle cells.

The mineral copper and the green matter in plants are also essential for iron activity.

For iron to be absorbed effectively, protein and vitamin C must be present. Excess cooking depletes iron in foods. A deficiency of the mineral iron often shows up as weariness, regular colds and inflammations, and lack of energy.

10. CELLULAR SYSTEM

As discussed above, iron is vital for the transport and storage of oxygen in the body. Because oxygen is required in the metabolism of all bodily cells, iron is linked to the health of all cells.

Some iron supplements are well balanced, but nothing can beat the balance of natural foods. If you do choose to supplement with iron, know that chelated iron tablets are three times more effective than nonchelated. For iron deficiencies such as anemia, it is vital to balance your iron supplements with copper, vitamins E and B complex, manganese, calcium, and protein, all of which are required for the proper utilization of iron.

5. MUSCULAR SYSTEM

Iron is the delivery service for the supply of oxygen to the entire muscular system, where it is stored in the myoglobin molecule. Iron can have an electrical charge of two or three, which allows it to pick up an extra oxygen atom and then deposit the oxygen elsewhere. Iron is also vital for cleansing the body's cells of toxins.

MAGNESIUM (MG) – ALKALINE MINERAL

1. CIRCULATORY SYSTEM

Magnesium is vital for the transfer of nerve impulses to the heart muscles, which keeps the heart rate steady. A deficiency may lead to high blood pressure, hardened arteries, and chronic fatigue syndrome.

Magnesium assists with calcium balance, the action of vitamin D, and the metabolism of numerous minerals. Excess alcohol, stress, nervousness, and the fact that magnesium cannot be stored for long periods in the body all point to the need for magnesium foods in the daily diet.

2. DIGESTIVE SYSTEM

Magnesium is involved in numerous digestive enzymes. Along wtih calcium, it is required for the conversion of glucose into energy, which involves the hormone insulin. Magnesium is the natural "antacid" mineral and is also required for fat and protein metabolism.

5. MUSCULAR SYSTEM

Magnesium protects against muscular cramps by promoting a steady flow of impulses from the nerves to the muscle tissues. If you exercise hard, make sure to get enough magnesium to support your muscles.

6. NERVOUS SYSTEM

Magnesium promotes steady nerves by regulating the white nerve fibers, which control the central nervous system.

A magnesium deficiency can result in various nervous disorders, hyperactivity in children, irritability, heart attacks, neuralgia, and depression.

Magnesium is also vital for the nourishment of the white nerve fibers of the brain; it helps other nutrients enter brain cells, it promotes memory, and it protects against mental illness.

IRON | MAGNESIUM

MANGANESE (MN) – ALKALINE MINERAL

2. DIGESTIVE SYSTEM

Manganese assists in the digestion, absorption, and utilization of the three main food groups: protein, carbohydrates, and lipids. It is required for various digestive enzymes and reactions, including the production of bile, which aids in fat digestion, and insulin, which converts carbohydrate into an energy source and stabilizes blood glucose levels. The processing of wheat and other grains can reduce the manganese content by 90%. Animal foods such as meat are a poor source of this mineral.

3. GLANDULAR SYSTEM

Manganese is a vital nutrient for the glands: the thyroid gland needs manganese and iodine to produce thyroxine, for bodily growth and metabolism and for the active control of 20 sets of glands. Manganese is essential for regulating menstrual periods, and during pregnancy and lactation for the production of milk from the mammary glands. Manganese is required in numerous hormones of both the male and the female reproductive glands.

6. NERVOUS SYSTEM

Manganese foods improve the coordination of nerves and nerve impulses to the muscles and nervous system. Manganese is also vital for the brain, for memory, and for mental stability.

8. SKELETAL SYSTEM

Manganese is important for children's growth. As a component of connective tissues, it is required for the lengthening of bones to their normal shape and size during the growth process.

9. BLOOD SYSTEM

Manganese, in combination with iron, copper, and cobalt, is vital in the formation of healthy red blood cells.

PHOSPHORUS (P) – ACID MINERAL

1. CIRCULATORY SYSTEM

Phosphorus is required for proper blood circulation and normal blood pressure. Phosphorus foods improve a poor complexion by stimulating circulation.

2. DIGESTIVE SYSTEM

Phosphorus is required for the utilization of fats, proteins, and carbohydrates. The phosphorus in the outer portion of whole grains is termed phytic acid; it can reduce the absorption of calcium, zinc, and iron. But the enzyme phytase in the small intestine breaks down the phytic acid to allow its absorption. Breadmaking activates gluten in the grain to reduce the phytic acid content.

6. NERVOUS SYSTEM

Phosphorus is essential for the maintenance and repair of the entire nervous system.

Phosphorus foods such as almonds strengthen the nervous system.

8. SKELETAL SYSTEM

Approximately 90% of the body's phosphorus is contained in the bones, teeth, and nails. It is totally renewed over a three-year period. It is essential for the healing of bone fractures and bone growth. Phosphorus may prevent poor teeth formation and limited growth in children.

19. BRAIN SYSTEM

Phosphorus is required for a good memory, creativity, proper concentration, efficient mental activity, and transfer of nerve impulses.

A lack of phosphorus leads to mental exhaustion. Excess sugar causes a phosphorus deficiency.

Every cell and chemical reaction in the body needs the mineral phosphorus for the transfer of hereditary characteristics.

NOTE: DV refers to the daily value for women 25–50 years, refer to RDI tables on pages 95–96 for adult male and child values.

POTASSIUM (K) – ALKALINE MINERAL

1. CIRCULATORY SYSTEM

Potassium is vital for the circulatory system as it keeps the heart muscles healthy and strong. In combination with iron, potassium promotes the use of oxygen in the body and normalizes heart muscle action such as contractions and heart rate.

2. DIGESTIVE SYSTEM

Potassium is often destroyed by heat, cooking, and processing. Alcohol, caffeine, and salt also cause a loss of this alkaline mineral.

Potassium is vital for the alkaline balance in the blood; most diets are acid forming, due to a potassium deficiency.

Potassium is essential in the formation of glycogen, which is stored in the liver and converted to glucose when the body requires extra energy.

5. MUSCULAR SYSTEM

Potassium is the muscle mineral. It is required for stimulation of the nerves connected to muscles, repair of muscles, and blood supply to muscles. It is vital for the heart muscles and for a steady heartbeat, as it regulates the muscle tone during activity and assists with relaxation of muscles after exertion.

19. BRAIN SYSTEM

Potassium foods promote the supply of oxygen to the brain, improving mental function.

20. REPAIR SYSTEM

Potassium is a most effective healing mineral, especially for damaged heart muscles. It regulates water balance and assists with the elimination of blood impurities via the kidneys.

Cancer cells cannot live in a solution of potassium.

SILICON (SI) – ACID MINERAL

6. NERVOUS SYSTEM

Silicon provides an insulating surface around the individual nerve fibers, thereby protecting the nervous system, especially during stress.

14. JOINT SYSTEM

Silicon is vital for proper calcium metabolism, preventing the accumulation of inorganic calcium around the bone joints. Silicon crystals can break up the uric acid crystals that result from excess protein, meat, caffeine, and tea intake, to mention a few. The uric acid crystals are then small enough to be eliminated; otherwise they tend to build around the bones and moving joints, leading to the development of gout. In lettuce, the combination of a rich silicon content and fluoride makes it one of the best foods to eat regularly to offset arthritis.

17. SKIN SYSTEM

Silicon is vital for efficient cell growth, hair growth, and the removal of dead skin cells. It promotes healthy skin by opening pores to allow toxins and grime to be discharged. It promotes the formation of healthy red blood cells and blood circulation. For men concerned with the possibility of hereditary baldness, extra silicon-rich foods will help to cleanse the scalp and keep the skin cells open, allowing hair follicles to grow. Because silicon is the major mineral in the building of hair, lettuce is really the best hair tonic as it is rich in both silicon and chlorophyll, vital ingredients for hair growth. For women, silicon foods will promote a clear skin and the hair quality you dream about, as long as the diet is natural.

Silicon also protects against nervous exhaustion, mental fatigue, cancerous tissue formation, and infections.

POTASSIUM | SILICON

SODIUM (NA) – ALKALINE MINERAL

1. CIRCULATORY SYSTEM

Sodium is required for normal and consistent blood pressure. It is vital for keeping other minerals soluble within the bloodstream and for prevention of hardened arteries. The natural sodium (in the form of sodium phosphate and sodium sulfate) obtained from foods is balanced to provide a stable pressure within individual cells. Common table salt (sodium chloride) retains excess fluids in the body at a rate of about 1 g of salt to 70 g of water, thereby increasing body weight. The sodium/potassium balance is the main factor in the control of the body's fluid balance. Table salt is concentrated sodium without the essential balance of potassium to ensure correct cell pressure. It is advised to restrict adding salt to meals, avoid salty processed foods, and increase the intake of potassium-rich foods. The excess use of salt has led to an increase in blood pressure; research has confirmed the direct link between salt and the risk of hypertension.

2. DIGESTIVE SYSTEM

Sodium is required for the production of saliva, which is required for the initial digestion of carbohydrate foods. Natural sodium provides an alkaline balance to the entire body, preventing disorders such as arthritis, ulcers, and stomach acidity.

9. BLOOD SYSTEM

Natural sodium promotes normal blood pressure and protects against blood clots and thickening of the blood.

14. JOINT SYSTEM

Sodium preserves flexibility of joints and promotes movement of muscles. It keeps blood minerals soluble and protects against arthritis. Celery and kelp are the ultimate natural sodium foods, and celery is well balanced with potassium.

SULFUR (S) – ACID MINERAL

2. DIGESTIVE SYSTEM

Sulfur promotes the absorption of protein and the conversion of amino acids. It stimulates the liver to produce bile for fat digestion. It has a cleansing and antiseptic effect on the digestive system. It is necessary for the production of insulin, which is required for conversion of carbohydrates (glucose) into energy.

3. GLANDULAR SYSTEM

Sulfur is vital for cleansing the glands, production of enzymes, and protecting against blood impurities. In particular, it participates in production of the pancreas enzymes, which are essential for the metabolism of fats.

4. LYMPHATIC SYSTEM

Sulfur cleanses the vital network of the lymphatic system. Conditions such as glandular fever are often caused by a buildup of toxins.

7. RESPIRATORY SYSTEM

Sulfur is a heat-sensitive nutrient. In winter people tend to eat more cooked meals. That's unfortunate, because winter is also when those nasty respiratory ailments seem to thrive. The common cold, bronchitis, and tuberculosis have been successfully treated with garlic (which contains sulfur) for years.

9. BLOOD SYSTEM

Sulfur is an excellent blood purifier; it provides oxygen to the blood and is required in the formation of blood plasma. It is contained in all bodily tissues and forms a part of hemoglobin. Insulin is a sulfur compound, making this mineral most valuable for diabetics.

17. SKIN SYSTEM

Sulfur is a vital ingredient of keratin, a protein substance contained in the outer skin layer. Sulfur foods promote a good complexion by cleansing the skin and scalp of toxins that can cause acne and dandruff.

NOTE: DV refers to the daily value for women 25–50 years, refer to RDI tables on pages 95–96 for adult male and child values.

ZINC (ZN)

2. DIGESTIVE SYSTEM

Zinc is required as a component of numerous digestive enzymes. It is vital in the production and proper action of insulin. A deficiency of zinc can show up as poor appetite and loss of taste and flavor in foods. Zinc is also required to break down alcohol; excess alcohol can lead to a zinc deficiency.

3. GLANDULAR SYSTEM

Zinc is essential for the prostate gland, the manufacture of various male reproductive hormones, and the development of the genital organs in children.

8. SKELETAL SYSTEM

Zinc is vital for the development of bones and teeth in children, for prompt repair of fractures, general growth, and the formation of cell proteins and bones, which need a constant supply of zinc-rich foods.

16. REPRODUCTIVE SYSTEM

Zinc is essential for the development of the reproductive organs. It is also required for the synthesis of DNA, the master cell code for life.

17. SKIN SYSTEM

Zinc is vital for the production of keratin; fingernails are composed mainly of keratin. Zinc is important for the healing of burns; zinc cream is used to protect from sunburn.

MOLYBDENUM

2. DIGESTIVE SYSTEM

Molybdenum is required for the metabolism of fats. It is used for the proper elimination of waste and for the manufacture of genetic enzymes such as DNA enzymes. Molybdenum may also be required for the utilization of iron.

Legumes are full of molybdenum.

COBALT

9. BLOOD SYSTEM

The essential trace mineral cobalt is especially important for the blood system; in combination with iron, manganese, and copper, it is required for the development of red blood cells.

A lack of cobalt can occur in a diet without seafood or fish as most soils do not contain this trace element. A prolonged deficiency of cobalt can lead to impaired red blood cell production and anemia.

Cobalt is part of the vitamin B12 structure. Cobalt also activates enzymes, body growth, and nerves, and is required for body healing.

SELENIUM

10. CELLULAR SYSTEM

Selenium has numerous body functions. Possibly its most important and best-known function is its antioxidant quality when combined with vitamin E, to assist in the body's use of oxygen and promote cell life. It delays the rate of oxidation of polyunsaturated fatty acids, which helps preserve the condition of cells and skin tissues. It protects against the development of cancerous cells, promotes the production of thyroxine for regulating body metabolism, and protects against premature aging. Refined and cooked foods are depleted in their supply of selenium.

One Brazil nut a day will easily supply all of your selenium needs.

VANADIUM

1. CIRCULATORY SYSTEM

Vanadium is an essential trace mineral. It promotes blood circulation and assists to inhibit the formation of cholesterol in the blood vessels, brain, and central nervous system. Seafoods are the best source of vanadium, and trace amounts are available from vegetables, depending on the soil condition.

ZINC | MOLYBDENUM | COBALT | SELENIUM | VANADIUM

NOTE: Nutrient amounts are listed as milligrams (mg) per 100 grams (g), unless otherwise stated.

MINERAL FOOD SOURCE TABLE

CALCIUM – ALKALINE MINERAL

Nutrients for effective absorption: essential fatty acids, inositol, Iron, magnesium, phosphorus, protein, vitamins A, C, D, E

Nutrient inhibiting factors: Alcohol, antibiotics, chocolate, diuretics, oxalic acid, refined foods, rhubarb, salt.

RDA: See page 95.

Almonds, bran, Brazil nuts, broccoli, carob powder, cheddar cheese, chickpeas, corn tortillas, dried apricots, dried figs, hazelnuts, milk, nuts, parmesan cheese, parsley, peanuts, prunes, salmon, sardines, soft cheese, spinach, sunflower seeds, swiss cheese, tahini, tofu, walnuts, wheat germ, yogurt.

CHLORIDE – ACID MINERAL

Nutrients for effective absorption: Potassium and sodium.

Nutrient inhibiting factors: Cooking, high temperatures.

No RDA established.
Adults safe level: 3,600 mg

Natural chloride: Asparagus, avocado, bananas, beets, berries, cabbage, carrot, celery, cucumber, dates, kelp, leeks, lettuce, mango, parsnip, pineapple, radish, raisins, tomato, turnip, watercress.
Added chloride: Bread, cheese, olives, peanut butter, tuna.

CHROMIUM

No RDA established.
AI: See page 95.

Apples, beef, butter, cheddar cheese, egg yolks, oysters, pasta, potatoes, rye bread, whole-grain bread, wine.

COBALT

Cheese, fish, milk, seafood, yogurt.

COPPER – ACID MINERAL

Nutrients for effective absorption: Cobalt, iron, zinc.

Nutrient inhibiting factors: Excess zinc (oysters).

RDA: See page 95.

Almonds, Brazil nuts, cashews, coconut, dried fruits, fruits, hazelnuts, macadamia nuts, oats, oysters, parsley, peanuts, pepitas, pine nuts, soybean, sunflower seeds, tahini, vegetables, walnuts, wheat germ.

FLUORINE – ALKALINE MINERAL

Nutrients for effective absorption: Calcium.

Nutrient inhibiting factors: Cooking in aluminum pots and saucepans.

No RDA established.
AI: See page 95.

Apples, asparagus, barley, beets, cabbage, cheddar cheese, citrus, fish, garlic, goat's milk, millet, oats, rice, rice bran, seafood, spinach, sweet corn, tea, watercress, wheat.

IODINE – ACID MINERAL

Nutrients for effective absorption: Selenium.

Nutrient inhibiting factors: Brussels sprouts, cabbage, turnips.

RDA: See page 95.

Asparagus, bell pepper, berries, blueberry, bread, butter, cheese, clams, cucumber, dairy, dried fruits, fish, kelp, lettuce, nuts, onion, peach, peanut, pineapple, rice, seafood, seeds, spinach, strawberry, vegetables, watermelon, wheat.

IRON – ALKALINE MINERAL

Nutrients for effective absorption: Vitamins B12, C, E, folate.

Nutrient inhibiting factors: Excess aspirin, antacids, antibiotics, caffeine and tannin, codeine.

RDA: See page 95.

Aroccoli, carob, cashews, chickpeas, clams, coconut, dried fruits, kelp, lentils, liver, miso, mussels, parsley, peanuts, peas, pepitas, raisins, rice bran, rolled oats, rye, salmon, spinach, sunflower seeds, tahini, tofu, tuna, vegetables, walnut, wheat bran, wheat germ.

NOTE: DV refers to the daily value for women 25–50 years, refer to RDI tables on pages 95–96 for adult male and child values.

MINERAL FOOD SOURCE TABLE

MAGNESIUM – ALKALINE MINERAL

Nutrients for effective absorption:
Calcium, phosphorus, protein, and vitamins B6, C, D.

Nutrient inhibiting factors:
Alcohol, antibiotics, caffeine, diuretics, nicotine.

RDA: See page 95.

Almonds, Brazil nuts, brown rice, carob powder, cashews, corn taco shells, dates, figs, hazelnuts, kelp, kelp, legumes, parsley, peanuts, pecans, pepitas, pine nuts, rolled oats, rye bread, soy flour, spinach, sunflower seeds, sweet corn, tahini, tofu, walnuts, wheat bran, wheat germ, whole wheat.

MANGANESE – ALKALINE MINERAL

Nutrients for effective absorption:
Calcium, copper, phosphorus, vitamins B1, E, zinc.

No RDA established.
AI: See page 95.

Almonds, beets, berries, bran, Brazil nuts, chestnuts, garlic, grapes, hazelnuts, legumes, oats, peanuts, pepitas, pineapple, rice, rye bread, tahini, tomato, walnuts, wheat germ.

MOLYBDENUM

RDA: See page 95.

Apricots, beans, carrots, cauliflower, cheese, coconut, corn, garlic, kidney beans, peas, soybeans, sprouted foods.

PHOSPHORUS – ACID MINERAL

Nutrients for effective absorption:
Calcium, essential fatty acids, manganese, vitamins A and D, protein.

Nutrient inhibiting factors:
Excess antacids, magnesium, refined foods, stress, sugar.

RDA: See page 95.

Almonds, Brazil nuts, cashews, cheddar cheese, legumes, milk, nuts, parmesan cheese, peanuts, pumpkin seeds, pine nuts, pistachios, rice bran, salmon, sardines, scallops, soybeans, sunflower seeds, tahini, vegetables, walnuts, wheat bran, wheat germ, whole grains.

POTASSIUM – ALKALINE MINERAL

Nutrients for effective absorption:
Chloride, phosphorus, sodium, sulfur, vitamin B6.

Nutrient inhibiting factors:
Excess alcohol, antibiotics, coffee, diuretics, laxatives, salt, stress.

No RDA established.
AI: See page 95.

Almonds, avocado, bananas, dates, dried apricots, figs, fruits, garlic, hazelnuts, legumes, mushrooms, nuts, parsley, parsnip, peaches, peanuts, pine nuts, potatoes, raisins, snapper, spinach, sunflower seeds, trout, tuna, vegetables, walnuts.

SELENIUM

Essential associated nutrients: Iodine, vitamin E.

RDA: See page 95.

Beef, Brazil nuts, chicken, eggs, fish, liver, oysters, seafood, sunflower seeds, tuna, wheat germ, whole-meal bread, whole grains.

SILICON – ACID MINERAL

No RDA established.

Asparagus, cabbage, cucumber, fruits, lettuce, onions, parsnip, spinach, strawberry, sunflower seeds, vegetables.

SODIUM – ALKALINE MINERAL

Nutrients for effective absorption:
Chloride, potassium, vitamin D.

Nutrient inhibiting factors:
Antibiotics, diuretics, excess salt, laxatives.

No RDA established.
AI: See page 95.
Adults safe level: 2,300 mg

Natural sodium:
Beets, broccoli, Brussels sprouts, cabbage, carrots, cashews, celery, coconut, eggs, fruits, garlic, kale, legumes, lentils, parsley, raisins, scallops, spinach, tahini, turnip, watercress.

Added sodium:
Butter, cheese, feta cheese, olives, tuna.

(cont'd.)

NOTE: Nutrient amounts are listed as milligrams (mg) per 100 grams (g), unless otherwise stated.

MINERAL FOOD SOURCE TABLE (CONT'D.)

SULFUR – ALKALINE MINERAL

Nutrients for effective absorption: Vitamin B group, especially thiamin and biotin. *Nutrient inhibiting factors:* Cooking, high temperatures. No RDA established.	Almonds, asparagus, avocado, berries, Brazil nuts, cabbage, carrots, cauliflower, celery, cheddar cheese, corn, crab, crayfish, cucumber, eggs, fruits, horseradish, lemon, lettuce, lime, melon, mussels, peaches, peanuts, prawns, radish, sardines, scallops, spinach, tomato, vegetables, watercress.

VANADIUM

	Fish, kelp, seafood, some vegetables.

ZINC

Nutrients for effective absorption: Calcium, copper, phosphorus, vitamins A, D, B group. *Nutrient inhibiting factors:* Alcohol, caffeine, HRT therapy, oral contraceptives, tea. RDA: See page 95.	Almonds, beef, bran, Brazil nuts, cashews, cheddar cheese, crab, egg yolk, garlic, hazelnuts, kelp, liver, mackerel, maple syrup, millet, miso, oats, olives, oysters, parmesan cheese, pumpkin seeds, rye, sardines, scallops, sunflower seeds, tahini, walnuts, wheat, wheat germ.

ALCOHOL (C_2H_5OH)

Alcohol is defined as a colorless, volatile, intoxicating, and flammable liquid. After entering the digestive system, a portion of the ethyl alcohol is absorbed through the stomach lining directly into the bloodstream. A special enzyme in the liver, alcohol dehydrogenase, is designed to convert alcohol; however, this is a slow process. In addition, some people may lack the enzyme and be intolerant to alcohol. The liver converts ethyl alcohol into aldehyde, a colorless, volatile fluid of suffocating smell. Another enzyme converts aldehyde into a form of vinegar, and once that is oxidized, the end product is carbon dioxide, a colorless heavy gas. The main body parts that are affected by alcohol are the brain and liver. Alcohol relaxes the brain but also destroys brain cells within the cerebellum, pineal gland, and cerebral cortex. Alcohol destroys liver cells.

ALCOHOL AND SMOKING—PROBLEMS

Problems	Nutrient To Counteract	Beneficial Foods
Cardiac damage, impaired learning, mental problems	Vitamin B1	Brazil nuts, peanuts, wheat germ, yeast extracts
Arthritis, baldness, mouth sores, nervous disorders, poor skin condition, ulcers, weak eyesight	Vitamin B2	Almonds, bran, cashews, cheese, wheat germ, yeast extracts
Depression, fatigue, headaches, indigestion, poor skin condition, nervous disorders	Vitamin B3	Fish, nuts, peanuts, rice bran, sunflower seeds, wheat germ, yeast extracts
Depression, chronic fatigue, heart problems, poor liver function	Vitamin B5	Almonds, peanuts, sunflower seeds, yeast extracts
Depression, headaches, nervousness, poor digestion, poor memory	Vitamin B6	Oats, rice bran, walnuts, wheat bran, yeast extracts
Arthritis, blood clots, mental illness, nervousness	Magnesium	Almonds, sunflower seeds, wheat bran, wheat germ
Fatigue, prostate problems, sterility	Zinc	Brazil nuts, oysters, sunflower seeds

NOTE: DV refers to the daily value for women 25–50 years, refer to RDI tables on pages 95–96 for adult male and child values.

CAFFEINE – TANNIN
COFFEE ARABICA
(Camellia sinensis)

Over one-third of the world's population regularly drink a caffeinated beverage. The average daily intake of caffeine is about 600 mg, that contained in about four cups of coffee, or eight cups of tea, or two cans of soft drink. The average 12-ounce soft drink contains at least five teaspoons of sugar. The combination of caffeine and sugar is a recipe for health problems. The nervous system is dependent on a regular supply of B vitamins. Caffeine restricts the absorption of B1 and B3 and inositol. Sugar depletes the reserves of B1, B2, B3, biotin, and the minerals calcium, phosphorus, and potassium. An excess of caffeine increases blood fatty acids, blood pressure, and cholesterol. It causes an irregular heartbeat and may inhibit DNA repair and transfer, leading to infertility. It may increase the risk of osteoporosis in women and worsen the symptoms of PMS. It affects fetal brain development and may cause breast cancer, insomnia, irritability, and nervousness.

On the other hand, research has shown positive factors in coffee, chocolate, and tea—but not in sugar! This is mainly due to the antioxidants contained in coffee and chocolate. In addition, the compound that gives coffee its aroma, trigonelline, promotes antibacterial activity. Caffeine increases the levels of cortisol, the antistress hormone, and endorphins, the natural painkiller, which may help to relieve headaches.

Green tea is a rich source of the polyphenol EGCG, or epigallocatechin gallate. It is a powerful antioxidant that may inhibit the growth of cancer cells, lower LDL cholesterol, and protect against blood clots. Green tea may reduce the risk of heart disease in smokers. It may also protect against rheumatoid arthritis, infection, impaired immune function, and cancer. Nearly 40% of the green tea leaf comprises polyphenols; the most important one is termed flavan-3-ols, or catechin, or flavonols.

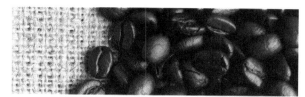

SMOKING – NICOTINE ($C_{10}H_{14}N_2$)

Nicotine is a very addictive drug.

After entering the lungs, nicotine enters the bloodstream and stimulates the adrenal glands. This causes an increased heartbeat, constriction of the arteries, and an increased conversion of glycogen, from the liver, thereby providing an energy burst. Nicotine also relaxes the muscles of the bronchi and lungs, causing "lazy lungs." The smoke and other chemicals in the cigarette damage lung tissues and arteries. Smokers may develop emphysema, heart problems, circulatory problems, poor eyesight, nervous disorders, recurrent colds, excess mucus, irritability, exhaustion, and nervousness.

Cigarette smoke contains, on average, at least 12 harmful compounds, including carbon monoxide, cyanide, and potassium nitrate. Nicotine can remain in the body and mind for many months—even years after a person has quit smoking. There are many nicotine alternatives and they can be very helpful while quitting. A cleansing diet of fresh fruit and vegetable juices will promote the release of nicotine from the body and reduce the urge for nicotine.

Smoking is a habit you will wish you never took up. It takes over your life, and quitting is so tough it's not worth it. If you don't smoke, don't start!

SMOKING—HEALTH PROBLEMS		
Problems	**Nutrient to Counteract**	**Foods**
Poor eyesight, infections, increased cholesterol, skin problems, poor blood condition, wrinkly skin, cancer, weak arteries, colds and flus	Vitamin C	Guava, red bell pepper, green bell pepper, currants, chili pepper, berries, parsley, lemon, oranges, papaya, kiwifruit, pineapple, broccoli
NUTRIENTS AND FOODS TO HELP PROTECT AGAINST SMOKING		
Cleanses the respiratory system	Sulfur	Garlic, carrot juice
Protect respiratory system from infections	Beta-carotene	Carrot juice, sweet potato
Decreases risk of lung cancer	Beta-cryptoxanthin	Pumpkin
Antioxidant, protects cells	Vitamin E	Wheat germ oil, sunflower seeds
Antioxidant, protects arteries	Vitamin C	Bell pepper, guava

NOTE: Nutrient amounts are listed as milligrams (mg) per 100 grams (g), unless otherwise stated.

MINERALS: SUMMARY OF FUNCTIONS

BROMINE: Glands, emotional stability, antidepressant, menopause, youthfulness.

CALCIUM: Bone growth, bone repair, digestion, glands, muscle action, teeth, blood clotting, nerves, tissue development, pregnancy, metabolism, sleep, skin, cellular growth.

CHLORINE: Protein digestion, heart action, blood pressure, cleansing, weight control, reproduction, acid–alkaline balance, fat digestion, skin, liver, pancreas, bile, hormones, hair.

CHROMIUM: Glucose metabolism, fat and protein synthesis, insulin effectiveness.

COBALT: Vitamin B12 structure, blood development, activates enzymes, body cell function, anemia, nerves, activate vitamin E, vitamin B12, healing, growth, energy.

COPPER: Iron utilization, blood development, skin/elastin production, healing, digestive system, tissue respiration, skin and hair pigment, nerve fiber protection, bones, cartilage, vitamin C absorption, anti-anemia.

FLUORINE: Eyes, skin, growth, blood, anti-infection, calcium metabolism, spine, iris, eyes.

IODINE: Thyroid gland, growth, energy production, fat and protein metabolism and oxidation, heartbeat, glands, mental stability, arteries, nerves, hair, nails, skin and teeth condition, vitamin A conversion, concentration, activate hormones, carbohydrate absorption.

IRON: Blood development, healing, respiratory system, anti-stress, anti-inflammatory, antibacterial, anti-viral, pregnancy, protein metabolism, growth, strength, childbirth, cell development, tissue repair, cleansing, menstruation, muscle power.

MAGNESIUM: Nervous system, bones, teeth, tissue development, digestion, acid–alkaline balance, mineral metabolism, blood pressure, arteries, brain, spine, memory, energy conversion, body temperature, muscular energy.

MANGANESE: Glands, blood development, memory, nervous system, metabolism, activates enzymes and vitamins, lactation, brain, skeletal system, sex hormone production, blood sugar control, iron effectiveness, insulin manufacture, bile and thyroxine production.

MOLYBDENUM: Iron utilization, oxidation of fats.

PHOSPHORUS: Nerves, blood circulation, energy distribution, bone growth, carbohydrate metabolism, strength, immune system, repair, concentration.

POTASSIUM: Muscular system, heart action, liver, brain, nerves, blood circulation, water balance, kidney function, growth, skin, digestion, glucose conversion, waste elimination, anti-stress, strength, alkalinity, blood pressure.

SELENIUM: Vitamin E effectiveness, fertility, antioxidant, elasticity of skin tissue, anti-premature aging, growth.

SILICON: Hair growth, skin and cell rejuvenation, calcium metabolism, strong bones and teeth, body cleansing, nervous system, blood circulation, perspiration, brain function, anti-infection, clear vision, skin repair, thyroid gland.

SODIUM: Acid–alkaline balance, saliva, carbohydrate digestion, blood pressure, arteries, lymphatic system, blood, elimination, calcium solubility, water balance, kidneys, youthfulness, pancreas, joint system.

SULFUR: Cleansing, purifying, liver, heart, muscles, growth, hair, skin, nerves, cell growth, insulin manufacture, metabolism.

VANADIUM: Blood circulation, low cholesterol, nervous system.

ZINC: Bone development, healing of bone fractures, children's growth, digestion of carbohydrates and protein, skin, hair and teeth condition, insulin action, vitamin action, tissue growth, reproduction, healing of burns and wounds, cell life, prostate gland, male hormone development, B-complex vitamin action, fatigue, low cholesterol, acne, diabetes, anti-infection.

NOTE: DV refers to the daily value for women 25–50 years, refer to RDI tables on pages 95–96 for adult male and child values.

Vitamins were determined to be essential nutrients over a century ago, but some vitamins have only recently been discovered. The word "vitamin" is derived from combining "vita," Latin for "life," plus "amine," from the word for a nitrogen-containing compound. Not all vitamins are amines, but that fact wasn't ascertained until the name had been established. The term was first introduced in 1912 by a Polish chemist, Casimir Funk, who recognized vitamins' existence and necessity for prevention of certain diseases.

Individual vitamins were mostly discovered by their availability from foods. Vitamins are the most intricate food substances. They exist in minute portions yet provide enormous benefits for protection from specific diseases and for activating numerous bodily functions.

Food processing, heat, and cooking deplete many vitamins, and the effects of stress, illness, and various risk factors greatly increase the need for vitamins to be obtained regularly from a variety of natural foods.

Vitamins are added to many processed foods to prevent against the development of well-recognized deficiency diseases, and many people purchase vitamin supplements in an effort to balance an inadequate dietary intake. However, one survey showed that 80% of people do not effectively absorb the vitamins from supplement tablets because the small intestine may create a barrier against such chemically isolated substances.

Only naturally produced vitamin supplements provide any benefits, and only natural foods provide these "essential food substances" in combinations with other vital ingredients to effectively activate their unique abilities to protect the human body from illness. There is no life without vitamins.

Over 200 common ailments are directly related to prolonged vitamin deficiency. This chapter lists numerous recognized functions associated with the various vitamins.

With 17 vitamins known to be essential for life, it is pushing the limits of nature to expect good health from a diet lacking in natural foods but full of processed foods, cooked foods, and canned foods. The results are evident in the increasing number of illnesses, hospital stays, and sick days.

Vitamins are absolutely required to transform your health into a positive state. Let your diet be full of the healing benefits afforded by the wide variety of natural foods. Just add exercise and fresh water!

NOTE: THE BODY SYSTEM NUMBERS CORRESPOND TO THE NUMBERS USED ON PAGES 177–191.

VITAMINS INTRODUCTION

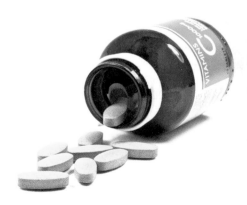

NOTE: *Nutrient amounts are listed as milligrams (mg) per 100 grams (g), unless otherwise stated.*

VITAMIN A – RETINOL/CAROTENE (FAT SOLUBLE)

13. IMMUNE SYSTEM

Vitamin A is most important in fighting infections as it provides strength to cell walls, which protect the inner parts of cells from attack by pollution and other toxins, and from viruses, bacteria, and other pathogenic organisms.

Vitamin A improves the functions of the white blood cells. Vitamin A increases immunity to disease and decreases the symptoms of colds and flu by retarding the spread of infection.

Carotenoids from plant sources provide powerful antioxidant action to protect cells from the effects of free radicals from cooked oils and processed foods. Beta-carotene is the most potent antioxidant carotenoid. Smoking depletes the store of carotenoids in the body.

Carotenoids improve cellular connections and may therefore prevent the development of cancerous cells. The antioxidant action of carotenoids may also prevent cancer formation.

17. SKIN SYSTEM

A prolonged deficiency of carotenoids increases the risk of diseases. Vitamin A is vital for the growth of healthy skin and hair and especially for the repair of damaged skin tissues and reduction of scar tissue.

Vitamin A is required for the removal of dead skin cells.

Teenage acne is usually due to changing hormonal balance, especially in the pituitary gland. However, such factors as emotional stress and a poor diet rich in cooked fats or chocolate and processed foods all contribute to the temporary problem. Vitamin A can assist in balancing hormonal function, cleansing skin tissues, and rebuilding damaged tissues.

A regular intake of carrot juice is hard to beat for skin benefits, especially as it is the sweetest source of organic sulfur, the ultimate skin-cleansing mineral.

16. REPRODUCTIVE SYSTEM

Vitamin A is required for the synthesis of RNA, a nucleic acid that assists in the transmission of hormones and chemical messengers for the reproduction of hereditary characteristics.

A deficiency of vitamin A can lead to impaired reproduction.

12. GROWTH SYSTEM

Vitamin A is essential for all cellular and bone growth. Vitamin A is also required for the effective use and metabolism of the minerals calcium and phosphorus, thereby promoting growth.

15. OPTIC SYSTEM

Vitamin A is essential for good eyesight, especially in dim lighting. The retina stores vitamin A within four optic pigments; the one used in dim lighting is termed "rhodopsin," or visual purple. The other three optic pigments are collectively termed iodopsins and are required for normal daylight vision.

Vitamin A is also required for peripheral or side vision and for correct color vision. A deficiency of vitamin A can lead to poor vision and cornea disorders, and a prolonged deficiency may cause blindness.

2. DIGESTIVE SYSTEM

Vitamin A is required for the secretion of gastric juices, which are required for protein digestion. Low-protein diets may restrict the effective use of vitamin A.

For people having difficulty in digesting fats, a deficiency of this vitamin may persist.

Alcohol consumption causes a loss of vitamin A via the liver.

Sweet potato, winter squash, and pumpkin are excellent sources of vitamin A carotene.

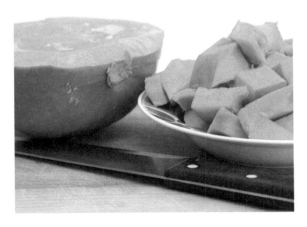

NOTE: DV refers to the daily value for women 25–50 years, refer to RDI tables on pages 95–96 for adult male and child values.

VITAMIN A

VITAMIN A — RETINOL/CAROTENE (FAT SOLUBLE)

7. RESPIRATORY SYSTEM

Vitamin A protects the delicate linings of the throat, mouth, trachea, nose, and lungs from infection, pollution, dust, and smoke. Vitamin A increases resistance of these mucus membranes against infections from bacteria and viruses.

There are three forms of conversion from food-based vitamin A (retinyl palmitate) into usable vitamin A, which is a fat-soluble compound. The most effective form for the respiratory system is retinoic acid, which is essential for the health of tissues within the lungs and trachea. These mucosal tissues protect against invading airborne pathogens.

The other forms of retinyl palmitate are retinol and retinal.

Research has shown that beta-cryptoxanthin provides great benefit to the respiratory system, in particular the lungs. A decreased risk of lung cancer for smokers was traced to an increased supply of beta-cryptoxanthin.

Pumpkin and winter squash are the best sources of beta-cryptoxanthin, with over 2,000 mcg/100 g serving.

Carrots supply 75 mcg of beta-cryptoxanthin, over 5,500 mcg of beta-carotene, and over 2,500 mcg of alpha-carotene.

5. MUSCULAR SYSTEM

Vitamin A is required for the growth of muscular tissues and for the repair of damaged tissues.

Retinoic acid from food-based vitamin A is required for the synthesis of glycoproteins to assist the joining of cells within tissues.

Vitamin A is a fat-soluble vitamin that can be stored in the liver for a few days or weeks, depending on conditions of stress and illness.

There are two main forms of vitamin A:
Preformed vitamin A — retinol (animal sources)
Proformed vitamin A — carotenoids (plants)

In 1974, the USDA introduced a way to calculate both forms of vitamin A:

RETINOL ACTIVITY EQUIVALENTS (RE)
1 RE = 1 mcg retinol
1 RE = 6 mcg beta-carotene
1 RE = 3.333 International Units (IU)

There are a few forms of carotenoids from plants that the body can convert into vitamin A; the most easily converted is beta-carotene.

About one-third of the carotene content in food is converted into usable vitamin A.

When starch foods are cooked, the carotene content is easier to absorb, meaning more vitamin A is obtained.

There are five main types of carotene:
1. alpha-carotene
2. beta-carotene
3. beta-cryptoxanthin
4. lutein
5. zeaxanthin

Diabetics may be unable to convert carotene from plant foods into usable vitamin A.

Cod liver oil, fish oils, liver, butter, and cheese all provide vitamin A (retinol).

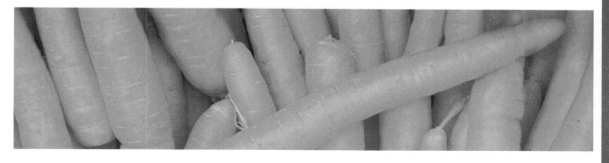

NOTE: Nutrient amounts are listed as milligrams (mg) per 100 grams (g), unless otherwise stated.

VITAMIN C – ASCORBIC ACID (WATER SOLUBLE)

17. SKIN SYSTEM

A daily intake of vitamin C is required for numerous functions—for example, the development of collagen, the substance that holds skin cells together. Conditions such as dry skin, wrinkles, easy bruising, and splitting hair may all be caused by a prolonged vitamin C deficiency, or to intermittent supplies that cause the body to go without for a few days.

Vitamin C is vital for prevention of and relief from skin infections that are caused by burns, wounds, and sports injuries.

13. IMMUNE SYSTEM

Vitamin C is the most active water-soluble antioxidant. To maintain a strong immune system, daily intake of vitamin C-rich foods is essential, especially for people who smoke or suffer from stress-related conditions. Vitamin C is the best known vitamin, especially to offset colds and winter viruses. Human cells, when subjected to a solution of vitamin C, were able to produce increased amounts of interferon, a substance that the body produces to protect cells from viruses.

Vitamin C increases the number and activity of white blood cells with normal intake from natural foods. Ideally vitamin C needs bioflavonoids, such as the white pith of citrus fruits and bell peppers to be fully active and effective.

Vitamin C protects cells from oxygen-based damage due to ailments such as cancer and cardiovascular disease. When children are scheduled to have vaccinations, ensure that their vitamin C levels are adequate. Vitamin C promotes the absorption of iron, and for body cleansing and elimination of toxins, both vitamin C and iron-rich foods are essential. Medications and drugs can diminish the body's store of precious vitamin C.

3. GLANDULAR SYSTEM

Vitamin C is essential for the health of the adrenal glands, and during conditions of stress, vitamin C is released from the adrenal glands. The liver requires vitamin C for elimination of toxins. Vitamin C protects against glandular infections such as tonsillitis, glandular fever, and mumps.

15. OPTIC SYSTEM

Vitamin C is required daily for the health of the optic system. The lens of the eye needs vitamin C, and a prolonged deficiency may cause poor vision.

2. DIGESTIVE SYSTEM

Vitamin C is required to convert cholesterol into bile acids. It is also vital for effective absorption of the mineral iron and for storage of iron in the bone marrow. Vitamin C protects against excess acidity and promotes the storage of folate for blood development and prevention of anemia. Ideally, vitamin C foods are obtained at most meals of the day, especially breakfast. Fat molecules that are transported around the body require vitamin C for protection from oxidation.

OTHER SYSTEMS

Vitamin C is required for the health of the nervous system. It has been called the "youth vitamin" because it preserves skin tissue. The older we are, the more vitamin C we need. Vitamin C can last in the body for 10–20 hours under normal conditions. Stress, smoking, injury, viruses, disease, colds, and infections can reduce vitamin C levels. Vitamin C and bioflavonoids are vital for the strength of arteries and capillaries. Vitamin C is important for children's growth and for the proper formation of their teeth.

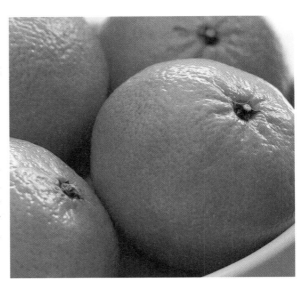

NOTE: DV refers to the daily value for women 25–50 years, refer to RDI tables on pages 95–96 for adult male and child values.

VITAMIN E – D-ALPHA-TOCOPHEROL (FAT SOLUBLE)

Vitamin E is the common name for a group of fat-soluble substances known as tocopherols and tocotrienols.

There are four main types of each: alpha, beta, delta, and gamma. The most potent forms of vitamin E are natural *d*-alpha and d-gamma tocopherol and tocotrienol. Numerous types of vitamin E supplements are available, but to be sure that it is natural vitamin E, the label must read: *d*-alpha-tocopherol or tocotrienol.

1. CIRCULATORY SYSTEM

Vitamin E assists with blood circulation by enlarging blood vessels and arteries, which provide both oxygen and nourishment to all body cells. Vitamin E (tocotrienols in particular) lowers blood cholesterol.

10. CELLULAR SYSTEM

Every cell in the body lives by burning oxygen to produce energy and warmth. Vitamin E regulates this action and prevents cells from burning out too quickly. The normal life of a healthy red blood cell is 120 days; a deficiency of vitamin E can reduce cell life to 70 days.

Vitamin E improves the number, activity, and potency of male sperm cells. Vitamin E preserves the walls of the red blood cells and prevents their destruction from oxidative stress.

Vitamin E is also essential for the transfer of cellular information within cells and to other cells. Because vitamin E is fat soluble, it links to fat membranes within and outside cells to protect against oxidation, thereby promoting life and (gaining the title "antiaging vitamin").

3. GLANDULAR SYSTEM

Vitamin E promotes the function of the pituitary and adrenal glands in the production of hormones.

5. MUSCULAR SYSTEM

Vitamin E increases the power and activity of muscles and improves their endurance by increasing the supply of oxygen and the lifespan of muscular cells. Vitamin E strengthens the heart muscles.

7. RESPIRATORY SYSTEM

Vitamin E strengthens the heart muscles. In combination with vitamin C, selenium, and vitamin B3, it protects the lungs from pollution due to the powerful antiperoxidase action of tocopherols and tocotrienols.

2. DIGESTIVE SYSTEM

Vitamin E helps regulate the body's use of dietary fats and proteins. Daily use of margarine and polyunsaturated fats greatly increases the need for vitamin E. Low vitamin E levels may lead to diseases of the pancreas, gallbladder, liver, and bladder, and to nervous disorders and celiac disease.

16. REPRODUCTIVE SYSTEM

Vitamin E promotes the activity of the ovaries and assists the body with normal menstruation. Vitamin E promotes blood supply to the unborn baby. It improves the potency of the male sperm cell. It is vital for normal fertility in both men and women.

The synthetic female hormone estrogen is a vitamin E antagonist.

The name tocopherol is derived from the Greek words *tocos,* meaning "childbirth," and *pherin*, meaning "to bring forth."

17. SKIN SYSTEM

Natural vitamin E foods protect the skin from ultraviolet radiation from sunlight and also promote the healing of burns and damaged skin tissues.

NOTE: Nutrient amounts are listed as milligrams (mg) per 100 grams (g), unless otherwise stated.

VITAMIN D – LUMISTEROL CALCIFEROL (FAT SOLUBLE)

8. SKELETAL SYSTEM

Vitamin D is produced by the action of sunlight on skin cells, which converts cholesterol into a form known as cholecalciferol, or provitamin D. It is transferred to the liver and converted into the form of calcitriol, or active vitamin D. The parathyroid glands use calcitriol to control calcium metabolism.

Vitamin D also assists in the absorption of phosphorus.

During winter adequate sunlight is required, preferably at least 15 minutes per day. In summer, especially in tropical areas, it is best to avoid sunlight during the hours of 11 a.m. and 3 p.m., due to the intense ultraviolet radiation.

Vitamin D can be stored in the body for many days, but during times of constant indoor work, clouds, rain, or snow, it is best to obtain vitamin D from cod liver oil, fish, or eggs.

2. DIGESTIVE SYSTEM

Vitamin D is essential for good digestion and the metabolism of numerous minerals and vitamins. The thyroid gland requires vitamin D for the control of digestion.

12. GROWTH SYSTEM

Vitamin D is essential for children's growth. Children require nearly twice as much vitamin D as adults, but beware of midday sun, and have kids wear hats during summer whenever they're outside.

3. GLANDULAR SYSTEM

The thyroid, parathyroid, pituitary, pineal, and adrenal glands require vitamin D for their activity.

6. NERVOUS SYSTEM

The nervous system requires nutrients that are activated by the effects of vitamin D, such as phosphorus, calcium, and magnesium.

VITAMIN K – PHYLLOQUINONE (FAT SOLUBLE)

9. BLOOD SYSTEM

Vitamin K is the key factor in the processes of blood coagulation and clotting. A substance in the blood known as prothrombin is formed by the action of vitamin K. At the site of abrasion or bleeding, the converted form of thrombin acts on the fibrinogen of plasma and converts it into the substance fibrin, which traps the red cells into a mesh, forming clots. Vitamin K has proved effective in reducing blood loss during menstruation. Vitamin K is required for blood circulation, and it assists the functions of the liver and heart.

2. DIGESTIVE SYSTEM

Vitamin K is required for the conversion of carbohydrates into glycogen, which is stored in the liver and converted into glucose when activity levels increase.

Vitamin K is absorbed from the upper section of the small intestines and in combination with bile it is transferred to the liver until required for blood clotting.

OTHER FACTORS

Vitamin K is best obtained from fresh green leafy vegetables, especially lettuce. Freezing and prolonged cooking deplete the supply of vitamin K. The older we are, the more vitamin K we need. Vitamin K protects the liver from lead pollution.

Regular use of aspirin, antibiotics, mineral oils, and exposure to X rays can destroy the vitamin K intestinal bacteria within the human body. Acidophilus yogurt helps to restore natural bacteria to the intestines and promotes the production and synthesis of internal vitamin K. Babies are given vitamin K at birth to promote healthy development of blood cells.

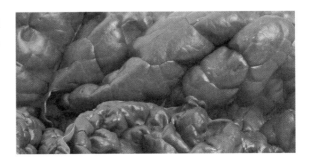

VITAMIN D | VITAMIN K

NOTE: DV refers to the daily value for women 25–50 years, refer to RDI tables on pages 95–96 for adult male and child values.

VITAMIN F – OMEGA-3 (ALPHA-LINOLENIC ACID),OMEGA-6 (LINOLEIC ACID)

Vitamin F was the original term for the essential fatty acids (EFAs): alpha linolenic acid, or omega-3, and linoleic acid, or omega-6. Some people still use the term "vitamin F," but most prefer "esssential fatty acids."

Neither omega-3 nor omega-6 can be produced by the body and *must be supplied through the diet. That's why they're called "essential."* They are crucial to life and must be balanced to ensure good health. Excess intake of omega-6 is fairly common, mainly from margarine and vegetable oils, but the intake of omega-3 is often inadequate. Excess omega-6 interferes with the unique functions of omega-3. The ideal dietary intake is one part omega-3 to two parts omega-6. The average diet may consist of 1 part omega-3 to 25 parts omega-6. This huge imbalance is due to a few factors: the big increase in consumption of margarine and other omega-6 foods, and the limited natural sources of omega-3. Foods such as pumpkin seeds (pepitas), walnuts, flaxseed oil, and canola oil are excellent sources of omega-3. Fish, seafood, egg yolk, pecans, and hazelnuts are good sources.

17. SKIN SYSTEM

Omega-3 helps to maintain resilience and lubrication of skin cells. Omega-3 foods promote healthy hair and hair growth and supple, youthful skin. The cellular system requires omega-3 in particular to retain water and vital nutrients. The types of fats contained in the diet greatly dictate the condition of individual cells. Excess saturated fats cause cells to become hard and to lack fluidity, and inhibit the storage of nutrients.

10. CELLULAR SYSTEM

Omega-3 protects against tumors and breast cancer by retarding the action of enzymes that damage cells. Omega-3 is vital for the cells of the nervous system, for development of sex hormones, and for healthy intestinal bacteria.

13. IMMUNE SYSTEM

Omega-3 is the key nutrient to offset inflammatory conditions such as back pain, asthma, bowel inflammation, rheumatoid arthritis, autoimmune diseases, joint stiffness, swelling, chronic fatigue, and atherosclerosis.

Omega-6 fats promote inflammatory reactions in molecules; in contrast, omega-3 helps to produce hormones known as prostaglandins that reduce inflammation.

19. BRAIN SYSTEM

Omega-3 is vital for brain development, especially DHA omega-3. No wonder fish is termed a "brain food." The brain is composed of 60% fat. It requires large amounts of DHA omega-3, especially in the first two years of life. Research shows that infants from mothers who have a high omega-3 blood level have advanced levels of learning and attention spans. Mother's milk transfers DHA to the baby when the mother's dietary intake includes omega-3 foods. Postnatal depression may be linked to a deficiency of DHA omega-3, as the baby will obtain as much as necessary from the mother. In addition, mental health conditions such as depression, mood swings, bipolar disorder, schizophrenia, and dementia can be traced to a deficiency of omega-3. Brain cell receptors require omega-3 to help direct a smooth and efficient neuron signal connection within a very complex brain system and integrated nervous system. Omega-3 promotes concentration.

1. CIRCULATORY SYSTEM

Omega-3 promotes low cholesterol levels, a regular heartbeat, reduced blood pressure, and protection from coronary disease. Omega-3 also helps thin the blood, preventing blood clots and strokes. Meat supplies no omega-3, except for venison and buffalo meat.

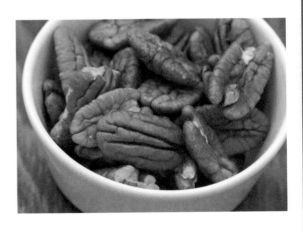

VITAMIN P – FLAVONOIDS

Vitamin P was the original term for the substances known as flavonoids (or bioflavonoids). The term has mostly fallen out of use. Nearly all brightly colored red, orange, blue, and yellow fruits and vegetables contain flavonoids. There are a few groups of flavonoids: flavonols, anthocyanins, anthocyanidins, dihydroflavonols, flavanones, and isoflavones. Within these groups there are numerous other forms of flavonoids; for example, within the group of flavonols the common forms are hesperidin, rutin, and quercetin.

Most flavonoids provide antioxidant activity and help prevent cellular damage.

13. IMMUNE SYSTEM

The immune system's functions are greatly enhanced by flavonoids, mainly due to the fact that they increase the antioxidant activity of vitamin C. The white pith of citrus fruits and bell peppers is full of flavonoids. Bottled orange juice may contain vitamin C, usually added, but the supply of flavonoids is often lacking. During conditions of stress and inflammation due to injury, flavonoids regulate the activity of the immune system to protect against over-activity of cells, which can lead to excess inflammation. In conditions such as joint inflammation, back injuries, spinal inflammation, various allergies, viruses, and tumors, flavonoids reduce the pain and symptoms by decreasing reactive cell activity.

The flavonoid quercetin, contained in apples, may help alleviate allergies by retarding histamine production. Flavonoids protect against high blood pressure by blocking the action of the enzyme angiosten. In addition, flavonoids such as rutin, found in buckwheat, are most beneficial for strengthening blood capillaries. They may protect against varicose veins and aid the entire vascular system by helping to develop strong cells.

15. OPTIC SYSTEM

Flavonoids may provide protection from cataracts (clouding of the eyes), especially in diabetics. Excess blood sugar levels produce alcohol sugars that can cause cataracts.

17. SKIN SYSTEM

The flavonol anthocyanidin is known to help strengthen and connect strands of collagen (skin protein).

Flavonoids can also protect against skin infections, bacteria, and fungus.

10. CELLULAR SYSTEM

Isoflavones such as genistein, found in soy products and some legumes, can block enzymes that cause tumor growths in uterine, breast, and prostate cancer, reducing the risk of ovarian and breast cancer.

Flavonoids can protect against recurrent nose bleeding, easy bruising, and platelet aggregation. They may also be required to prevent the development of leukemia and hemophilia. Flavonoids regulate the permeability of blood capillaries.

Flavonoids regulate the activity of immune system cells such as B cells, T cells, NK cells, and others, thereby aiding in the proper functioning of the immune system. Flavonoids provide antiviral activity; they may help in cases of HIV and herpes by retarding the activity of other infections that attempt to develop. Flavonoids also provide antibiotic action, protecting the body against harmful bacteria. Flavonoids protect LDL cholesterol from possible oxidation by the action of free radicals.

Flavonoids, in addition to vitamin C and the mineral iron, may protect against the common cold.

Flavonoids are destroyed by the processing of foods.

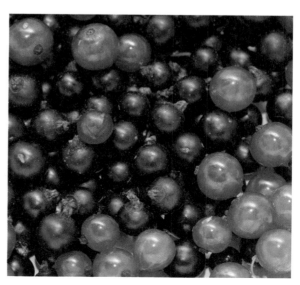

NOTE: DV refers to the daily value for women 25–50 years, refer to RDI tables on pages 95–96 for adult male and child values.

VITAMIN P

VITAMIN B1 – THIAMINE (WATER SOLUBLE)

6. NERVOUS SYSTEM

A sufficient daily intake of vitamin B1 is required for the health of the nervous system. The body can only store limited amounts of the vitamin; during conditions of stress, physical exercise, and depression, increased intake of B1 is essential. The nervous system requires B1 for the development of the myelin sheaths, the fat layer covering nerve endings. A deficiency of B1 can result in damage to the nerve endings.

In addition, B1 is essential for the production of a neurotransmitter called acetylcholine, which activates muscle action. A deficiency may lead to sciatica, muscle cramps, poor coordination, tiredness, lack of concentration, and compromised learning ability.

Alcohol depletes the reserves of this vitamin; excess alcohol intake can increase the need for B1 by a factor of 10 to 100.

2. DIGESTIVE SYSTEM

The process of digestion is dependent on B1; it is required for the conversion of glucose into energy and for the production of hydrochloric acid for protein digestion. The substance allicin, contained in garlic and onions, increases the absorption of thiamine.

A deficiency of B1 can lead to loss of appetite, anorexia, accumulation of fat in the arteries, constipation, and stomach ulcers.

Vitamin B1 is vital for children's growth because it helps to increase their appetite and enhances the absorption of nutrients from foods. It is essential to increase the intake of vitamin B1 during pregnancy and lactation, and it is vital for adult fertility.

Thiamine increases oxygen absorption within blood, which promotes mental function and physical activity. Intake of caffeine, antibiotics, and the contraceptive pill deplete vitamin B1 by acting as diuretics, which remove water-soluble vitamins.

VITAMIN B2 – RIBOFLAVIN (WATER SOLUBLE)

15. OPTIC SYSTEM

Vitamin B2 is vital for the optic system because it promotes cell respiration and the body's use of oxygen. It also aids in the recycling of enzymes that protect the body from oxidation.

A deficiency of B2 may result in cataracts, sensitivity to light, blurred vision, itching eyes, burning sensation in the eyes, and dimness of vision.

17. SKIN SYSTEM

Vitamin B2 is required for healthy skin by promoting cell respiration and cellular growth. A deficiency of B2 may result in conditions such as cracked skin near the corners of the mouth, dermatitis, acne, oily skin, peeling skin, and sore lips, tongue, and mouth.

A deficiency may also contribute to baldness and weight loss. Alcohol, stress, and excess physical exertion can lead to a deficiency, while antibiotics, the pill, and various drugs cause a loss of vitamin B2.

2. DIGESTIVE SYSTEM

Vitamin B2 is required for the secretion of protein-digestive enzymes and the absorption of numerous nutrients. Vitamin B2 promotes the supply and conversion of other vitamins such as B3, B6, folate, and vitamin K into active forms.

Vitamin B2 is essential for the production of energy from carbohydrates, proteins, and lipids. It attaches to protein enzymes and promotes oxygen and energy production, especially in the heart and skeletal muscles. Riboflavin is stable to heat, cooking, acids, and air, but it is destroyed by light and alkalis. Processing destroys over 70% of a food's B2 content.

B2 protects against baldness, anemia, migraine, and lack of energy. It is vital during pregnancy and lactation and for children's growth and development.

VITAMIN B1 | VITAMIN B2

VITAMIN B3 – NIACIN (WATER SOLUBLE)

17. SKIN SYSTEM

Vitamin B3 is important for healthy skin, but an excess intake of B3 supplements can cause a red skin rash.

2. DIGESTIVE SYSTEM

Vitamin B3 is essential for the conversion of fats. It controls the release of fats for energy and for production of cell membranes. It is also required for the production of cholesterol within the liver and for the efficient use of protein.

A deficiency of B3 may lead to indigestion, constipation, diarrhea, and other digestive disturbances. A deficiency can also show as muscular weakness and poor appetite, and can lead to dermatitis, cataracts, and skin allergies.

Vitamin B3 is a most stable B vitamin; it is not destroyed by cooking, heat, acids, alkalis, air, or light. Conditions of stress, trauma, fever, intake of the contraceptive pill, and excess alcohol consumption can lead to a vitamin B3 deficiency.

Vitamin B3 assists the functioning of the digestive enzymes. It is vital for conversion of all food groups into usable energy and for the storage of starch glucose in the liver as glycogen.

Vitamin B3 is vital for the brain and normal mental functions; a prolonged deficiency may lead to Alzhiemer's disease and other age-related mental conditions. Vitamin B3 is also obtainable via the conversion of the amino acid tryptophan.

OTHER FACTORS

The hormone insulin is dependent on a regular supply of vitamin B3 for blood sugar regulation and proper insulin activity. B3 is an essential ingredient in the production of both male and female hormones for reproduction. Vitamin B3 promotes a peaceful night's sleep, and it is required for the production of DNA (deoxyribonucleic acid).

VITAMIN B5 – PANTOTHENIC ACID (WATER SOLUBLE)

2. DIGESTIVE SYSTEM

Vitamin B5 is essential for the transport of fatty acids within body cells. It is required for the release of energy from stored fats and for the synthesis of cholesterol.

The word "panto" means "everywhere," and without a doubt vitamin B5 is located in every cell. It is essential for white blood cell production, for the utilization of carbohydrates and proteins, and for the functioning of vitamin B2. A deficiency of vitamin B5 may lead to abdominal pains, kidney damage, and ulcers.

3. GLANDULAR SYSTEM

Vitamin B5 is essential for the health of the adrenal glands and for the production of the hormone adrenaline, which kicks in during an acute stress response. Vitamin B5 is destroyed by cooking and processing; frozen foods may lose up to 70% of their B5 content. Vitamin B5 may protect against chronic fatigue syndrome and arthritis.

6. NERVOUS SYSTEM

Vitamin B5 is essential for the growth and development of the nervous system. A deficiency of vitamin B5 often shows as fatigue and weakness because nerve disorders produce weak muscle action along with pins and needles in the hands and feet. Vitamin B5 has beneficial effects in conditions such as insomnia, psychosomatic disorders, cramps, depression, apathy, and unstable heart action.

Vitamin B5 is required for the production of antibodies to fight infection; it protects cells against radiation and is essential for the development of healthy fats in cells. Vitamin B5 assists chemical processes in cells—such as with hormone production—and helps to protect cells from chemical breakdown. Vitamin B5 promotes healthy skin and hair and also assists the functions of the liver.

VITAMIN B3 | VITAMIN B5

NOTE: DV refers to the daily value for women 25–50 years, refer to RDI tables on pages 95–96 for adult male and child values.

VITAMIN B6 – PYRIDOXINE, PYRIDOXAL, PYRIDOXAMINE (WATER SOLUBLE)

6. NERVOUS SYSTEM

Vitamin B6, also referred to as the "vitality vitamin," participates in the activity of over one hundred enzyme reactions and is vital for the transfer of nerve responses throughout the nervous system. A deficiency of B6 can lead to headaches, poor memory, irritability, convulsions, nervousness, depression, confusion, and oversensitivity. It has been used effectively in the treatment of Parkinson's disease. Vitamin B6 is a vital component in the production of the nerve transmitters epinephrine, seratonin, norepinephrine, and melatonin. Excess vitamin B6 supplementation can be detrimental to the nervous system.

2. DIGESTIVE SYSTEM

Vitamin B6 assists in the production of gastric juices for protein digestion. In addition, vitamin B6 is required in the construction of amino acids, for the conversion of tryptophan into niacin, for the absorption of vitamin B12, and for the metabolism of carbohydrates, especially the conversion of glycogen (the form of glucose stored in muscle cells and the liver) into usable energy. A prolonged deficiency of vitamin B6 may contribute to acne, eczema, and dermatitis. The master gland of the body, the pituitary gland, requires vitamin B6 to promote normal metabolism. The contraceptive pill, estrogen therapy, and some medications can deplete the body's reserves of vitamin B6. Processing and cooking can cause up to a 95% reduction in a food's B6 value.

9. BLOOD SYSTEM

The development of white blood cells, hemoglobin, and adrenaline all require vitamin B6.

Vitamin B6 is vital during pregnancy to offset nausea. It helps to rid the blood of harmful toxins and is required for DNA manufacture.

VITAMIN B12 – COBALAMIN (WATER SOLUBLE)

9. BLOOD SYSTEM

Vitamin B12 is stored in the liver, kidneys, and various body tissues. It is vital for the proper formation of blood. The mineral cobalt has a central role in the development of vitamin B12, hence the name cobalamin.

Foods rich in folate and iron, such as parsley, protect against red cell retardation and anemia.

2. DIGESTIVE SYSTEM

Within the stomach a special mucoprotein termed "intrinsic factor" is essential for vitamin B12 to be absorbed later in the small intestine. Excess use of antacids and stomach ulcer medications can deplete the intrinsic factor. Vitamin B12 is also required for the metabolism of carbohydrates and fats and the utilization of amino acids throughout the body.

6. NERVOUS SYSTEM

Vitamin B12 is an important component in the formation of the protective layer of nerve cells, the myelin sheaths.

Vegan mothers need to be aware that infant and children can develop nerve and muscular problems from a deficiency of vitamin B12 foods.

OTHER FACTORS

Plants, animals, and humans cannot produce vitamin B12; it is made by bacteria, algae, molds, yeasts, and fungi.

For vegetarians, foods such as yogurt and cheese provide a good supply of vitamin B12.

Seafood such as clams, oysters, and fish are an excellent source of B12. Vitamin B12 is heat sensitive; up to 80% can be lost in cooking.

Vitamin B12 can be recycled in the body for several years.

VITAMIN B6 | VITAMIN B12

NOTE: Nutrient amounts are listed as milligrams (mg) per 100 grams (g), unless otherwise stated.

VITAMIN B15 – PANGAMIC ACID (WATER SOLUBLE)

1. CIRCULATORY SYSTEM

Vitamin B15 has not been classified as an essential vitamin; however, it participates in certain vital functions, such as blood circulation and the improved utilization of oxygen. Vitamin B15 helps to protect against carbon monoxide pollution. It has helped to improve conditions of angina, hypertension, arteriosclerosis, and heart disease due to its ability to lower cholesterol and improve cell life. Vitamin B15 has proved effective in the treatment of hypoxia, a shortage of oxygen.

Excessive perspiration causes a loss of B15.

13. IMMUNE SYSTEM

Vitamin B15 functions as a detoxifying agent against cancer-causing chemicals, especially against environmental pollutants. Vitamin B15 was discovered in 1951 by Dr. Ernst Krebs in apricot kernels. It extends cell life and works as an antioxidant. It may also provide benefit in cases of hepatitis, cirrhosis of the liver, and emphysema.

19. BRAIN SYSTEM

Vitamin B15 helps to stabilize emotional and mental problems, and as a supplement it has proved beneficial in cases of autism. One study showed a considerable improvement in the speech of mentally impaired children, as well as better concentration and greater interest in toys and games. It has been used in the treatment of Alzheimer's disease, diabetes, liver disease, alcoholism, trauma, stress, senility, and athletic injuries. Vitamin B15 assists in protein synthesis, is beneficial for the prevention of premature aging, and helps to neutralize alcohol cravings.

BIOTIN – COENZYME R, VITAMIN H, VITAMIN B7 (WATER SOLUBLE)

17. SKIN SYSTEM

Biotin is essential for the production of healthy skin cells and tissues. It assists in the maintenance and repair of bones. During pregnancy and lactation, additional intake of biotin foods is vital to protect against sudden infant death syndrome (SIDS) and various birth defects. One study showed that nearly 50% of pregnant women were deficient in biotin. Raw egg white, which contains the glycoprotein avidin, inhibits the absorption of biotin, and a deficiency of vitamin B5 can also lead to a biotin deficiency. Baldness may also result from a prolonged biotin deficiency.

2. DIGESTIVE SYSTEM

Biotin is essential for the conversion of fatty foods into individual cells, as it activates the enzyme that is vital for cell construction. Biotin also promotes the conversion of blood sugar—glucose—into a usable form of energy. It protects against digestive disorders such as irritable bowel syndrome, ulcerative colitis, and diarrhea.

Biotin can be synthesized by intestinal bacteria in favorable conditions. Antibiotics and mineral oils may upset the intestinal bacteria. Most processed cereals have no biotin. Such nutrients as folic acid, vitamins B5 and B12, protein, and carbohydrates need biotin for their full effectiveness and utilization.

A biotin deficiency may contribute to overweight because it is essential for the conversion of fats.

6. NERVOUS SYSTEM

Biotin is vital for the nervous system and may protect against the development of poor muscle and nerve coordination, seizures, muscle cramps, and poor muscle tone. Biotin is stable to oxygen, cooking, and light.

VITAMIN B15 | BIOTIN

NOTE: DV refers to the daily value for women 25–50 years, refer to RDI tables on pages 95–96 for adult male and child values.

CHOLINE (WATER SOLUBLE)

2. DIGESTIVE SYSTEM

Choline is usually classed among the B vitamins. It converts fats into smaller water-soluble substances, a role similar to that of bile. This function promotes the distribution of fat-soluble nutrients into the bloodstream and into developing cells, which are primarily made of fats. The name comes from "chole," which is taken from the Greek word for "bile."

Choline needs the other B-complex vitamins to be effective, especially folate and vitamin B3.

6. NERVOUS SYSTEM

Choline is essential for the nervous system; it is vital for the prevention and treatment of such conditions as Parkinson's disease, attention deficit disorder, Alzheimer's disease, autism, poor memory, hyperactivity, and various other nervous conditions. Most processed foods are deficient in choline.

The substance known as lecithin, made from corn or soybeans and available as a supplement, is vital for the replenishment of choline reserves. The body can only produce lecithin when it has sufficient choline.

19. BRAIN SYSTEM

The brain needs lecithin to function properly; over 28% of brain matter is composed of lecithin. Research has shown that in mentally impaired persons lecithin content in the brain is often as low as 19%. Stress and nervousness rapidly use up lecithin reserves. Lecithin is a natural tranquilizer; it promotes a good night's sleep and protects against fatigue and insomnia.

A deficiency of choline can lead to cardiovascular disease, renal failure, hardened arteries, high blood pressure, weak blood capillaries, high cholesterol, infertility, liver disorders, and obesity.

Choline can be made with healthy intestinal bacteria.

FOLATE – FOLIC ACID (VITAMIN B9)

9. BLOOD SYSTEM

Folate is essential for the development of red blood cells; it shares this role with cobalt, iron, manganese, and vitamins B12 and C. Increased folate intake is vital during pregnancy; it is required for reproduction and in the formation of genetic material such as DNA and RNA, which cannot divide properly without folate. It is vital for the prevention of blood disorders such as cardiovascular disease, anemia, and poor circulation.

A folate deficiency may contribute to childhood leukemia.

Folate reduces blood levels of harmful homocysteine and protects against such conditions as dementia and Alzheimer's disease. One report showed a fourfold increase in those ailments when folate levels were low and homocysteine levels were high.

Folate is destroyed by high temperatures, cooking, and lengthy storage. Antibiotics, alcohol, the contraceptive pill, and excess acids also reduce folate levels. Increased folate intake is required during periods of infection, mental fatigue, depression, insomnia, and irritability.

10. CELLULAR SYSTEM

Folate is vital for the correct transfer of nerve messages and for cellular growth and reproduction. It is vital for the production of new cells; a deficiency can cause skin conditions such as vitiligo, gingivitis, and cleft palate.

Various forms of cancer are related to a folate deficiency, including lung, cervical, intestinal, and esophageal cancer.

"Folate" is derived from the Latin word for "foliage" or "leaf." Green leafy vegetables are good dietary sources of folate. Folate is vital for children's growth; infants require more folate than adults. Protein is required for proper folate absorption.

INOSITOL – MYO-INOSITOL (WATER SOLUBLE)

1. CIRCULATORY SYSTEM

Inositol, a B-complex vitamin, is required for the health of arteries; it increases their elasticity, thereby protecting against hardened arteries. Inositol is important for the metabolism of fats and cholesterol and may help to reduce blood cholesterol levels. Similar to choline, inositol assists in the movement of fats from the liver and muscles; it is a component of the cell membrane and is required for the transfer of hormones and nerve impulses within cells.

6. NERVOUS SYSTEM

Inositol is often considered a nonessential vitamin because it can be made by the body from intestinal bacteria and glucose. Howevere, for people who regularly consume caffeine, including tea, chocolate, cola drinks, and coffee, it really is an essential vitamin as caffeine destroys inositol.

A deficiency can lead to a deteriorating nervous system including conditions of anxiety, insomnia, and nervousness. Inositol is required within fat cells to assist in nerve transmission.

10. CELLULAR SYSTEM

Inositol is an essential component in the proper formation and construction of new cells.

Inositol is necessary for hair growth; a prolonged deficiency may contribute to baldness. Diabetics excrete an elevated amount of inositol.

16. REPRODUCTIVE SYSTEM

Inositol is essential for reproduction. A prolonged deficiency may cause infertility in males or females. Inositol is required for the control of estrogen levels; it provides protection against the development of breast lumps. Inositol is required for uterine contractions and hormone–cell transfer.

PABA – PARA-AMINOBENZOIC ACID (WATER SOLUBLE)

17. SKIN SYSTEM

PABA, a component of folic acid, is a vitamin within a vitamin and can be made by intestinal bacteria. It is therefore not considered an essential vitamin. However, such factors as the intake of antibiotics and sulfa drugs can destroy the natural bacteria that are required to produce PABA and other B-complex vitamins.

Various skin and hair conditions may be due to a prolonged deficiency of PABA, as it protects natural hair and skin color, prevents premature graying of the hair, aging, and wrinkling of the skin. A general deficiency of B-complex vitamins also contributes to these factors.

PABA is famous for its role as a sunblock. It protects against sunburn and, as a cream, may be used to treat conditions of sunburn. It protects the skin from ultraviolet radiation and promotes the repair of skin blotches caused by excess sunlight or ultraviolet lamps. (Be aware that excess use of sunscreens may reduce the production of vitamin D within the skin's surface.)

OTHER FACTORS

PABA can be stored in tissues. When the body has no further stores, due to excessive use of antibiotics or sulfa drugs, conditions such as fatigue, irritability, nervousness, and depression may develop.

PABA is required for the metabolism of individual amino acids, and it helps promote the use of protein.

PABA promotes the effects of cortisone; it may prevent the development of abnormal fibrous tissues, connective tissue disorders, and eczema.

VITAMIN FOOD SOURCE TABLE

BIOTIN – COENZYME R/VITAMIN H OR B7

Nutrients for effective absorption: B complex.	Beef, broccoli, fish, organ meats, peanuts, soybean oil, spinach.
Nutrient inhibiting factors: Food processing, avidin (egg white).	

CHOLINE

Nutrients for effective absorption: B complex vitamins, inositol.	Barley, cabbage, cauliflower, corn, dried yeast, eggs, lecithin, legumes, potatoes, soy, spinach, tahini, wheat germ.
Nutrient inhibiting factors: Alcohol, processing.	

COENZYME Q10

	Beef, broccoli, fish, organ meats, peanuts, soybean oil, spinach.

FOLATE – FOLIC ACID/VITAMIN B9

Nutrients for effective absorption: Vitamins C, B12, and B6.	Almonds, asparagus, cashews, corn, dried yeast extracts, green vegetables, hazelnuts, legumes, mint, oat bran, parsley, spinach, sunflower seeds, wheat germ.
Nutrient inhibiting factors: Heat, light, air, antibiotics, alcohol, oral contraceptives.	

INOSITOL / PABA

INOSITOL	PABA
Grapefruit, lecithin, melons, onions, oranges, peanuts, peas, pecans, whole grains.	Citrus fruits, oats, wheat germ.

VITAMIN A – RETINOL/CAROTENE

Nutrients for effective absorption: Calcium, phosphorus, zinc, vitamins C, E, F, B group.	Apricots, apricots (dried), broccoli, cantaloupe, carrot juice, carrots, chives, collard greens, dandelion greens, endive, kale, lettuce, mango, papaya, parsley, peach (dried), prune, pumpkin, spinach, sweet potato, turnip greens, watercress, winter squash.
Nutrient inhibiting factors: Strenuous exercise, stress, alcohol, antibiotics, low fat intake.	

VITAMIN B1 – THIAMINE

Nutrients for effective absorption: Vitamins C and B complex, sulfur.	Brazil nuts, breakfast cereals, cashews, chestnuts, legumes, macadamia nuts, malt, oat bran, peanuts, pine nuts, pistachios, rice bran, rye, sunflower seeds, tahini, walnuts, wheat germ, whole-meal bread, yeast extracts.
Nutrient inhibiting factors: Alcohol, tobacco, stress, refined foods and drinks, processing, cooking, antibiotics, tannin, caffeine, antacids.	

VITAMIN B2 – RIBOFLAVIN

Nutrients for effective absorption: Vitamins C and B group.	Almonds, apricot, avocado, bran, cashews, cheese, dates, eggs, legumes, liver, millet, nuts, oats, parsley, peach, soy flour, sprouts, wheat germ, yeast extracts.
Nutrient inhibiting factors: Alcohol, light, tobacco, drugs, stress, processing, the pill, antidepressants.	

VITAMIN B3 – NIACIN

Nutrients for effective absorption: Vitamins C and B group.	Dates, fish, legumes, millet, mushrooms, nuts, peanuts, pumpkin seeds, rice bran, salmon, sunflower seeds, tahini, tuna, wheat bran, wheat germ, wild rice, yeast extracts.
Nutrient inhibiting factors: Alcohol, stress, tobacco, processing.	

VITAMIN B5 – PANTOTHENIC ACID

Nutrients for effective absorption: B-complex vitamins.	Almonds, cashews, eggs, liver, mushrooms, nuts, peanuts, pumpkin seeds, sunflower seeds, wheat bran, wheat germ, yeast extracts.
Nutrient inhibiting factors: Processing, cooking, caffeine, drugs, alcohol.	

VITAMIN B6 – PYRIDOXINE

Nutrients for effective absorption: B-complex vitamins, especially B1, B2, and B5.	Bananas, dates, dried yeast, liver, mackerel, oats, peanuts, peas, pecans, pumpkin seeds, rice bran, salmon, soy, sunflower seeds, tuna, walnuts, wheat bran, wheat germ, yeast extracts, hazelnuts.
Nutrient inhibiting factors: Alcohol, smoking, light, oxidation, processing.	

(cont'd.)

NOTE: Nutrient amounts are listed as milligrams (mg) per 100 grams (g), unless otherwise stated.

VITAMIN FOOD SOURCE TABLE (CONT'D.)

VITAMIN B12 – COBALAMIN

Nutrients for effective absorption: Cobalt, folate, iron. *Nutrient inhibiting factors:* Antacids, air, alcohol, laxatives, light, oral contraceptives.	Cheese, clams, egg yolk, fish, kidney, liver, meat, milk, oysters, salmon, seafood, skim milk, tuna, yogurt.

VITAMIN B15

	Apricot kernels, dried yeast, grains, oats, pumpkin seeds, rice bran, rye, tahini, wheat germ.

VITAMIN C – ASCORBIC ACID

Nutrients for effective absorption: Calcium, magnesium, vitamins P and A. *Nutrient inhibiting factors:* Heat, oxidation, smoking, pollution, aspirin, alcohol.	Acerola cherry, berries, broccoli, Brussels sprouts, cantaloupe, chili pepper, collard greens, currant, dock, guava, kale, lemon, lime, lychee, mango, mustard greens, oranges, other fresh fruits, parsley, red and green bell pepper, spinach, strawberry, turnip greens, watercress.

VITAMIN D – LUMISTEROL CALCIFEROL

Nutrients for effective absorption: Calcium, phosphorus, vitamins A, C, F, B group.	Butter, cod liver oil, eggs, halibut, margarine, outdoor living, salmon, sardines, sunshine.

VITAMIN E – D-ALPHA TOCOPHEROL

Nutrients for effective absorption: Manganese, sulfur, vitamins C, B group. *Nutrient inhibiting factors:* Processing, freezing, cooking, laxatives.	Almond oil, almonds, canola oil, corn oil, hazelnuts, nuts, olive oil, safflower oil, sesame oil, soybean oil, sunflower oil, sunflower seeds, tahini, walnuts, wheat germ oil, wheat sprouts.

VITAMIN F - ESSENTIAL FATTY ACIDS

OMEGA-3	OMEGA-6
Good sources: Anchovies, canola oil, egg yolk, fish, flaxseed, flaxseed oil, herring, mackerel, mullet, pecans, pepitas, prawns, salmon, sardines, seafood, soybean oil, sunflower oil, sunflower seeds, trevally, trout, tuna, walnuts.	Almonds, Brazil nuts, canola oil, cashews, dairy foods, hazelnuts, macadamia nuts, margarine, meat, olive oil, peanuts, pecans, pumpkin seeds, poultry, soybean oil, soybeans, sunflower oil, sunflower seeds, tahini, walnuts.

VITAMIN K – PHYLLOQUINONE

Nutrients for effective absorption: Vitamin C. *Nutrient inhibiting factors:* Freezing, heat, X rays, warfarin, radiation, pollution.	Asparagus, berries, broccoli, cabbage, celery, cucumber, legumes, lettuce, oats, parsley, peas, spinach, sprouts, vegetables, watercress, wheat germ.

VITAMIN P – FLAVONOIDS

Nutrients for effective absorption: Vitamin C. *Nutrient inhibiting factors:* Processing, heat, cooking, oxygen, light.	Apricots, berries, blackcurrants, blueberries, buckwheat, cherries, citrus pith and peel, grapes, mulberries, pepper pith.

VITAMIN T | VITAMIN U

VITAMIN T	VITAMIN U
Egg yolks, sesame seeds tahini.	Cabbage, coleslaw, sauerkraut.

NOTE: DV refers to the daily value for women 25–50 years, refer to RDI tables on pages 95–96 for adult male and child values.

This chapter on the human body systems includes:

MAIN BODY SYSTEMS

1. circulatory
2. digestive
3. glandular
4. lymphatic
5. muscular
6. nervous
7. respiratory
8. skeletal

SUB SYSTEMS

9. blood
10. cellular
11. elimination
12. growth
13. immune
14. joint
15. optic
16. reproductive
17. skin
18. urinary
19. brain
20. repair

Within each section, a basic guide to the main function of the system is provided, as well as the vital nutrients required and their natural food source. It will be clear from this information that numerous minerals and vitamins are required by each body system.

The human body is a very complex structure and only the basic body functions are outlined in this chapter.

By understanding these functions we can be encouraged to help the body obtain the nutrients that support the numerous needs of individual body systems and sub systems.

This information is provided as a guide only; it is not to be used for personal diagnosis of any condition. Seek the advice of a qualified medical practitioner or naturopath.

In each table on pages 194–198, ailments are listed in the left column. The second column is body systems. The numbers listed there refer to the numbers assigned on this page to each body system or sub system. Those are the systems that are affected by the particular illness. As you read through the chart, refer back to the descriptions of body systems in this section to gain information on the nutrients required for each ailment and the best food sources of those nutrients.

Various factors can lead to the onset of illness, sometimes taking many years to be noticed. It is likely that without risk factors, there would be a significant decrease in numerous common ailments. Page 194 lists nearly 50 risk factors, with abbbreviations assigned to each.

The charts on pages 194–198 also contain a list of the risk factors, indicated by their abbeviations, that are commonly associated with specific ailments. Some risk factors are hard to overcome as they are part of the daily lifestyle, or they may be passed on via hereditary traits. Other risk factors are caused by habit-forming drugs or substances. Ideally, for any ailment, it is best to eliminate or at least reduce all the risk factors and to increase the intake of foods that may benefit the individual body systems. The human body works hard to keep in a healthy state, but when the risk factors continue eventually illness may develop.

Fortunately, natural foods can provide an abundance of specific nutrients, antioxidants, and other substances to help overcome some illnesses. With this information we can improve our diet, which may help us avoid illness. Exercise is also an important factor in the whole equation of health.

NOTE: Nutrient amounts are listed as milligrams (mg) per 100 grams (g), unless otherwise stated.

CIRCULATORY SYSTEM

1 - superficial temporal -
  occipital - maxillary -
  vertebral
2 - facial
3 - lingual
4 - common carotid
5 - subclavian
6 - arch of aorta
7 - superior vena cava
8 - heart
9 - superior mesenteric
10 - inferior vena cava
11 - liver
12 - renal
13 - kidneys
14 - spleen
15 - radial
16 - ulnar
17 - common iliac
18 - hypogastric
19 - external iliac
20 - femoral
21 - saphenous
22 - popliteal
23 - post. tibial
24 - anterior tibial
25 - saphenous
26 - dorsalis pedis
27 - dorsalis venous
28 - arcuate

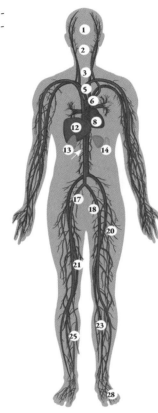

MAIN FUNCTIONS

HEART The heart pumps blood at 72 beats per minute for an adult, 90 beats per minute for a child, and 110 beats per minute for an infant. The heart pumps about 7,500 liters of blood every 24 hours. It takes about 10 seconds for the heart to pump blood throughout the entire body in a complete cycle.

LIVER The liver removes toxins from the bloodstream at a rate of at least 1.5 liters every minute.

KIDNEYS The kidneys are a pair of filters comprised of millions of tiny tubes called nephrons. They have a remarkable ability to regulate the amount of blood salt and acid levels. The kidneys filter blood at a rate of 1.3 liters per minute.

SPLEEN The spleen destroys old red blood cells and blood platelets and provides lymphocytes for new blood.

ARTERIES The blood leaves the heart via the pulmonary artery and enters the lungs where oxygen is added. Arteries then carry oxygenated blood throughout the body.

VEINS Veins transport blood from which the oxygen has been spent back to the heart to be reoxygenated and then recirculated via the arteries. The combined network of arteries and veins within the circulatory system measures approximately 96,000 kilometers (60,000 miles).

VITAL NUTRIENTS

Calcium regulates and assists the smooth functioning of the heartbeat. Magnesium and calcium nourish the circulatory system.

Phosphorus is essential for proper blood circulation, regulation of blood pressure levels, and heart muscle contractions.

Potassium is essential for the heart muscles, proper blood circulation, heart muscle contractions, and regular heartbeat.

Iron is required to carry oxygen.

Magnesium assists nerve impulses for the heart.

Silicon assists with blood circulation.

Iodine protects against heart palpitations.

Sodium maintains blood pressure.

Vanadium regulates blood circulation.

Vitamin E promotes the ability of red blood cells to carry oxygen; it also assists the heart muscles to use oxygen more efficiently and protects against blood clots.

Vitamins C and P promote strong blood capillaries.

Vitamin B15 protects against hardened arteries.

BENEFICIAL NATURAL FOODS

tahini, cheese, almonds, hazelnuts, sunflower seeds, dried apricots, spinach	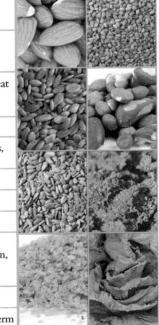
pumpkin seeds (pepitas), sunflower seeds, tahini, Brazil nuts, cashews, walnuts, almonds, lecithin	
dried apricots, dried fruits, fresh wheat germ, legumes, almonds, sunflower seeds	
pumpkin seeds, tahini, parsley	
Brazil nuts, tahini, almonds, cashews, lettuce, spinach, strawberries	
kelp, watermelon, bell peppers	
celery, olives, spinach, cheese	
fresh fish, tuna, kelp, seafood	
sunflower seeds, tahini, almonds, hazelnuts, fresh wheat germ, peanuts, apples, lettuce, walnuts, Brazil nuts	
guava, bell peppers, citrus fruits	
pumpkin seeds, tahini, oats, wheat germ	

NOTE: DV refers to the daily value for women 25–50 years, refer to RDI tables on pages 95–96 for adult male and child values.

MAIN FUNCTIONS

SALIVARY GLANDS The three pairs of salivary glands produce the enzyme ptyalin, required for the initial conversion of cooked starch into the form of maltose.

STOMACH The stomach produces an enzyme, pepsin, from a combination of the enzyme pepsinogen and hydrochloric acid, for the initial conversion of protein foods.

PANCREAS, GALLBLADDER, DUODENUM The pancreas produces an enzyme, trypsin, for the conversion of protein (proteoses and peptones) into peptides, assisted by the gallbladder, which produces bile. This takes place within the duodenum. Fats and oils (lipids) are converted by bile and the enzyme lipase (pancreas) into fatty acids and glycerol.

SMALL INTESTINE, LIVER, COLON In the small intestine, the enzyme amylase converts uncooked starch into maltose, and maltase converts maltose into glucose. Also within the small intestine, the jejunum converts peptides into amino acids; they pass into the bloodstream and go to the liver. The colon collects all the unused food materials and disposes of the waste via the rectum.

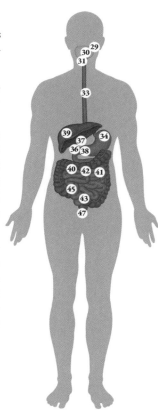

29 - parotid gland
30 - submandibular
31 - sublingual gland
32 - mouth/tongue
33 - esophagus
34 - stomach
35 - pylorus
36 - duodenum
37 - gallbladder
38 - pancreas
39 - liver
40 - jejunum
41 - ileum
42 - small intestine
43 - colon
44 - cecum
45 - appendix
46 - sigmoid
47 - anus

BENEFICIAL NATURAL FOODS

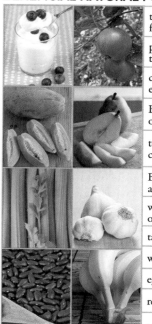

	tahini, yogurt, almonds, hazelnuts, sunflower seeds, dried apricots, walnuts
	pumpkin seeds, sunflower seeds, tahini, Brazil nuts, cashews, garlic
	celery, olives, spinach, cheese, eggs, beets, carrots, pears
	Brazil nuts, scallops, crustaceans, garlic, onions, spinach
	tomato, celery, lettuce, cabbage, papaya, radish
	Brazil nuts, tahini, pumpkin seeds, almonds, cashews, bananas
	wheat germ, hazelnuts, other nuts, oats, garlic, seeds, apples
	tahini, sunflower seeds, cashews
	wheat germ, sunflower seeds
	eggs, whole grains, cheese
	regular moderate sunlight
	refer to nutrient tables

VITAL NUTRIENTS

Calcium is essential for the involuntary muscular movements of the digestive system, termed peristaltic action.

Phosphorus is required for the movement of fatty acids and phospholipids and the distribution of fats.

Sodium stimulates the production of carbohydrate digestive enzymes such as saliva.

Sulfur keeps the digestive system clean, for production of pancreatic enzymes and insulin, and for protein digestion.

Chlorine is essential for the production of the protein enzyme pepsin, in the stomach.

Magnesium is an ingredient of enzymes for protein and carbohydrate digestion and glucose conversion.

Manganese is involved in production of bile and insulin and is essential for metabolism.

Copper is involved in protein metabolism and is an enzyme component.

Iodine is crucial to the thyroid gland, digestion, metabolism.

Zinc is a component of insulin and many enzymes.

Chromium required for glucose conversion, insulin activity.

Vitamin D is essential for digestion and metabolism.

Vitamins B complex, vitamins A and K.

NOTE: Nutrient amounts are listed as milligrams (mg) per 100 grams (g), unless otherwise stated.

GLANDULAR SYSTEM

48 - pineal
49 - pituitary
50 - lacrimal
51 - ceremonius
52 - ebner
53 - thyroid
54 - parathyroid
55 - thymus
56 - mammary
57 - adrenal
58 - fundus
59 - mucus
60 - ovaries
61 - prostate
62 - testes
63 - sweat
64 - sebacious
65 - epithelium
66 - digestive

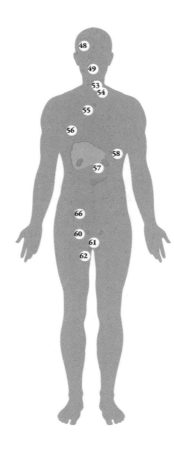

MAIN FUNCTIONS

51 - PINEAL coordinates sensory consciousness.

52 - PITUITARY controls metabolism, lactation, sex hormones, para- and thyroid glands, and the pancreas.

53 - produces moisture for the eyes and tears.

54 - produces wax to protect the ears.

55 - produces water solution for the tongue.

56 - THYROID produces the hormone thyroxine, which controls growth, mental development, nervous activity, and general metabolism.

57 - PARATHYROID controls calcium metabolism.

58 - early childhood development/reproductive organs.

59 - produces colostrum during lactation.

60 - ADRENALS secrete adrenaline for digestion, stress control, glucose production, and heart rate.

67 - produces hydrochloric acid/stomach.

68 - assists excretion of toxins from digestion.

69 - estrogen hormone for fertilization/menstruation.

70 - prostatic fluid for production of semen.

71 - produces the male hormone testosterone.

72 - produces the fluids apocrine and eccrine for sweating.

73 - produces sebum for healthy skin and hair.

74 - produces enzymes to assist with digestion.

75 - absorbs nutrients, water, and enzymes.

VITAL NUTRIENTS

Calcium blood levels and storage of calcium are regulated by the parathyroid glands, dependent on supply of vitamin D.

Sulfur is vital for the function of the pancreas gland, for insulin production, and for the fat-digestive enzymes lipase and trypsin.

Chlorine is required by the reproductive organs and is an essential mineral for cleansing.

Manganese is required by the mammary glands for lactation, and by the thyroid gland (along with iodine) for production of the hormone thyroxine. With zinc, it is required for the manufacture of insulin.

Iodine is essential for the thyroid gland to produce the hormone thyroxine, required for metabolism, growth, nerves, skin, hair, and energy levels.

Bromine levels are controlled by the pituitary gland. This trace mineral is required for stable emotions, especially during menopause and the "mid-life crisis."

Vitamin C protects against glandular infections.

Vitamin D activates the glandular system.

Vitamins E and *B-complex* are vital for all the body's glands.

BENEFICIAL NATURAL FOODS

tahini, cheese, almonds, hazelnuts, sunflower seeds, dried apricots, walnuts, spinach
carrot juice, carrots, spinach, garlic, onions, cucumber, lettuce, celery, tomato, figs
tomato, celery, lettuce, cabbage, mango, carrots, peach
hazelnuts, pecans, walnuts, pine nuts, pumpkin seeds, beets, pineapple, grapes, parsley, lettuce, tahini, garlic, legumes
fish, seafood, kelp, spinach, iodized salt, watermelon, cucumber, spinach, berries
watermelon, rockmelon, honeydew melon, cucumber, celery, asparagus, tomato, lettuce, carrots, garlic, peach
berries, tomato, peach, orange
regular moderate sunlight
tahini, almonds

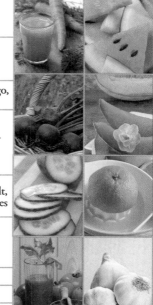

NOTE: DV refers to the daily value for women 25–50 years, refer to RDI chart on pages 95–96 for adult male and child values.

GLANDULAR SYSTEM

MAIN FUNCTIONS

The lymphatic system is best described as the body's processing, protection, and filtration system. Think of it as the body's secondary circulatory system. The lymphatic glands process fats, expel worn-out blood corpuscles, and protect against bacterial invasion.

SPLEEN The spleen is the largest organ of the body's lymphatic system. It is not considered "essential" to life; however, it functions to eliminate old red blood corpuscles and blood platelets. It stores iron from the worn-out cells and produces bilirubin, required as a part of bile, to break down fats. The spleen also participates in producing antibodies and fighting infections; it also produces some of the blood lymphocytes.

MESENTERIC The lymphatic glands of the small intestine are termed mesenteric glands. They are vital for absorption of fats from the diet, which are then conveyed via the lymphatic system to the liver, which removes the hydrogen from fats and then returns the "unsaturated fats" to the fat stores of the body. When the lymph glands become clogged, illness results.

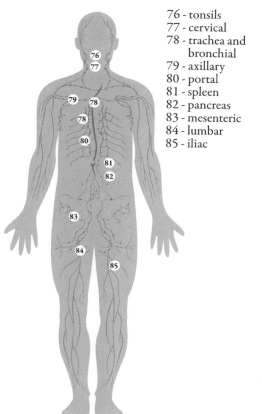

76 - tonsils
77 - cervical
78 - trachea and bronchial
79 - axillary
80 - portal
81 - spleen
82 - pancreas
83 - mesenteric
84 - lumbar
85 - iliac

BENEFICIAL NATURAL FOODS

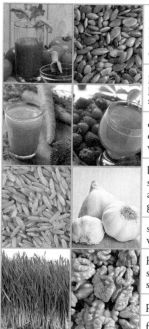

tomato, celery, lettuce, cabbage, watercress, cucumber, carrots, berries, beets, mango, pineapple, lime, guava, dates
pumpkin seeds, wheat germ, kelp, parsley, tahini, wheatgrass, sunflower seeds, almonds
carrots, figs, dates, garlic, onions, cabbage, pineapple, celery, tomato, wheatgrass
bran, pumpkin seeds, wheat germ, sunflower seeds, Brazil nuts, tahini, almonds, peanuts, walnuts, lecithin granules, oats, hazelnuts
sprouts, parsley, garlic, wheat germ oil, tahini, almonds
hazelnuts, wheatgerm, seeds, sunflower seeds, almonds, avocado, strawberry, nuts, tahini
peanuts, fish, walnuts
fresh fish, tuna, kelp, seafood

VITAL NUTRIENTS

Chlorine is involved in regulating the blood's acid–alkaline levels. It also stimulates the functions of the liver and is vital for cleansing the blood and reducing fatty deposits.

Iron is required to eliminate toxic waste from the bloodstream, thereby protecting the lymphatic system from impurities and inflammation.

Sulfur provides a cleansing and antiseptic effect on the digestive system and the lymphatic glands of the small intestines (mesenteric glands).

Phosphorus is found in every cell and is required for the transfer of nutrients through cell walls. Lecithin is a phosphorus compound and is used for the conversion and movement of fats throughout the lymphatic system.

Vitamin E reduces oxidation of fats, thereby protecting the lymphatic system from toxins.

Vitamin F, in particular linoleic acid, is required for cholesterol control and protection from high blood pressure.

Biotin and other B-complex vitamins are required for fat metabolism.

Choline is vital for the control of cholesterol and fats.

86 - frontalis
87 - temporal
88 - occipitalis
89 - facial
90 - orbicularis oculi
91 - buccinator
92 - masseter
93 - digastric
94 - levator
95 - scalene
96 - omohyoid
97 - sternomastoid
98 - trapezius
99 - deltoid
100 - pectoralis major
101 - biceps
102 - brachialis
103 - pronator
104 - brachioradialis
105 - flexor carpi radialis
106 - flexor carpi ulnaris
107 - sublimis
108 - thenar
109 - hyponar
110 - acromion process
111 - pectoralis minor
112 - serratus anterior
113 - latissimus dorsi
114 - serratus anterior
115 - linear alba
116 - external oblique

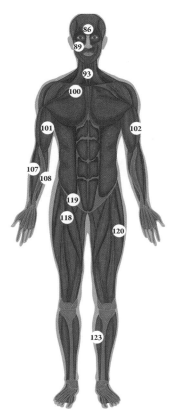

MAIN FUNCTIONS

A muscle is described as an organ that produces motion by the action of the nervous system and contraction of muscle fibers. The two main types of muscle fibers are striated and smooth. The muscular system covers most parts of the body; about 40% of body mass is muscle. Muscles are made from millions of fibers and covered by tissues called fascia. Muscles are connected to the skeletal system by tendons. Nearly all muscles have an opposite: one to lift and the other to lower. There are about 650 muscles in the adult human body. The three main types of muscles are: heart muscles (cardiac muscles), visceral muscles (stomach and bloodstream), and skeletal muscles (legs, arms, and spine). Large voluntary muscles are composed of about 80% water and 20% protein. Muscles require heat to perform; about 75% of the energy used by muscles is for heat production, 25% for muscle action.

117 - gluteus medius
118 - gluteus maximus
119 - rectus femoris
120 - vastus externus
121 - vastus internus
122 - tibialis anterior
123 - soleus
124 - peroneus longus
125 - transversus
126 - internal intercostal

VITAL NUTRIENTS

Potassium, the "muscle mineral," is required for stimulating the nerves connected to the muscles. It is also vital for repair and conditioning of muscles.

Calcium is needed for regulating the heartbeat, muscular growth, and muscle contraction.

Iron is the foundation mineral of myoglobin; it supplies oxygen to the muscle cells and activates muscular contractions.

Magnesium provides the connection between muscles and nerve stimuli. It helps protect against cramps and assists with muscular contractions.

Manganese is required for muscular strength and muscular coordination by stimulating proper transfer of nerve impulses to the muscular tissues.

Copper is required for elastin, a protein involved in muscle stretching and contracting.

Selenium preserves muscular elasticity.

Sodium is required for muscular enlargement.

Vitamin E is the "muscle vitamin"; it promotes oxygen supply and endurance to muscles and promotes blood circulation.

Vitamins A and B complex are vital for the muscular system.

BENEFICIAL NATURAL FOODS

wheat bran, pumpkin seeds, wheat germ, sunflower seeds, almonds, hazelnuts, tahini, Brazil nuts, cashews, banana, rice bran	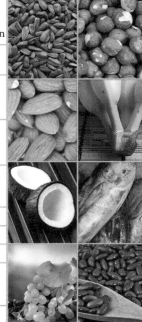
tahini, acidophilus yogurt, almonds, nuts, sunflower seeds	
pumpkin seeds, almonds, parsley, tahini, sunflower seeds, kelp, rice bran, wheat germ, tofu	
Brazil nuts, tahini, pumpkin seeds, almonds, sunflower seeds, wheat germ, bananas	
wheat germ, hazelnuts, oats, garlic, peanuts, tahini, sunflower seeds, coconut	
tahini, cashews, sunflower seeds	
Brazil nuts, wheat germ, tuna	
celery, olives, spinach, cheese	
wheat germ oil, tahini, almonds, sunflower seeds, hazelnuts, wheat germ, peanuts, pecans	
refer to nutrient tables	

NOTE: DV refers to the daily value for women 25–50 years, refer to RDI chart on pages 95–96 for adult male and child values

MAIN FUNCTIONS

There are three main parts to the nervous system: the central nervous system (spinal cord and brain), the peripheral nervous system (organs and muscles), and the sympathetic nervous system (brain and nerves). The nervous system works constantly to coordinate every movement, conscious and subconscious. During sleep the nervous system relaxes, thereby allowing nerve endings to repair, to receive nutrition, and to be ready for when we wake. When we are awake, the nervous system provides the many actions and reactions from physical, subconscious, and emotional involvement, including the functions of the brain: memory, thought, speech, vision and sight interpretation, and sense awareness such as pain, excitement, and pleasure. There are 31 pairs of spinal nerves, each connecting to different parts of the body. Nerve cells (neurons) transmit messages. The brain is the master controller of nearly all nervous system interactions and the speed of message transfer varies from over 125 miles per hour to less than 2.5 miles per hour.

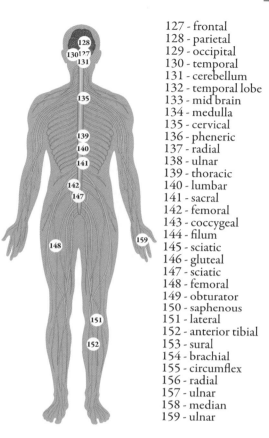

127 - frontal
128 - parietal
129 - occipital
130 - temporal
131 - cerebellum
132 - temporal lobe
133 - mid brain
134 - medulla
135 - cervical
136 - pheneric
137 - radial
138 - ulnar
139 - thoracic
140 - lumbar
141 - sacral
142 - femoral
143 - coccygeal
144 - filum
145 - sciatic
146 - gluteal
147 - sciatic
148 - femoral
149 - obturator
150 - saphenous
151 - lateral
152 - anterior tibial
153 - sural
154 - brachial
155 - circumflex
156 - radial
157 - ulnar
158 - median
159 - ulnar

BENEFICIAL NATURAL FOODS

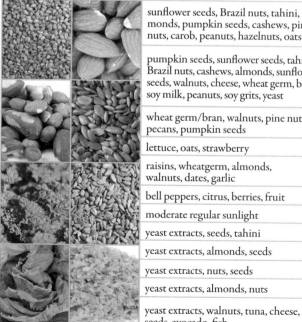

sunflower seeds, Brazil nuts, tahini, almonds, pumpkin seeds, cashews, pine nuts, carob, peanuts, hazelnuts, oats	
pumpkin seeds, sunflower seeds, tahini, Brazil nuts, cashews, almonds, sunflower seeds, walnuts, cheese, wheat germ, bran, soy milk, peanuts, soy grits, yeast	
wheat germ/bran, walnuts, pine nuts, pecans, pumpkin seeds	
lettuce, oats, strawberry	
raisins, wheatgerm, almonds, walnuts, dates, garlic	
bell peppers, citrus, berries, fruit	
moderate regular sunlight	
yeast extracts, seeds, tahini	
yeast extracts, almonds, seeds	
yeast extracts, nuts, seeds	
yeast extracts, almonds, nuts	
yeast extracts, walnuts, tuna, cheese, seeds, avocado, fish	

VITAL NUTRIENTS

Magnesium is the "nerve mineral"; it regulates the white nerve fibers and the central nervous system. It protects against nervous exhaustion.

Phosphorus is vital for conditioning the responses of the nervous system and protects against nervous stress. The gray matter of the brain is composed of phosphorus compounds called lecithin and phospholipids.

Manganese nourishes the nerves, maintains nerve impulses, and coordinates nerve transmission.

Silicon insulates nerve fibers and protects from stress.

Potassium assists to coordinate nerves and muscles and impulses and stimulation to the brain.

Vitamin C protects against nervous stress.

Vitamin D maintains a healthy nervous system.

Vitamin B1 promotes memory and concentration.

Vitamin B2 protects against nervous stress.

Vitamin B3 nourishes the nervous system.

Vitamin B5 promotes strong nerves.

Vitamins B6, B12, and *choline* protect the nerves.

NOTE: Nutrient amounts are listed as milligrams (mg) per 100 grams (g), unless otherwise stated.

160 - nose
32 - mouth
33 - esophagus
161 - pharynx
162 - larynx
163 - trachea
164 - bronchi
165 - lungs

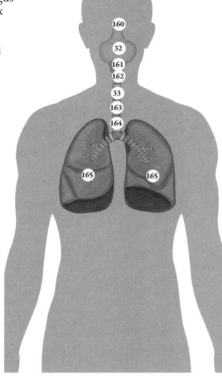

MAIN FUNCTIONS

NOSE The nose contains membranes that are full of blood; they allow the inhaled air to warm to body temperature before reaching the lungs. Tiny nostril hairs help to filter, warm, and humidify the air.

MOUTH The mouth is primarily for ingesting food and drink and for speech. Air can be inhaled through the mouth but it is less protected from dust than air inhaled via the nose.

ESOPHAGUS The esophagus is a muscular tube, about 10 inches long, lined with mucus membranes, extending from the pharynx to the stomach. It is for food intake.

PHARYNX The pharynx is divided into three parts: the naso, oral, and laryngeal pharynx. The nasopharynx is positioned at the back of the nasal cavity and includes the tonsils; their function is to protect against bacteria.

LARYNX The larynx is for speech and air passage.

TRACHEA/BRONCHI The trachea, or windpipe, is about five inches long. It separates into two tubes that pass into the bronchi, which are similar in structure to the trachea.

LUNGS The lungs absorb oxygen from the inhaled air for transport in the blood to cells throughout the body. They also exhale carbon dioxide.

VITAL NUTRIENTS

Sulfur is required for cleansing the respiratory system and for tissue respiration in the process of new cell development. Garlic oil contains about 80% sulfur content.

Iron is essential for the transfer of oxygen throughout the body in the form of hemoglobin, and for storing oxygen in the muscles in the form of myoglobin.

Potassium, combined with the mineral phosphorus, is required for the supply of oxygen to the brain, which sends impulses to the diaphragm and the muscles surrounding the rib cage to inhale and exhale. In a 24-hour period the lungs inhale/exhale about 14,000 liters of air.

Vitamin A is essential for the protection of the internal linings of the mouth, throat, nose, and lungs from infection, dust, and smoke. Mucus is produced to eliminate toxins from the respiratory system.

Vitamin C is essential for tissue respiration and to defend the respiratory system from bacteria.

Vitamin E is required for repair of damaged lung tissues. It also promotes the function of oxygen within body cells.

B complex vitamins: See pages 169–172.

BENEFICIAL NATURAL FOODS

garlic, onions, horseradish, radish, carrot juice, carrots, raw cabbage, coleslaw, scallops, Brazil nuts, crustaceans, peanuts, figs, dates, spinach, tomato	
pumpkin seeds, almonds, parsley, tahini, sunflower seeds, kelp, wheat germ, tofu, rice bran	
rice bran, wheat bran, pumpkin seeds, wheat germ, sunflower seeds, almonds, hazelnuts, tahini, Brazil nuts, cashews, peanuts, walnuts, parmesan cheese, raisins, parsley, pine nuts, garlic	
carrot juice, carrots, parsley, guava, mango, pumpkin, papaya, sweet potato, cheese, butter, apricots, cantaloupe	
guava, bell peppers, parsley, mango, currants, papaya, citrus	
wheat germ oil, tahini, almonds, sunflower seeds, wheat germ	
B-complex tablet daily	

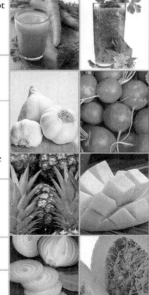

NOTE: DV refers to the daily value for women 25–50 years, refer to RDI chart on pages 95–96 for adult male and child values.

MAIN FUNCTIONS

The human skeleton is the body's frame. It is made up of about 200 bones in adults and 350 bones in infants. The name "skeleton" comes from the Greek word for "dried up"; however, bones contain approximately 30% water. The skull along comprises over 20 different bones.

The inner part of bones is made from a protein, collagen. The outer layer is composed mainly of the minerals calcium, phosphorus, silicon, fluorine, and magnesium.

SPINAL COLUMN The spinal column is the central part of the skeletal system, supporting the head and consisting of 33 bones with two main groups: flexible (seven cervical are at the top, 12 dorsal, five lumbar) and fixed (five sacral, four coccyx).

RIBS The ribs are arranged in twelve pairs; the "true" ribs are the top seven pairs. The ribs protect the vital organs such as the heart, liver, and lungs.

TEETH By the age of two the first set of 20 "milk teeth" or "baby teeth" has formed; progressively from the age of six to 25 the 32 permanent teeth are formed. Teeth are made from calcium, phosphorus, magnesium, and zinc.

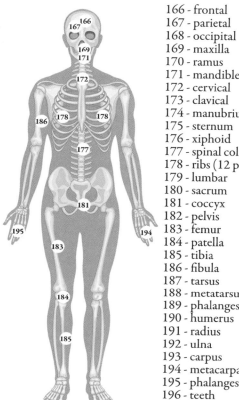

166 - frontal
167 - parietal
168 - occipital
169 - maxilla
170 - ramus
171 - mandible
172 - cervical
173 - clavical
174 - manubrium
175 - sternum
176 - xiphoid
177 - spinal column
178 - ribs (12 pairs)
179 - lumbar
180 - sacrum
181 - coccyx
182 - pelvis
183 - femur
184 - patella
185 - tibia
186 - fibula
187 - tarsus
188 - metatarsus
189 - phalanges
190 - humerus
191 - radius
192 - ulna
193 - carpus
194 - metacarpals
195 - phalanges
196 - teeth

BENEFICIAL NATURAL FOODS

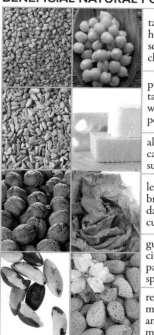

tahini, acidophilus yogurt, almonds, hazelnuts, walnuts, sunflower seeds, dried apricots, cheese, milk, chickpeas
pumpkin seeds, sunflower seeds, tahini, cheese, cashews, almonds, walnuts, wheat bran, oats, rice bran, peanuts, wheat germ
almonds, wheat germ, rice bran, cashews, Brazil nuts, tahini, walnuts, sunflower seeds
lettuce, oats, barley, asparagus, rice bran, spinach, parsnips, onions, dates, strawberries, sunflower seeds, cucumber
guava, blackcurrants, bell peppers, citrus fruits, rockmelon, broccoli, parsley, papaya, berries, kiwi, mango, spinach, tomato
regular direct sunlight in winter; moderate direct sunlight in autumn and spring; in summer, caution with midday direct sun

VITAL NUTRIENTS

Calcium is the main bone mineral. The total calcium content of the body is renewed over a six-year period. About 90% of the calcium within the body is in the skeletal system.

Phosphorus is essential for repair of bone fractures. To function efficiently calcium (2.5 parts) must be balanced with phosphorus (1 part). Eighty percent of the body's phosphorus is contained within the skeletal system.

Magnesium is essential for proper absorption of both calcium and phosphorus. About 70% of the body's magnesium is stored within the skeletal system.

Silicon is essential for calcium metabolism. It also provides strength to the bones. It protects bones from uric acid crystals by assisting in their elimination from around the joints.

Vitamin C is essential in the formation of collagen, the protein substance within every bone. Vitamin C is required daily to assist in the growth and maintenance of bones.

Vitamin D and sunlight are vital for strong bones and bone growth in children. It is essential to ensure an adequate amount of sunlight, especially in winter.

NOTE: Nutrient amounts are listed as milligrams (mg) per 100 grams (g), unless otherwise stated.

9 BLOOD SYSTEM

MAIN FUNCTIONS

The blood system is the carrier of all nutrients in the form of oxygen, glucose, amino acids, minerals, water, vitamins, and enzymes. Blood is our lifeline, and over a period of two months the entire inventory of the body's blood cells is renewed. The main functions of blood are to:

1. remove waste via the liver and kidneys
2. transfer chemical messages as hormones
3. supply antibodies to areas of infection
4. convey oxygen to all body tissues and organs
5. defend the body via the action of white cells
6. carry all nutrients for body nourishment
7. maintain physical and mental abilities.

Blood is composed of 55% plasma, 45% cells. Plasma contains 90% water and 10% solids in the form of minerals and protein. Blood cells are 95% red cells, 3% platelets, and 2% white cells. Blood contains 16 mineral elements; the average human body holds six liters of precious blood.

BENEFICIAL NUTRIENTS

Potassium eliminates blood impurities, reduces high blood pressure, improves blood circulation.

Sodium keeps minerals soluble within the bloodstream and controls blood pressure.

Sulfur provides oxygen to the blood, which is required for the development of blood hemoglobin.

Chlorine purifies the blood and regulates blood pressure.

Fluorine increases the number of blood cells.

Iron is vital for blood hemoglobin production.

Manganese, with iron and copper, assists in the formation of red blood cells.

Cobalt maintains red blood cells.

Other essential nutrients for the blood system are chromium, vanadium, and vitamins C, F, K, P, and B complex.

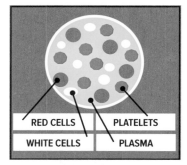

RED CELLS | PLATELETS
WHITE CELLS | PLASMA

NATURAL FOODS

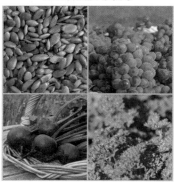

10 CELLULAR SYSTEM

MAIN FUNCTIONS

The diagram on the right shows the six main types of cells. A cell is defined as a small mass of protoplasm containing a nucleus and having the following abilities:

1. assimilation of nourishment
2. growth and repair
3. reproduction
4. excretion of waste
5. power of movement.

Protoplasm consists of the following substances: organic compounds as protein, fatty substances, carbohydrates, inorganic salts, and water.

Within the structure of every living cell there is a code stored in the DNA molecule with the unique ability to issue instructions for the reproduction of identical new cells via the RNA (ribonucleic acid) at the outer boundary of cells. (The exception is red blood cells, which don't have a nucleus.) There is a constant flow of nutrients within each cell that occurs millions of times a day throughout the body. All cells require a combination of glucose, minerals, vitamins, oxygen, and water.

BENEFICIAL NUTRIENTS

Sodium regulates fluids from either side of cell walls.

Sulfur is for cell respiration, new cells.

Chlorine is for cell membranes.

Fluorine increases red blood cells.

Iron is in the nucleus of every cell and transports oxygen to muscle cells.

Magnesium activates protein and carbohydrates within cells.

Silicon is vital for cell growth in the hair, skin, and eyes, promotes red blood cell and bone development.

Cobalt maintains body cells.

Chromium is involved in movement of glucose (blood sugar) into cells.

Vitamin A is for skin, digestive, respiratory, bone, and urinary cells, and for the transfer of genetic material.

Vitamin C is vital for skin cells.

Vitamin E promotes cell life and cell respiration.

Vitamins F, K, and B complex are also needed.

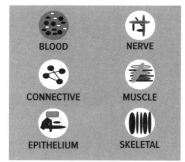

BLOOD | NERVE
CONNECTIVE | MUSCLE
EPITHELIUM | SKELETAL

NATURAL FOODS

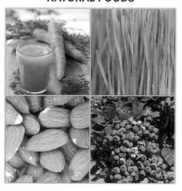

NOTE: DV refers to the daily value for women 25–50 years, refer to RDI chart on pages 95–96 for adult male and child values.

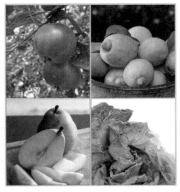

NATURAL FOODS

MAIN FUNCTIONS

There are two main parts to the elimination system: digestive system and excretory fluids system. After the process of digestion occurs within the stomach and small intestine, the remaining food chyme passes into the large intestine, which is about five feet long and has five main parts: cecum, transverse colon, descending colon, pelvic colon, and rectum. Digestive elimination requires a fair portion of roughage to function efficiently. Such foods as fruits, vegetables, legumes, and whole grains are ideal for assisting with elimination.

The excretory fluids system includes the kidneys, skin, liver, and lungs. The kidneys remove excess urea (protein) via the urine. The skin removes excess moisture via perspiration. The liver removes nitrogen, old red blood cells, and toxic substances. The lungs expel carbon dioxide and water. Mucus is produced within the body to expel toxins from the respiratory system and the digestive system. Fasting is beneficial.

11 ELIMINATION SYSTEM

BENEFICIAL NUTRIENTS

Sodium eliminates carbonic acid from the lungs and inorganic waste elements from the body.

Chlorine removes toxins from the liver, blood, and respiratory system.

Sulfur eliminates toxins from digestion and from skin and blood.

Iron in combination with copper eliminates waste from the blood.

Silicon cleanses the skin and removes uric acid from the blood.

Potassium assists the colon, and kidneys, and skin to remove waste.

Magnesium removes kidney stones.

Manganese removes excess sugar from the blood, via the urine.

Phosphorus assists the kidneys and the elimination of excess acids.

Choline eliminates excess fats.

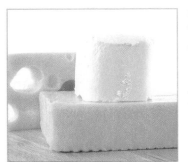

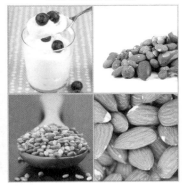

NATURAL FOODS

MAIN FUNCTIONS

The growth system has numerous stages throughout the human life span:

1. From conception to three months, when all cells are formed. 2. In the first year the baby will triple in weight and double in height and brain size. 3. From ages 2 to 10, the child grows in height on average three inches per year. 4. From 11–20 years the rapid growth stage occurs, with over three inches height increase per year in boys during adolescence, and 2.5 inches height increase in girls per year.

The pituitary gland is the most important controller of growth. It produces a hormone for body growth, somatotropin, as well as other hormones to stimulate the growth of the thyroid gland, which produces thyrotrophic hormone to increase the body's metabolism rate. The adrenal glands and the sex glands are stimulated by various hormones produced by the pituitary gland. The thymus gland functions from birth till about age seven, for development of the reproductive and immune systems.

12 GROWTH SYSTEM

BENEFICIAL NUTRIENTS

Calcium is the main growth mineral; however, it requires numerous other minerals and vitamins to function efficiently. Calcium is required for growth of bones, skin, teeth, blood, and hormone development.

Phosphorus is required in a ratio of 2.5 parts calcium to one part phosphorus for growth of bones and nerves.

Potassium is for muscle growth.

Iodine is essential for the thyroid gland, which controls both body and mental growth.

Fluorine assists in strong bone growth.

Magnesium assists the development of strong bones, teeth, and nerves.

Iron is required for blood hemoglobin, which aids growth by transporting oxygen to bodily cells.

Other essential factors are the daily supply of protein, vitamin A, and sunlight.

NOTE: Nutrient amounts are listed as milligrams (mg) per 100 grams (g), unless otherwise stated.

13 IMMUNE SYSTEM

MAIN FUNCTIONS

The immune system is constantly on the alert for any invading bacteria, viruses, and other pathogens. The first line of defense are the white cells of the blood, one type of which are called phagocytes. They multiply rapidly to destroy the pathogen, bacterium, or virus. The second line of defense comes from the lymphatic system, which produces lymphocyte cells. These produce antibodies that attempt to prevent bacteria and viruses from reproducing. The phagocytes ingest the captured pathogens and dispose of them. The spleen plays a major role: it produces antibodies and lymphocytes and destroys worn-out blood cells. The most common ways for bacteria and viruses to enter the body are through diet, water, and inhaled air. The lymphatic system consists of a wide-ranging network of lymph nodes in the neck, groin, armpits, digestive system, and spleen. The lymph nodes are like filters, collecting infectious agents for the white cells and antibodies to destroy.

BENEFICIAL NUTRIENTS

Iron (in combination with copper and manganese) strengthens the immune system by replacing worn-out blood cells.
Potassium assists the kidneys to remove fluid waste and infections.
Calcium increases the body's ability to fight infections.
Chlorine removes toxic waste.
Vitamin A promotes the immune system's ability to fight infections and increases resistance to toxins.
Sulfur prevents infections.
Vitamin C protects against toxins and infections by increasing the supply of white blood cells.
Vitamin P activates vitamin C.
Vitamin D activates all nutrients.
Vitamins B5 and B6 assist in the production of antibodies.

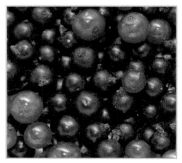

NATURAL FOODS

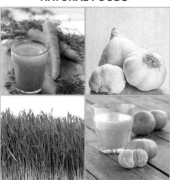

14 JOINT SYSTEM

MAIN FUNCTIONS

The joint system performs an incredible variety of movements. The three main types of joints are: fixed joints (skull bones); slightly movable (pelvis, collarbone); and freely movable (hands, feet, knees, spine, hip, neck, shoulders, wrist, elbows, jaw, and ankles).

The most common problem with the joint system is the condition of arthritis. There are two main types of arthritis: osteoarthritis and rheumatoid arthritis. Osteoarthritis involves a loss of cartilage linings around the moving joints, often caused by years of wear and tear, incomplete nutrition, insufficient rest, work under stessful conditions, and excess bodily acidity. Rheumatoid arthritis causes the joints to become inflamed and painful; the exact cause is uncertain, but conditions of prolonged emotional stress, anger, and resentment may trigger the condition.

Excess intake of refined foods may cause inorganic calcium to build up around joints, replacing tissues and resulting in the deterioration of joint flexibility.

BENEFICIAL NUTRIENTS

Sodium—from natural sources such as celery, not table salt—keeps calcium soluble in the blood, preventing a buildup around the joints. It also reduces acidity in the blood.
Potassium helps to balance the acid–alkaline levels of the blood.
Chlorine maintains healthy joints as it purifies the blood of toxic waste.
Sulfur eliminates body toxins.
Vitamin C is essential for production of collagen and synovial fluid; plus it protects against inflammation.
Vitamin E repairs damaged tissues and improves circulation, cell nourishment, and body flexibility.
Vitamin F repairs damaged tissues.
Vitamin S repairs damaged tissues and promotes cellular growth.
Salicylic acid in grapefruit reduces the build-up of inorganic calcium.

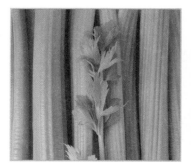

NATURAL FOODS

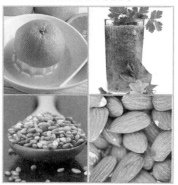

NOTE: DV refers to the daily value for women 25–50 years, refer to RDI chart on pages 95–96 for adult male and child values.

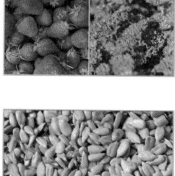

NATURAL FOODS

MAIN FUNCTIONS

The optic system provides the view to the world and reveals the incredible range of colors, shapes, and objects. Light enters the eyes through the cornea, and then enters the lens through the pupil. The pupil changes size to regulate the amount of light admitted to the retina.

Muscles within the eye (ciliary muscles) cause the lens to bulge or flatten during the transfer of light to the retina. Within the retina, millions of light receptors called cones (for color) and rods (for black and white) build an image that is then transferred to the brain for final evaluation, via the optic nerve. The eyes are protected by the eyelid. Blinking keeps the eye moist and clean, eyebrows keep sweat from the eyes, and eyelashes keep dust away from the eyes. The optic system can become strained by poor lighting, excessive use of computers and television screens, and excess exposure to ultraviolet sunlight. Protection of the eyes is vital to maintain good vision for many years.

BENEFICIAL NUTRIENTS

Vitamin A is essential for correct peripheral (side) vision, color vision, and night vision. It protects against eye infections; a prolonged deficiency can lead to blindness.

Fluorine assists with the function of the iris and promotes a sparkle to the eye.

Silicon repairs damaged tissues.

Zinc is stored within the eyes; a deficiency can lead to poor sight.

Calcium assists in preventing cataracts.

Vitamin C is essential for the lens of the eyes and the nourishment of the eyes.

Vitamin P assists vitamin C functions.

Vitamin B2 promotes clear vision.

Vitamin B5 nourishes the eyes.

Vitamin B6 protects against eye strain and cataracts.

Choline protects from glaucoma.

16 REPRODUCTIVE SYSTEM

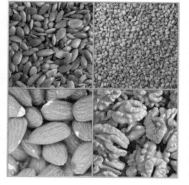

NATURAL FOODS

MAIN FUNCTIONS

The reproductive system develops during puberty, approximately ages 12–15. From birth till age seven, the thymus gland initiates the development of the reproductive organs. At puberty, the pituitary gland produces a hormone (GTH) that stimulates the production of the male hormone (testosterone) and the female hormone (estrogen).

The female is born with all the eggs (ova) that are required during the reproductive years. It takes about 46 days for the male sperm to mature; millions are produced every day.

The combination of the male sperm and female egg create a transformation of life by combining two sets of 23 chromosomes into 46 chromosomes, producing a fertilized egg. Once pregnancy has occurred, gestation is about 37 weeks.

The reproductive life of the male can last for 70 to 80 years, but for the female, the onset of menopause during the late forties will be the end of the reproductive cycle.

BENEFICIAL NUTRIENTS

Chlorine assists in the distribution of the reproductive hormones.

Iron is essential during pregnancy and menstruation.

Manganese is vital for the glands of the reproductive system, for production of milk and sex hormones, and for menstrual cycles.

Zinc is essential for the reproductive organs and protects against sterility and prostate problems.

Chromium assists cell growth.

Selenium enhances vitamin E.

Vitamin E is the "life vitamin"; it is essential for cell division at conception and protects against sterility, miscarriage, and premature birth.

Vitamin A is required for the transfer of hereditary characteristics.

B-complex vitamins are vital; see pages 169–174.

NOTE: Nutrient amounts are listed as milligrams (mg) per 100 grams (g), unless otherwise stated.

17 SKIN SYSTEM

MAIN FUNCTIONS

The skin supports a number of important functions by providing the body with a protective layer that keeps out pathogens, water, and sunlight. The skin is sensitive to heat, cold, pain, and pressure, thereby providing a warning signal and temperature gauge. The outer layer of skin (epidermis) contains no blood vessels and is in fact dead skin. The next layer (dermis) is living skin and consists of fibrous and connective tissues, sweat glands, nerve fibers, oil glands (sebaceous), and blood vessels. The sebaceous glands produce sebum, which keeps the skin supple and the hair oiled. The body has about three million sweat glands, which balance body temperature via sweating (pores open) to cool the body. When cold, the sweat glands constrict through the contraction of blood vessels and muscles. The skin is also important in supplying the body wtih vitamin D. The skin contains a substance—a form of cholesterol—that, when it receives ultraviolet radiation from the sun, is transformed into vitamin D.

BENEFICIAL NUTRIENTS

Phosphorus is part of every skin cell and is vital for skin repair.
Sulfur cleanses the skin.
Chlorine rejuvenates the skin.
Fluorine preserves healthy skin and hair.
Silicon eliminates toxins from the dermis layer, repairs damaged skin, and removes dead skin.
Copper is required for skin and hair pigment.
Iron promotes a healthy complexion.
Selenium preserves skin elasticity and assists the action of vitamin E.
Vitamin E assists in the growth and repair of skin.
Vitamins C, P, and F help to develop collagen.
Vitamin E promotes healthy skin life and is essential for healing of skin tissues.
Vitamins B2, B3, B5, and PABA.

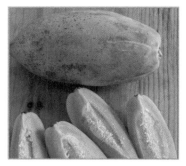

NATURAL FOODS

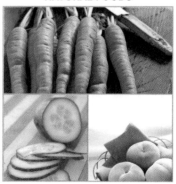

18 URINARY SYSTEM

MAIN FUNCTIONS

The urinary system filters and eliminates waste liquids. The kidneys, a pair of highly efficient filters, cleanse approximately one liter of blood per minute in adults. Blood enters the kidneys via the renal arteries, which transfer blood via millions of capillaries (glomeruli) under high pressure into the Bowman's capsules. Red and white blood cells, fat and protein molecules, and platelets are too large to pass into the Bowman's capsule; they bypass and re-enter the bloodstream via the renal vein.

Plasma, containing water, amino acids, glucose, salts, and urea, passes into the capsule and then through the long system of tubes (tubules), the next filtration stage of the kidneys. Nearly 99% of the water and all the nutrients are reabsorbed into the bloodstream. The remaining substances are mainly water (96%); solids (2%); chlorides, phosphates, sulfates, and oxalates; and urea (2%), the end product of protein digestion. All these substances, plus toxins and some drugs, are passed from the kidneys via the urine.

BENEFICIAL NUTRIENTS

Potassium cleanses the kidneys and regulates the body's water balance.
Magnesium maintains minerals in a soluble state, preventing kidney stones.
Sodium works with potassium to regulate the body's water balance.
Manganese is involved in the formation of urea.
Vitamin A protects against kidney stones and inflammation of the prostate gland.
Vitamin B6 protects against kidney stone formation.
Choline is required for healthy kidneys.
Vitamin C protects against inflammation of the urinary system by phosphatic crystals, which it can dissolve.
Vitamin E stimulates the elimination of urine and may aid in the reduction of edema.

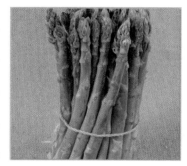

NATURAL FOODS

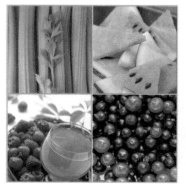

NOTE: DV refers to the daily value for women 25–50 years, refer to RDI chart on pages 95–96 for adult male and child values.

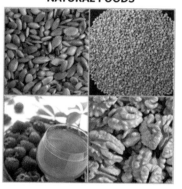

NATURAL FOODS

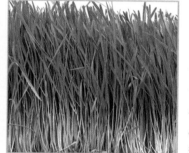

MAIN FUNCTIONS

The brain is the control center for actions, reactions, and sensations. The brain has two main parts: the higher center and the lower center. The cortex or cerebral hemisphere is the main part of the brain (80%); it consists of gray matter, or 10 million nerve cells, and is the center of thoughts, intelligence, memory, speech, hearing, vision, and the direction of physical actions. The lower center (cerebellum) controls unconscious actions such as balance, posture, and movement. The brain stem controls respiration, heart rate, blood vessel size, swallowing, and production of saliva and digestive enzymes. Also contained within the brain are four main glands. The pituitary produces growth hormones, sex hormones, milk hormones, and, as the "master gland," controls other glands: thyroid, adrenal, pancreas, and sex glands. The pineal gland is the spiritual center of the brain. The thalamus gland is responsible for feelings of pain. The hypothalamus gland regulates body temperature, blood, and water and salt balance.

19 BRAIN SYSTEM

BENEFICIAL NUTRIENTS

Phosphorus transfers nerve impulses and is essential for brain function.

Magnesium is required for memory, nourishment, regulating the white nerve fibers of the brain and spinal cord, and steady nerves.

Manganese nourishes the nerves and brain and promotes memory.

Iodine is essential for speech and mental functioning. During pregnancy it promotes mental and physical development of the child.

Bromine protects against mental depression and emotional stress.

Vitamin T promotes a good memory and concentration.

Vitamins B1, B3, B5, B6, B12, B15, and folic acid promote memory, concentration, mental stability, sleep, and emotional stability.

20 REPAIR SYSTEM

BENEFICIAL NUTRIENTS

Calcium assists bone repair in combination with vitamins D, A, and C, plus the minerals phosphorus, magnesium, fluorine, and zinc.

Iron repairs the blood.

Fluorine strengthens bone repairs.

Zinc is vital for repair of burns or wounds by combining with white cells to remove injured tissues.

Copper is essential for repair of bones, skin, muscles, and nerves.

Vitamin A is essential for repair of damaged skin, tissues, and bones.

Vitamin C is vital for repair of wounds, varicose veins, bruises, fractures, acne, and all tissues.

Vitamin D is essential for general body repair and bone fractures.

Vitamin E is vital for skin, tissue, and general repairs.

MAIN FUNCTIONS

The repair system is constantly working to rebuild cuts, abrasions, and damage to the various internal organs, such as the liver. The body is usually able to repair itself when adequate time is allowed and suitable treatment is obtained (depending on the severity of the condition). The process depends on an adequate supply of essential healing nutrients. Generally speaking, all the bodily systems are in a constant state of repair. For some conditions that have developed over many years of hard living and lack of suitable nutrition, the benefits derived from increased nutrition, rest, and proper treatment will provide relief—and sometimes a complete cure. For children, healing occurs at a faster rate compared to adults, provided they are given a proper diet. The human body has a genuine interest and ability to repair: even if nobody else cares, your body will relish proper daily nutrition. Refer to the ailment charts for help on healing specific body parts. Let nature be your true healer.

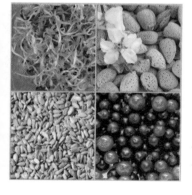

NATURAL FOODS

NOTE: Nutrient amounts are listed as milligrams (mg) per 100 grams (g), unless otherwise stated.

AILMENTS AND HEALING INTRODUCTION

This section, on ailments and healing, is designed to cover a wide range of common ailments and to list the most suitable natural foods, supplements, and other factors to assist with either the prevention or healing of the specific ailment.

The information is provided as a guide only. It should not be interpreted as a cure for any ailment or condition. Obtain advice and guidance from a qualified medical practitioner, naturopath, or therapist for a diagnosis and suitable treatment.

A key index appears on pages 192–194. Use it as a guide to the tables on pages 194–198.

The tables list many different ailments and the bodily systems that are affected by them; for example, abscess (see table excerpt below): number 17 (skin system), number 13 (immune system). Refer back to the sections dealing with the skin system (page 190) and immune system (page 188) for detailed information on the functions of the specific body system, the essential nutrients required to maintain it, and the foods that supply the required nutrients.

Every ailment affects at least one bodily system. Usually, at least two or three systems are in need of repair, correct food intake, specific nutrients, and other factors. These are all summarized in the far-right column of the charts, under the heading "Nutritional Needs." Most ailments can benefit from natural foods, supplements, and nutrients. Let nature protect and heal your body.

The main causes of nearly all ailments are the Health Risk Factors, listed and assigned an abbreviation in the key index on page 194. For example, abscess, *risk factors*: infection, bacteria, and poor hygiene. For effective healing, the risk factors must be eliminated or controlled by suitable treatment. Again, refer to the Nutritional Needs column, and/or obtain proper medical advice.

AILMENT	BODY SYSTEMS	RISK FACTORS	NUTRITIONAL NEEDS
ABSCESS	17, 13	I, B, H	41 42 148 227

Body systems: skin system and immune system
Risk factors: infection, bacteria, hygiene – poor
Nutritional needs: 41 Vitamin A, 42 Vitamin C, 148 Wheatgrass Juice, 227 Tea Tree Oil

BS	BODY SYSTEMS						
1	CIRCULATORY	13	IMMUNE	25	CHLORINE	38	VANADIUM
2	DIGESTIVE	14	JOINT	26	SODIUM	39	BROMINE
3	GLANDULAR	15	OPTIC	27	SILICON	40	CHROMIUM
4	LYMPHATIC	16	REPRODUCTIVE	28	SULFUR	VIT	VITAMINS
5	MUSCULAR	17	SKIN	29	MAGNESIUM	41	A
6	NERVOUS	18	URINARY	30	MANGANESE	42	C
7	RESPIRATORY	19	BRAIN	31	COPPER	43	D
8	SKELETAL	20	REPAIR	32	IODINE	44	E
9	BLOOD	MN	MINERALS	33	ZINC	45	F
10	CELLULAR	21	CALCIUM	34	COBALT	46	K
11	ELIMINATION	22	PHOSPHORUS	35	FLUORINE	47	P
12	GROWTH	23	POTASSIUM	36	SELENIUM	48	T
		24	IRON	37	MOLYBDENUM	49	U

50	B1	92	BROCCOLI	133	HAZELNUT	170	FLOUNDER
51	B2	93	BR. SPROUTS	134	PECAN	171	HADDOCK
52	B3	94	CABBAGE	135	PISTACHIO	172	HERRING
53	B5	95	CARROTS	136	WALNUT	173	MACKEREL
54	B6	96	BELL PEPPER	SEED	SEEDS	174	PERCH
55	B12	97	CAULIFLOWER	137	PUMPKIN (PEPITA)	175	PIKE
56	B15	98	CELERY	138	SESAME	176	SALMON
57	BIOTIN	99	CUCUMBER	139	SUNFLOWER	177	SARDINE
58	CHOLINE	100	GARLIC	SPR	SPROUTS	178	SNAPPER
59	FOLIC ACID	101	LEEK	140	ALFALFA	179	SHARK
60	INOSITOL	102	ONION	141	BEAN	180	TROUT
61	PABA	103	LETTUCE	142	BUCKWHEAT	181	TUNA
FRU	FRUITS	104	PARSLEY	143	LENTIL	SFO	SEAFOOD
62	APPLE	105	PARSNIP	144	MUNG	182	CAVIAR
63	APRICOT	106	POTATO	145	SESAME	183	CLAMS
64	AVOCADO	107	PUMPKIN/SQUASH	146	SUNFLOWER	184	CRAB
65	BANANA	108	RADISH	GJ	GRASS JUICE	185	LOBSTER
66	BERRIES	109	WATERCRESS	147	BARLEY	186	OYSTERS
67	CHERRIES	110	CHARD	148	WHEAT	187	PRAWNS
68	CURRANTS	111	SPINACH	DR	DAIRY	188	SCALLOPS
69	DATES	112	ZUCCHINI	149	BUTTER	189	SHRIMP
70	FIGS	GR	GRAINS	150	CHEESE HARD	SPL	SEA PLANTS
71	GRAPEFRUIT	113	BARLEY	151	CHEESE SOFT	190	AGAR
72	GRAPES	114	CORN	152	CREAM	191	KELP
73	GUAVA	115	MILLET	153	MILK – COW'S	192	SPIRULINA
74	KIWI	116	OATS	154	MILK – GOAT'S	SUP.	SUPPLEMENTS
75	LEMON	117	RICE	155	YOGURT	193	APPLE CIDER VINEGAR
76	LIME	118	RYE	POU	POULTRY	194	ACIDOPHILUS
77	MANGO	119	WHEAT	156	CHICKEN	195	ASCORBIC ACID
78	MELON	LEG	LEGUMES	157	DUCK	196	B COMPLEX
79	NECTARINE	120	CAROB	158	EGGS	197	BREWER'S YEAST
80	OLIVES	121	CHICKPEA	159	EGG YOLK	198	COCONUT MEAL
81	PAPAYA	122	GREEN BEAN	160	TURKEY	199	CORN FLOUR
82	ORANGE	123	KIDNEY BEAN	MT	MEAT	200	DANDELION COFFEE
83	PEACH	124	LENTIL	161	BACON	201	DRIED FRUITS
84	PEAR	125	LIMA BEAN	162	BEEF	202	ECHINACEA
85	PINEAPPLE	126	MUNG BEAN	163	HAM	203	EUCALYPTUS OIL
86	PLUM	127	PEANUTS	164	LAMB	204	HONEY
87	TOMATO	128	PEAS	165	PORK	205	LECITHIN
88	WATERMELON	129	SOYBEAN	166	RABBIT	206	LICORICE
VEG	VEGETABLES	NUT	NUTS	167	VEAL	207	MAPLE SYRUP
89	ARTICHOKE	130	ALMOND	FISH	FISH	208	MISO
90	ASPARAGUS	131	BRAZIL NUT	168	BASS	209	MUESLI
91	BEETS	132	CASHEW	169	COD		

(cont'd.)

210	MOLASSES
211	MUSHROOMS
212	MUSTARD
213	NORI
214	OATMEAL
215	PASTA
216	PECTIN
217	PITA BREAD
218	PROPOLIS
219	PUMPERNICKEL
220	RICE BRAN
221	RICE FLOUR
222	ROYAL JELLY
223	SOY FLOUR
224	SOY MILK
225	SOY SAUCE
226	TAHINI
227	TEA TREE OIL
228	TEMPEH
229	TOFU
230	VINEGAR
231	WHEAT BRAN
232	WHEAT GERM
233	YEAST
HB	HEALTH BENEFITS
234	BALANCED DIET
235	EXERCISE
236	FASTING

237	RELAXATION
238	SLEEP
239	SUNSHINE
240	SWIMMING
241	WATER
242	YOGA
RF	HEALTH RISK FACTORS
A	ALCOHOL
AB	ANTIBIOTICS
AG	ALLERGY
B	BACTERIA
C	CAFFEINE – EXCESS
CH	CHEMICALS
CG	CONTAGIOUS
D	DIET – DEFICIENT
DS	DISEASE
DR	DRUGS
E	EXERCISE – LACK
F	FATS – EXCESS
FE	FEVER
Z	FOOD ADDITIVES
FP	FOOD POISONING
FG	FUNGUS
G	GLUTEN
HR	HEREDITARY
H	HYGIENE – POOR
I	INFECTION

IF	INFLAMMATION
IJ	INJURY
J	JUICE – LACK
M	MEAT – EXCESS
K	MILK – EXCESS
U	MINERALS – LACK
O	OBESITY
OA	OLD AGE
OE	OVEREATING
PR	PRESERVATIVES
P	PROTEIN – LACK
RA	RADIATION
R	REFINED FOODS
Q	SALT – EXCESS
T	SMOKING
BS	STINGS/BITES
SB	STRESS – PHYSICAL
S	STRESS – NERVOUS
X	SUGAR – EXCESS
SU	SUNLIGHT – LACK
TX	TOXINS – AIR
TF	TOXINS – FOOD
TO	TOXINS – OILS
N	UNKNOWN
VR	VIRUS
V	VITAMINS – LACK
L	VITAMIN B – LACK
XR	X RAYS

YS	YEAST INTOLERANCE
HRB	HERBS
292	ALOE VERA
293	ANISEED
294	BASIL
295	CALENDULA
296	CHAMOMILE
297	COMFREY
298	DANDELION
299	GINGER
300	GINSENG
301	LAVENDER
302	MINT
303	PENNYROYAL
304	ROSEHIP
305	ST. JOHN'S WORT
NOL	NATURAL OILS
306	CORN OIL
307	OLIVE OIL
308	SAFFLOWER OIL
309	SESAME OIL
310	SUNFLOWER OIL
311	SOY OIL
312	WHEAT GERM OIL

AILMENT	BODY SYSTEMS	RISK FACTORS	NUTRITIONAL NEEDS
ABSCESS	17, 13	I, B, H	41 42 148 227
ACNE	17, 3, 4	H, D, R, X, F	33 196 41 VEG FRU(JCE) 100
ADENOIDS	3, 4, 7, 13	D, I, L, E, R,	95(JCE) 239 100 HYDROGEN PEROXIDE*
ANEMIA	9, 2	D, U, R, P, L	137 24 42 139 91 196
ANGINA PECTORIS	1, 9, 7	S, T, F, Q, A	44 205 312 85 142 103
ARTERIOSCLEROSIS	1, 9, 2, 11	E, S, T, O, F	205 41 42 44 36
ARTHRITIS	14, 8	S, R, Q, G, D	44 FISH 71 240 98 234
ASTHMA	7, 6, 13	YS, K, L, R, S	95 100 85 136 203 130

* hydrogen peroxide gargle

AILMENT	BODY SYSTEMS	RISK FACTORS	NUTRITIONAL NEEDS
BAD BREATH	2, 7, 11	E, D, G, I, T	236 194 235 234 241
BALDNESS	17, 10, 20, 1	D, L, S, R, HR	103 235 148 196 116
BRONCHITIS	7, 13	YS, I, T, D, K	100 148 85 239 95 41
BRUISING	1, 20, 10	O, D, L, V, E	142 312 96 91 42
CANCER	13, 10, 9, 20	D, V, U, J, L	148 100 147 94 42 VEG
CHICKENPOX	13, 17, 20	V, H, J	238 196 42 95 237 81
CIRCULATION	1, 5, 9	E, D, F, J	235 312 205 240 226
CHOLESTEROL	9, 1, 2, 4	F, M, K, S, R	205 LEG VEG NUT
CELIAC DISEASE	2, 11	G, HR, R, D	LEG FRU NUT VEG 194
COLITIS	11, 2, 20	S, IF, I, AG, D	MN VIT 81 194 62
COMMON COLD	7, 13, 11, 4	K, V, IF, J, TX, S	95 239 96 202 42 146 304
CONSTIPATION	11, 2, 6	D, S, R, L, E	84 216 FRU 241 LEG
CROUP	7, 13, 11	I, V, K, R, D	85(JCE) 237 63 203 INHALE STEAM
CYSTIC FIBROSIS	3, 2, 7	HR, N, P, E	196 312 148 239
CYSTITIS	7, 11, 13	B, I, D	88(JCE) 66(JCE) 99(JCE) 241
DANDRUFF	17, 3, 10, 11	V, D, B, H, L	196 95(JCE) 139 100 227
DERMATITIS	17, 10, 6, 20	IF, S, CH, AG	241 96 196 237 42
DIABETES, TYPE 2	2, 3	X, OE, D, HR, R, S, K	196 42 LEG 312 40 116 33
DIARRHEA	11, 2, 3	B, S, H, D, Z	120 66 155 106 62 237 201
DIVERTICULITIS	2, 20, 11, 6	IF, B, D, R, H	220 62 201 LEG 214 241
ECZEMA	17, 6, 20, 13	S, CH, AG, HR, B, D	FISH 226 VEG 196 FRU 95(JCE)
EDEMA	18, 2, 1, 11	Q, L, E, D, O	98(JCE) 234 65 312 130 235
EMPHYSEMA	7, 11, 10	T, E, YS, I	95(JCE) 148 235 312 85(JCE)

(cont'd.)

AILMENT	BODY SYSTEMS	RISK FACTORS	NUTRITIONAL NEEDS
EPILEPSY	6, 19	IJ, TF, AG, K, HR, U	237 NUT 234 VEG FRU(JCE)
FEVER	13, 4, 1	I, V, B, TX	75(JCE) FRU(JCE) 195 238 202 209
GALLSTONES	2, 11, 4	F, X, AG, D, O	205 307 75(JCE) VEG
GASTRITIS	2, 11, 10	A, C, D, Z, B,	81 94 65 148 95(JCE)
GASTROENTERITIS	2, 13	B, TX, VR, AG, A	236 302(TEA) 100 238
GLAUCOMA	15, 3	HR, IJ, DS, IF	95(JCE) 195 FRU 66 FISH 196
GOITER	3, 2, 11, 4	U, TX, I, D	191 KELP TABLETS 139 131
GOUT	14, 9, 2, 11	M, A, D, O, C	241 122 FRU(JCE) 98 88
HEMORRHOIDS	11, 2, 5	SB, D, E, R, C	292 81 235 142 237
HAY FEVER	15, 6, 11, 13	AG, YS, CH, HR, TX	95(JCE) 75(JCE) 100 HORSERADISH
HEADACHE	19, 6, 9, 13, 11	S, SB, I, AG, E, TO	FRU(JCE) 130 237 62 235 137
HEART ATTACK	1, 6, 2	D, F, E, O, S	205 85(JCE) 100 42 136 312
INDIGESTION	2, 6,	OE, S, F, D, A	237 62 241 201
INFECTION	13, 4, 10, 20	IJ, DS, B, H	95(JCE) 148 227 42 204 295 (EYE) 218
INSOMNIA	6, 19	S, E, C, D, X	296 196 103 239 155 235
JAUNDICE (HEP. A)	9, 11, 17, 2	V, D, F, A, R, IF, H	91(JCE) 95(JCE) 238 87(JCE) 205 VEG
KIDNEY STONES	18, 2, 9, 3	M, A, R, D	241 VEG(JCE) FRU(JCE) 237
LEUKEMIA	9, 13, 10	RA, CH, X, R, D, VR	148 91(JCE) 95(JCE) VEG FRU
MEASLES	13, 7, 4, 17	IF, VR, FE, TX, CG	237 FRU(JCE) VEG(JCE)
MENINGITIS	19, 9, 13	VR, FE, B, IF	MEDICAL HELP 95(JCE)
MONONUCLEOSIS/ GLANDULAR FEVER	4, 3, 13, 9	D, IF, H, VR	238 95(JCE) VEG(JCE) 42 196
MULTIPLE SCLEROSIS	6, 19	VR, DS, R, S, D	196 130 136 312 FISH 137

AILMENT	BODY SYSTEMS	RISK FACTORS	NUTRITIONAL NEEDS
NEPHRITIS	18, 1, 20	IF, S, E, D, R	VEG FRU 241 LEG
NEURITIS	6, 13, 5	M, IF, L, IJ, FP	75(JCE) 196 VEG NUTS
OBESITY	2, 11, 3, 4, 1	E, OE, F, M, K	235 FRU(JCE) 241 VEG(JCE) 236
OSTEOARTHRITIS	14, 10, 8	SB, U, OA, E, R	71(JCE) 98(JCE) 312 239 65
OSTEOPOROSIS	8, 16, 20, 10	U, OA, E, A, T	239 NUTS 235 224 297 242
PARKINSON'S DIS.	6, 19, 5	SB, S, L, DS, TX	54 196 148 136 50 45 239 44
PNEUMONIA	7, 13, 10	IF, B, VR, V, T	95(JCE) VEG(JCE) 239 148 FRU
POLIO	6, 5, 13	VR, H, IF	VEG(JCE) 148 95(JCE) 196 239
PROSTATITIS	18, 16, 13, 3	S, H, IF, OA, C	137 91(JCE) 44 NUT 87
PSORIASIS	17, 10	HR, D, U, TX	239 139 FISH 95(JCE) 312
RSI/REPETITIVE STRAIN INJURY	5, 6, 14, 1, 19	SB, S, D	237 312 340 NUT 226 239
RHEUMATISM	5, 14, 13	IF, D, U, OA, S	98(JCE) 239 226 136 130
RHEUMATOID ARTHRITIS	14, 13, 5,	S, IF, OA, D, V	100 138 299 139 235 312
SCALDS/BURNS	17, 10, 13, 20	FIRE, HEAT	BATHE IN COLD WATER, SEEK MEDICAL HELP
SCIATICA	14, 5, 8, 6	SB, IJ, IF	237 226 240 196 65 242 FRU(JCE)
SHINGLES	6, 13, 17, 10	VR, D, S, OA	196 239 42 295 81 148
SINUSITIS	7, 13, 4, 11	K, D, B, R, V	100 111 95(JCE) VEG(JCE) 239 85(JCE)
SLIPPED DISC/ BACKACHE	14, 8, 5, 6	IJ, E, O	237 312 240 226 239 65 235
STOMACH ULCER	2, 6, 10	D, S, T, A, K, Q, C	81 94 241 194 237 95(JCE) 206 100
STRESS	6, 19, 3	E, L, C, T, X	237 238 196 235 239 130 240 62 88 137 103 296
STROKE	1, 19, 7, 5, 9	S, D, Q, E, T	205 237 196 312 FRU(JCE) 65 FISH

(cont'd.)

AILMENT	BODY SYSTEMS	RISK FACTORS	NUTRITIONAL NEEDS
SUNBURN/SUN STROKE	17, 10, 20	SUN EXP., W	241 81(GEL) 292 44 301 295 CALAMINE
SWOLLEN GLANDS/ GLANDULAR FEVER	3, 4, 9, 13	VR, V, D, J	95(JCE) 237 100 42 VEG(JCE) 85
STI/SEXUALLY TRANSMITTED INFECTION	16, 17, 3, 13, 9	I, H, CG, VR	148 100 42 147 202 218 96
THROMBOSIS	1, 9, 5	E, O, D, TX	142 85(JCE) 42 98(JCE) 235 71 312
THRUSH	2, 13, 16, 17	AB, DR, X, FG, YS	194 155 100 295 227
TINEA	17, 13, 10	FG, H, CG, B	239 227 301 196 234
TONSILITIS	4, 7, 13	VR, B, IF, J, D	85(JCE) 42 95(JCE) 204 HPG*
TUBERCULOSIS	7, 13, 4	I, VR, K, D, B, T	95(JCE) 75(JCE) 85(JCE) 148 100 FRU(JCE)
ULCERS	17, 20, 13	AG, H, S, D	81 312 155 292
URTICARIA/HIVES/ NETTLE RASH	17, 13, 10	DR, Z, S, AG, BS	42 191 102 295 296 96 100
VAGINITIS	16, 13, 20, 17	IF, B, YS, CH, D	194 155 193 100 227
VARICOSE VEINS	1, 5, 9, 7	E, O, HR, V, SB	142 98(JCE) 42 237 96 71
VENEREAL DISEASE	16, 18, 20, 13	DS, CG, I, H	148 202 96 42
VIRUSES	7, 13, 9, 4	CG, IF, K, D, J	85(JCE) 100 104 42 148 VEG(JCE)
WARTS	13, 9, 17	VR, S, X, CG	227 75(OIL)
WHOOPING COUGH	7, 13, 4	B, I, K, D	85(JCE) 96 95(JCE) 241 63 204 239
WORMS	2, 11	IF, H, M, CG	100 137 95(JCE)
WOUNDS	17, 9, 20, 10	IJ, I , IF	292 312 95 295 81(GEL) 296

* hydrogen peroxide gargle

The following pages provide a guide to various ideas for diet plans that are based on the benefits of natural foods. These diet plans are not remedies or treatments—please consult a medical practitioner for a diagnosis and advice. The main aim of the various suggestions is to show how natural foods in the daily diet contribute specific nutrients or ingredients that may provide improved health benefits, when taken regularly. In most cases, natural foods are recognized as being safe and essential for human health. As the research on natural foods continues, more benefits seem to be discovered.

In this era, factories manufacture food products that are nearly always based on natural foods. This food processing is basically all about profit (advertising costs are just a tax deduction). Colorful, shiny packages containing a single finely sliced potato, cooked oils, free radicals, salt, and flavorings provide no health benefits—and they cost the earth. Factory foods take the place of the real thing: properly prepared natural meals that can be quick, simple, cheap, nutritious, and delicious!

If we forget the art of using natural foods and let our tastebuds be dictated to by advertising, packaging, additives, flavorings, cooked oils, takeout, drive-ins, and fast food, our generation and future ones of processed-food addicts are likely to end up with recurrent health problems. Is that worth the temporary taste stimulation from a repetitive intake of two-minute meals and fast-acting sugar drinks? Natural foods provide all the human nutritional needs, and they are presented in unique packages. Natural foods are the undisputed king of nutrition and queen of generous health benefits.

This book provides over two hundred different meal ideas that are full of flavor, nutritional benefits, and health advantages. Put together a shopping list of natural foods based on some of the recipes on pages 216–221. Most recipes take less time to make than a trip to the drive-through. Tonight, skip the waiting in line, the car exhaust fumes, and the paying through the nose for fast food. Instead, be inspired by the world of real foods.

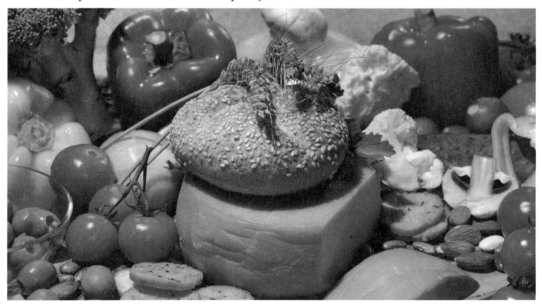

CUSTOM-MADE DIETS INTRODUCTION

ANTICANCER DIET IDEAS

This information is provided as a guide only. Please consult your medical practitioner for a proper diagnosis and treatment plan. Cancer comes in many forms; some of the ideas mentioned here may suit one type of cancer but be less helpful for other types. Natural foods in their natural state provide safe nutrition, and they offer numerous possible healing benefits if consumed regularly.

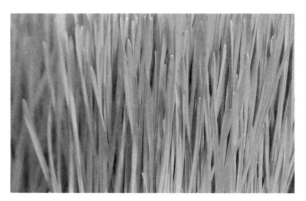

BREAKFAST

A papaya for breakfast provides benefits for colon cancer, due to its fiber, folate, vitamin C, and beta-carotene. The kiwi supplies a good amount of vitamin C antioxidant power, which reduces free radicals. Lemon and lime juice supply flavonoids (flavonol glycosides) that help to reduce cell division in many cancer cells; plus, they supply vitamin C. Grapefruit contains phytochemicals known as limonoids, which inhibit tumor formation by producing an enzyme that helps eliminate toxins from the liver. Pineapple juice provides manganese, vital for antioxidant defense against free radicals. Muskmelon or cantaloupe provides vitamins C and A, for antioxidant power and to counteract free radical activity. Berries, especially blueberries, are full of antioxidant power from their content of phenols, which promote anticancer action by preventing oxidative damage to organs. Blueberries and strawberries also supply ellagic acid, an antioxidant that can block cancer development. Blueberries are the ultimate source of phytonutrients that neutralize free radical cell damage and promote the action of vitamin C. A fresh fruit breakfast is a positive way to start a day.

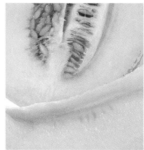

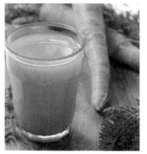

MORNING SNACK

Start with a freshly extracted carrot and parsley juice for an excellent dose of carotene to inhibit tumor growth and for help with lung and pancreatic cancer. Sulfur in carrots assists to eliminate toxins. Parsley supplies anticancer benefits in the form of myristicin, a volatile oil, and the flavonoid luteolin, an antioxidant. Furthermore, with its excellent vitamin C content, parsley heals. Try a juice of 90% carrot and 10% parsley every two days.

LUNCH

For colon cancer, try a legume meal (refer to the recipes on page 219). For other cancers, try steamed brown rice with broccoli, sliced Brussels sprouts, carrots, onions, corn, and red bell pepper. Rice is alkaline; it helps with healing. Add garlic in the last seconds and ground pepitas, especially for prostate cancer. Or, for a simple snack, try asparagus with soy mayonnaise and baked tofu, or a fresh salad with walnut oil.

AFTERNOON SNACK

Wheatgrass juice is the ultimate blood rebuilder and anticancer tonic due to its super beta-carotene power, super lycopene antioxidant power, and chlorophyll content (refer to page 112 for details). Without a regular wheatgrass juice, blood-based cancers are hard to beat.

EVENING MEAL

Try baked pumpkin or winter squash with broccoli and fish with lemon juice for help with lung cancer. Tabouli salad with grilled tofu for help with colon cancer. Pasta with lots of ground pumpkin seeds, chopped parsley, and parmesan cheese to help blood-based cancers. Serve with a sip of red wine. Enjoy Brussels sprouts with honey carrots plus salmon with red chilli peppers for help with skin cancer. For dessert, acidophilus yogurt with honey for colon health. Black cherries contain ellagic acid, flavonoids, and perillyl alcohol; they're anticarcinogenic and they stunt the growth of cancer cells.

NOTE: DV refers to the daily value for women 25–50 years, refer to RDI tables on pages 95–96 for adult male and child values.

ANTISTRESS DIET IDEAS

BREAKFAST

Watermelon juice and apple juice both provide alkaline balance to the blood; plus melons are full of bromine, which is vital for emotional stability and also as an anti-depressant. Try tahini on toast, as tahini is full of *magnesium* (320 mg), the nerve mineral, plus *calcium* (330 mg), for calming the nerves and peaceful sleep. Vegemite, or yeast extract, on toast, is a very good source of vitamins *B1*: nerves; *B2*: anti-stress, anti-fatigue; *B3*: nourishes the nerves, anti-depression, fatigue; *B5*: anti-stress, depression; *B6*: anti-stress, irritability, nervousness; folate: nerves, brain, anti-fatigue. Most of these B vitamins are water soluble and required daily. A B-complex tablet taken every day is beneficial.

MORNING SNACK

Try a handful of almonds—*phosphorus* (490 mg): increases strength and repairs nerves, improves concentration and memory; *magnesium* (260 mg): protects against hardened arteries and high blood pressure; and *calcium* (250 mg): promotes regular heart action and digestion. Have an apple or two peaches with the almonds.

LUNCH

Veggie sandwich—lettuce is an excellent source of *silicon:* (1,500 mg) protects against nervous exhaustion, mental fatigue, and baldness. Lettuce also supplies *folate* (15 mg): nerve functioning; *sulfur* (580 mg): brain functioning; and *chlorine:* regulates blood pressure. Add some sliced red bell pepper for an excellent supply of *vitamin C*, the anti-stress and headache vitamin. Add a few walnuts, rich in *omega-3:* nerve functioning; and *biotin:* for sleep, antidepression, and nervousness. Include a few slices of cheddar cheese (*protein:* nerve cell building, adrenaline production, brain hormone transfer) on rye bread for *potassium* (460 mg): strengthens the heart muscles and vital for mental function, nervous system, and brain.

AFTERNOON SNACK

A handful of cashews with a cup of tea. Cashews are rich in *zinc* (5.7 mg): protects against fatigue and is required for the action of B vitamins and for mental alertness. Cashews are a good source of *manganese* (0.8 mg) required for memory; *magnesium* (250 mg); *phosphorus* (530 mg) for energy production, concentration, nerves, and brain health. Cashews and a crisp apple are the perfect nourishing nerve snack.

EVENING MEAL

Pumpkin seed (pepita) pasta: Add 4 tablespoons of ground pepitas to your pasta sauce, or sprinkle on top of the pasta with cheese. Pepitas are an excellent source of *iron* (11.3 mg): protects against fatigue, promotes endurance and resistance to stress. Pepitas are also an excellent source of *zinc* (7.5 mg): required for the action of B vitamins, alcohol conversion, and protection from fatigue and mental stress; *magnesium* (535 mg): controls the central nervous system, protects against mental exhaustion and irritability. Also affords an excellent balance of *phosphorus* (1,174 mg): essential for the nervous system and brain function by promoting memory and concentration; copper (1.4 mg): promotes vitamin C absorption, protects the nerve fibers, promotes iron utilization. Add ground pepitas to soup or vegetable burgers for the ultimate regenerating balance to the nervous system. Pepitas are the greatest antistress food.

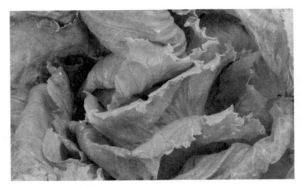

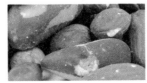
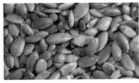

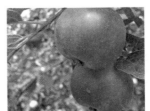
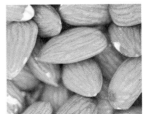

NOTE: Nutrient amounts are listed as milligrams (mg) per 100 grams (g), unless otherwise stated.

ATHLETE'S DIET IDEAS

BREAKFAST

Grape juice freshly extracted provides the ultimate source of *dextrose*, easily absorbed into the bloodstream, providing nearly instant energy for that early-morning workout.

Sunflower butter is easy to make. Grind 1 cup of sunflower kernels in a blender or grinder, place in a large bowl, add 1 tablespoon honey and 2 tablespoons soft butter, mix together with a fork into a smooth consistency, serve on rye toast. Sunflower butter provides an excellent source of *vitamin E* (34 mg): promotes the endurance, stamina, and power of muscles; *protein* (23 g): muscle growth (muscle fibers are collections of protein molecules), repair of damaged tissues, and hormones, which regulate body functions. *It also provides vitamin B1* (2.3 mg): essential during strenuous exercise for oxygen absorption and energy conversion; *iron* (6.8 mg): muscle endurance, tissue repair, and blood oxygen levels; *phosphorus* (705 mg): energy distribution and blood circulation; *zinc* (5.1 mg): tissue growth and insulin/glucose activity; *selenium* (60 mcg): vitamin E activity; *vitamin B3* (4.5 mg): protein effectiveness and energy production in muscle cells. Vitamin B3 is depleted during bouts of strenuous exercise.

MORNING SNACK

Have a banana smoothie. The banana is an ideal provider of *energy* (22 g) and a good source of *potassium* (358 mg), known as the muscle mineral because it is vital for repair of muscles, strength of muscles, and is the foundation mineral of muscular tissue. *Chlorine* (270 mg) for heart muscle action; *sulfur* (120 mg) for heart muscles, carbohydrate metabolism, and insulin manufacture. Milk provides a fair amount of *calcium* (115 mg) for muscle action, tissue development, heart muscle function, and bone strength and repair.

AFTERNOON SNACK

Two servings of hazelnuts with two apples, for an excellent supply of *protein* (30–42 g), vitamin E (30 mg), carbohydrate (34 g), magnesium (320 mg), calcium (220 mg), and unsaturated fats (100 g) for lasting energy.

LUNCH

Kidney bean tacos. Kidney beans provide excellent *carbohydrate* value (60 g) with a low GI and an energy supply to last all afternoon. Excellent *potassium* (1,406 mg) for muscles; *iron* (8 mg) for oxygen supply; *folate* (394 mcg) for physical endurance and protein formation; *calcium* (143 mg) for bone strength; *phosphorus* (407 mg) for bone strength and energy production; *magnesium* (140 mg) for muscle function and protection from muscular cramps; *copper* (1 mg) for heart muscles; *molybdenum* for iron-oxygen utilization. Add lettuce, carrot, onion, and tomato salsa to provide numerous nutrients, and cheese to increase the protein value of the kidney bean's already *complete protein* (24–40 g) and to add excellent *calcium* (700–900 mg) for bone strength and muscle action.

EVENING MEAL

Fish and chips. Fish supply excellent *protein* (20–25 g) for muscle growth; *cobalt* for body cell activity, growth, and energy; *selenium* for growth, skin elasticity; *vanadium* for blood circulation. Potato chips provide quick carbohydrate energy with the fat content providing a slower release of energy. About two to three hours after the fish meal, have a large serving of yogurt to promote a peaceful night's sleep and to relax your muscles, as yogurt helps to break down lactic acid, which builds up during strenuous exercise.

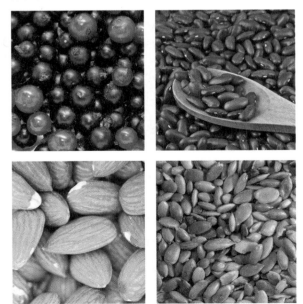

NOTE: DV refers to the daily value for women 25–50 years, refer to RDI tables on pages 95–96 for adult male and child values.

CHILDREN'S DIET IDEAS

BREAKFAST

- pineapple, strawberry, and mango juice in summer
- grape juice in autumn
- mandarin and strawberry juice in winter
- apple and peach juice in spring

Allow children to have a choice from a variety of in-season fruits to make a freshly extracted juice. Start with small serves of about 120 ml or half a cup, serve in a glass, and in hot weather, add a few cubes of ice. The fresh juice in the morning will provide children with a fair dose of *vitamin C,* depending on the juice, plus a variety of other vitamins and minerals that are lacking from cooked and processed foods. Freshly made fruit juices provide the natural sweetness that children crave, as fructose (fruit sugar) is converted into glucose. Over 90% of all glucose is used for the nervous system and for brain activity. Give your children a head start, every day.

Cereal, toast, pancakes, muffins, scrambled eggs, croissants, rolled oats, fruit salad, or yogurt: Allow children to choose from at least a few of these. Even set up a small blackboard/whiteboard on the kitchen wall and pretend it's a classy restaurant. Nearly every day, children have slightly different nutritional needs, and by giving them a choice, once a child has experienced a variety of foods, their body and tastebuds will go for the foods that may provide the specific nutrients that are required for their current development. Processed cereals of good quality are okay once or twice a week. Try the blackboard choice idea, and utilize natural foods and canned apricots or peaches on cereal, or a sprinkle of finely chopped macadamias or pecans, or pancakes with stewed apples and cream, or toast with honey or peanut butter. Breakfast is vital for growing children.

MORNING SNACK AT SCHOOL

Children are keen to run and play after a morning of sitting down. They have little time to eat, so give them quick snacks and make up for the nutrition factor at home. Make the servings small, to fit in their hand. A cheese sandwich cut into quarters is ample and excellent; crackers and cheese; a small tub of yogurt; a muesli bar or sesame bar; an apple juice; a fresh crisp small apple; dried apricots. Apples provide compact nutrition—time for the bell!

LUNCH

Give your children the choice: It's their lunch. Use the blackboard idea at home for lunch ideas. Depending on the season and temperature always give them pure water and a *choice* of sandwich: salad or cheese or chicken or ham or egg. Or crackers with cheese, or muffins, a snack bar, or tub of yogurt. In winter, a milk drink can last till after school; in summer a frozen fruit juice will be refreshing.

Lunch time is also play time!

AFTER SCHOOL AND EVENING MEAL

A milkshake and hummus on crackers, or a chocolate drink and pancake, or a toasted cheese sandwich will give children ample nourishment while they're doing their homework till the evening meal. For evening meal ideas, as a family, choose from the variety of recipe ideas on pages 216–221. For dessert, yogurt is ideal as it provides essential calcium during their sleep.

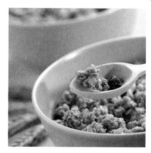
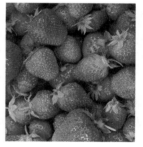
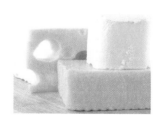
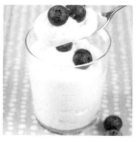

OUR HOME MENU

- ☐ pancakes with apple and cream
- ☐ scrambled eggs on toast
- ☐ rye toast with hummus
- ☐ toast with cheese
- ☐ rolled oats with peaches, apricots
- ☐ cereal with macadamia nuts
- ☐ yogurt with waffles and strawberries
- ☐ croissants with blueberry jam and cream

NOTE: Nutrient amounts are listed as milligrams (mg) per 100 grams (g), unless otherwise stated.

IRON-BOOSTING DIET IDEAS

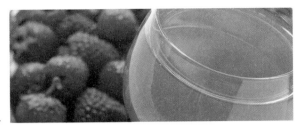

BREAKFAST

Apple (0.2 mg) and strawberry (0.6 mg) juice. *Total iron:* approximately 0.8 mg.

Rolled oats (3.7 mg) with ¼ cup raisins (2.2 mg) plus a tablespoon of wheat germ (2 mg). Serve with a cup of milk (0.05 mg) or soy milk (0.5 mg). *Total breakfast iron:* approximately 8.4 mg.

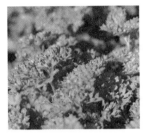
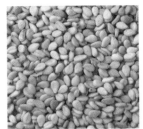

MORNING SNACK

Date dip: dried dates (2.6 mg) dipped into ¼ cup tahini (3 mg). Or walnuts (2.5 mg) on rye bread (2.7 mg) with honey, or ¼ cup sunflower seed butter (2 mg) on whole-meal bread (2.2 mg).

LUNCH

Tabouli salad: ¾ cup parsley (4.5 mg), ¼ cup chopped tomato (0.2 mg), ¾ cup chopped raw spinach (3.2 mg), 2 tablespoons tahini dressing (1.7 g) on rye bread (2.7 mg). *Total lunch iron:* 12.3 mg. Seafood mix with mussels (14 mg) or clams (8 mg). Hummus dip: chickpeas (2.5 mg) with 2 T tahini (1.8 mg) on rye cracker biscuits (2 mg). *Total lunch iron:* 6.3 mg.

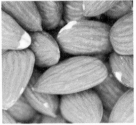
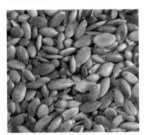

AFTERNOON SNACK

Carob milkshake: mix ¼ cup carob powder (2.3 mg) with 2 cups soy milk (1.1 mg). *Total iron:* 3.4 mg.

Carrot and parsley juice: 8 ounces carrot (2.2 mg) with ¾ cup parsley (4.7 mg). *Total iron:* 6.9 mg.

EVENING MEAL

Stir fry. Into the wok add tofu cubes (7.9 mg) with ⅓ cup peas (1.6 mg), broccoli (1 mg), ¾ cup parsley (4.7 mg), ⅓ cup chopped onions (0.27 mg), bell pepper (0.7 mg), and 2 ounces cashews (1.9 mg). *Total iron:* 18 mg.

Pumpkin seed burgers. In a bowl, mix ground pumpkin seeds (11.2 mg), ½ cup finely chopped parsley (3.2 mg), spinach (3.2 mg), and 2 T chopped onion (1.2 mg) with 100 g cooked rice (0.4 mg). Form into patties, fry with canola oil, and serve with garden fresh salad (3 mg). *Total iron:* 19.2 mg.

DAILY IRON INTAKE — RDA		
Gender/Stage	**Age**	**Iron (mg per day)**
Children	1–13	7-10 mg
Male	14–18	11 mg
Male	19–50	8 mg
Female	14–50	18 mg
Female	51+	8 mg
Pregnancy	19–50	27 mg
Lactation	19–50	9 mg
IRON-BOOSTING DIET DAILY SUPPLY VALUES		
Meal	**Total (mg)**	**Average (mg)**
Breakfast	8.4	8.4
Morning snack	5	5
Lunch	6.3–14	10
Afternoon snack	3.4–6.9	5
Evening meal	18–19.2	18.5
Total Daily Iron Average		**46.9 mg**

NOTE: DV refers to the daily value for women 25–50 years, refer to RDI tables on pages 95–96 for adult male and child values.

REJUVENATING DIET IDEAS

BREAKFAST

Papaya slices with a squeeze of lemon juice promote cleansing and healing. The papaya provides *lutein* and *zeaxanthin* for eyesight restoration, *carpain* for heart healing, *beta cryptoxanthin* for colon health, and *vitamin C* (62 mg), the youth vitamin, for supple skin, reduced skin cell oxidation, good eyesight, and collagen/skin formation. Lemon juice provides *vitamin C*, as well as *sulfur* (125 mg), for cleansing and elimination of bacteria.

MORNING SNACK

Walnuts and swiss cheese on rye with green tea. Walnuts are an excellent source of *omega-3* for healthy skin and eyes; *vitamin B6* (0.7 mg), the vitality vitamin, for antibody production and pituitary gland function; *copper* (2 mg) for skin pigment and vitamin C activity; *folate* (98 mcg) for reproduction of cells; *biotin* for cellular rejuvenation and conversion of fats into energy. Green tea provides *flavonoids,* which promote antioxidant benefits and healthy skin. Swiss cheese provides excellent *protein* for cellular production and excellent *calcium* to offset osteoporosis and for elasticity of the skin.

LUNCH

Tahini with sprout salad. Tahini is a very good source of *vitamin E* (40 mg), which protects cells from oxidation, promotes healing of damaged skin, and promotes normal cell life and skin nourishment; torulitine (*vitamin T*) for brain nourishment and improved memory; *zinc* (4.6 mg) for healing, healthy skin and hair; *calcium* (420 mg) for good sleep, skin cell and tissue development.

The sprouts provide numerous active enzymes to promote digestive, glandular, and immune system functions, plus vitamin C and numerous trace nutrients to rejuvenate the body.

For a super-rejuvenating sprout salad, add 2 tablespoons of ground pepitas to obtain an excellent supply of *iron* for cell development, tissue repair, and body cleansing; *protein* for cellular repair; and a wide variety of minerals for a complete balance of body needs.

AFTERNOON SNACK

Carrot and cucumber juice, the ultimate skin-cleansing and rejuvenating juice. The excellent carotene supply from carrots (11,000 mg) promotes soft skin and healing of damaged skin; the excellent sulfur content (445 mg) and chlorine content (318 mg) promote liver and skin cleansing like no other food. Carrot and cucumber are good sources of silicon, vital for healthy hair growth and a good complexion.

EVENING MEAL

Salmon with a fresh garden salad. Salmon is a very good source of omega-3, for improved skin condition and healing and protection from dry skin. The lettuce provides the ultimate source of silicon for hair growth and condition, plus chlorophyll for body cleansing, and numerous active enzymes for rejuvenation. Red bell pepper provides an abundance of vitamin C for skin rejuvenation and improved eyesight, and bioflavonoids for prevention of cell oxidation and premature aging. Asparagus provides an abundance of *fluoride* for skin and eye health and bladder cleansing, *folate (*120 mcg) for the cellular system and skin health, and *rutin* to strengthen blood vessels and protect against varicose veins. Later in the evening, have a serving of acidophilus yogurt for a peaceful sleep and to balance and cleanse the digestive system of bad bacteria and toxins.

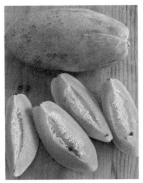
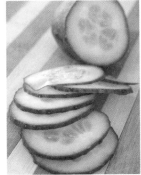
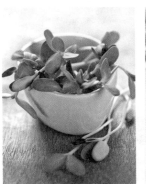
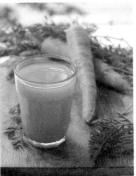

NOTE: Nutrient amounts are listed as milligrams (mg) per 100 grams (g), unless otherwise stated.

TEENAGER'S DIET IDEAS

BREAKFAST

Start the day with any freshly extracted fruit juice to kick off the brain power; the fruit sugar will quickly get to work, feeding the brain. And in case you have a hangover (naughty!) fructose will eliminate excess alcohol quicker than any other substance. Vitamin C eliminates toxins and boosts the immune system with antioxidant power. Try pineapple, orange, and strawberry juice for a delicious nonalcoholic cocktail! For further brain power, if you are a student, try some slivered almonds on your breakfast cereal; they're full of magnesium and brain minerals. Or try some tahini, the memory food, with rye toast for super brain power, or add a few lecithin granules to your scrambled eggs to feed the gray matter—28% of a healthy brain is comprised of lecithin. (Very few foods contain lecithin, and processed foods certainly don't.) If you are a physically hard-working teenager, check the athlete's diet on page 202 for breakfast ideas. Give your body the *breakfast habit:* it's the foundation for brain stability.

MORNING SNACK

Try a walnut cream bun, or an almond cake with a cup of mixed cereal, plus coffee and half-and-half, for a mild but steady caffeine hit. If you have an acne problem, have a glass of water, one apple or peach, and a handful of raw almonds, a rich source of vitamin E, which is an antioxidant and required regularly. Take a low-dose vitamin B-complex tablet to help the skin and brain; there are 12 B vitamins, 5 of which are required daily, and they are hard to get from takeout and cooked foods.

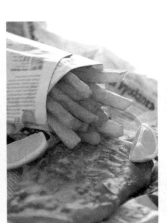
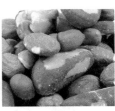
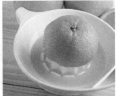

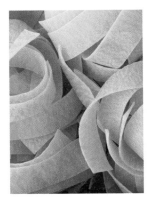
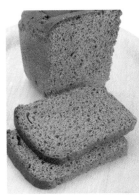

LUNCH

Depending on the climate, a serving of fish and chips will provide *protein* and *carbohydrate* energy, or try a kebab with lots of salad. If you have a skin problem, carrot juice is the best as it provides abundant *sulfur* for eliminating toxins from the skin plus loads of *carotene* for the skin. Have a carrot juice three times a week and watch zits disappear. A veggie sandwich is easy, cheap, and beneficial.

AFTERNOON SNACK

If you live in a city or near a big shopping center, the variety of snacks available to you is amazing, but choose wisely for true value. If you have not had any fresh juice, make it a priority, then add calories knowing your body will obtain great benefit from the juice: cleansing of the skin, antioxidant power, and brain energy. A handful of almonds, Brazil nuts, and cashews with an apple will keep you going for hours while providing excellent protein and nutrients. A turkey or roast beef sandwich provides 600 calories, about the same as the nuts, and will keep you going for three hours. You need 2,700–3,000 calories a day.

EVENING MEAL

Rice and pasta are simple to prepare and, depending on the additions, they can be a very good base for a complete meal. For a real protein and iron boost, add a tablespoon of ground pepitas to the pasta or stir-fry, and gain the best omega-3 and iron boost in the world; it will promote healthy skin and resistance to bugs, flus, infections, viruses, and fatigue. Tacos with veggies are easy and nutritious, or fish and baked vegetables, or check any of the recipe ideas on pages 216–221. It's the *natural foods you add* that make all the difference in flavor and nutrition.

NOTE: DV refers to the daily value for women 25–50 years, refer to RDI tables on pages 95–96 for adult male and child values.

ANTIAILMENT DIET IDEAS AND RECIPE GUIDE

The table below provides a list of dietary ideas that may help prevent particular ailments. The table is not to be used as a treatment guide for a specific ailment. Please consult a medical practitioner or naturopath for diagnosis and treatment of illness. The code system refers to the Nutrition and Diet Summary Tables on pages 216–221. The numbers refer to the left columns of the tables; the letters refer to the meal code across the top of each chart. For example, anti-aging diet, breakfast, 9PL (page 216, fruits): 9 = melons or papaya; PL = pre-lunch: fresh papaya entree.

These simple meal ideas afford numerous nutritional benefits from specific foods. Feed your nutritional appetite daily with natural foods!

Diet Ideas	Breakfast	Morning Snack	Lunch	Afternoon Snack	Evening Meal	Other Beneficial Factors	Possible Detrimental Factors
Antiaging	9 PL	57 B	21 L	12 AS	47 E	papaya, flax oil, swimming	excess sunlight, smoking, stress
Antiarthritis	8 B	1 M	23 L	33 E	60 E	celery, grapefruit, almonds	refined wheat, stress, worry, excess work
Antiasthma	1 B	1 PL	1 M	1 AS	1 ES	apples, pineapple, pumpkin/winter squash	pollen, dust, stress, strenuous work
Antibaldness	33 B	25 L	33 L	33 L	25 E	lettuce juice, cucumber juice, B-complex vitamins	hereditary factors, excess meat, smoking, stress
Antibowel cancer	30 B	9 M	35 L	59 B	30 L	pears, dates, legumes	refined foods, meat, chicken
Antihigh blood pressure	7 B	13 M	23 L	48 L	41 E	grapes, lecithin, pineapple, celery, flax oil	saturated fats, margarine, stress
Anticold	8 B 11 B	9 PL	21 21 E	13 M	28 E	sunlight, lemons, rest, bell peppers, garlic, chili peppers	milk, dairy foods, stress, processed foods
Antidiabetes	49 B	58 B	40 L	33 L	33 E	rolled oats, celery, pumpkin seeds	refined foods, sugar, soft drinks
Antiosteo-porosis	48 B	33 L	59 L	60 E	48 E	sunlight, almonds, cheese, yogurt	refined wheat, lack of exercise
Menopause	9 B	35 B	57 L	21 L	15 E	melons, rye, cantaloupe, pineapple	obesity, poor diet
Pregnancy/ lactation	57 B	6 AS	48 E	6 ES	57 L	walnuts, dates, sunlight	stress, obesity, poor diet, drugs, smoking, alcohol
Weight-loss	9 B	30 B	41 E	14 B	15 E	fresh fruits, rice, exercise, juices, water	animal fats, dairy products, big breakfast

FOOD-COMBINATION TABLE

MAIN FOOD GROUPS		SWEET FRUITS 1	SUB-ACID FRUITS 2	ACID FRUITS 3	MELONS 4	VEGETABLES 5	STARCHY VEGETABLES 6	GRAINS AND PRODUCTS 7	LEGUMES 8	NUTS AND SEEDS 9	MEAT, FISH, POULTRY 10	DAIRY PRODUCTS 11
SWEET FRUITS	1		✓✓		××	×	××		××	××	××	
SUB-ACID FRUITS	2	✓✓	✓✓✓	✓✓	×		×	✓	×			✓
ACID FRUITS	3	×	✓✓	✓✓	×		×	✓		✓		✓
MELONS	4	××	×	×	✓✓	××	××	××	××	××	××	××
VEGETABLES	5	×			××	✓✓✓	✓✓	✓✓✓	✓✓✓	✓	✓✓✓	✓✓
STARCHY VEGETABLES	6	××	×	×	××	✓✓	✓	×	×	××		✓
GRAINS AND PRODUCTS	7		✓	✓	××	✓✓✓	×		✓			✓
LEGUMES	8	××	×		××	✓✓✓	×	✓	✓	×	×	✓
NUTS AND SEEDS	9	××		✓	××	✓✓	××		×	××	×	
MEAT, FISH, POULTRY	10	××			××	✓✓✓			×	×		
DAIRY PRODUCTS	11		✓	✓	××	✓✓	✓	✓	✓			✓✓

Excellent Combo ✓✓✓	Very Good Combo ✓✓	Good Combo ✓	Fair Combo	Poor Combo ×	Bad Combo ××

This food-combination table provides guidance on how to combine foods from the various food groups. See page 210 for a table summarizing which foods belong to which group. Combining foods advantageously enhances foods' ability to promote proper digestion and thus provide a good supply of nutrients. The difference between a diet with good to excellent combinations and one with fair to poor combinations is remarkable.

A great increase in health benefits is possible just by understanding and utilizing proper food combinations at every meal. Obviously, simple meals composed of only one or two foods are usually easy to digest, but it really depends on the individual meal combinations.

More information about food combinations is provided on pages 209–210. Simply speaking, ongoing intake of meals with poor food combinations is one of the main reasons for obesity, or, more specifically, for the distended stomach image. This is due to the fact that poor combinations promote the formation of intestinal gas, which over many years causes the lower intestine area to expand. In addition, the loss of food value from meals may lead to overeating in order to satisfy the nutritional appetite. Also, once the body becomes used to large meals, it continually requires an intake that will support the additional fat cells even though they are not required.

To reverse the problem, proper natural food combinations and a strong willpower to offset hunger demands are required on a regular basis.

FOOD-COMBINING INFORMATION

SWEET FRUITS

Sweet fruits, especially all dried fruits, are a concentrated source of energy in the form of fruit sugars (fructose), and they require unique digestion. Simple combinations are best; a few dried fruits as a snack are ideal. However, when combining other fruits, it is best to have an apple or a peach. Bananas are a concentrated food and should not be combined with any dried fruit but can be combined with apple, apricot, peach, or pear. Do not combine dried fruits with nuts, peanuts, or any other food group as poor digestion and gas may develop.

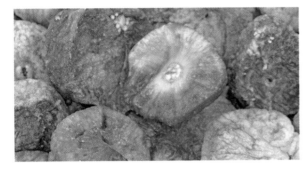

SUB-ACID FRUITS

Sub-acid fruits combine very well with one another; feel free to toss a variety of fruits into a nutritious fruit salad. Obviously some of the sub-acid fruits would not be included due to their unfavorable taste combinations. Avocado on toast, or in a salad with olives, is good. Apples or peaches with almonds is an excellent, delicious, simple snack. Papaya with banana is an excellent snack. Grapes are best eaten alone or just a few in fruit salad or muesli.

ACID FRUITS

Simple combinations of acid fruits are excellent, such as orange, pineapple, and mandarin. Or kiwi, strawberry, tangerine, and pineapple. The tomato is an acid fruit and is widely used in various combinations; however, these are not always nutritionally favorable. Ideally, tomato should not be combined with starches; in that case they may be replaced with red bell pepper. Acid fruits do combine well with small portions of sub-acid fruits, and combinations such as orange and almond are good.

MELONS

Melons require no digestion in the stomach and are basically the simplest food to assimilate due to their very high water content and very simple structure. Melons are best thought of as a drink and should not be eaten after a large meal, as fermentation and gas may develop. They are an ideal breakfast food.

LEAFY AND OTHER VEGETABLES

The variety of vegetables is abundant; they provide the widest range of very suitable food combinations. Fresh garden salads are optimum nutritionally and combine very well with all grains, or nuts and seeds, or animal proteins, or legumes. Ideally, avoid combining raw and cooked vegetables. Some vegetables mixed with dairy foods also combine very well. Ideally, you can combine any leafy vegetable with any single protein food, or with a grain and legume meal, for an excellent combination.

BRASSICA AND STARCHY VEGETABLES

Brassica vegetables combine very well with leafy vegetables, with simple meals such as pasta or rice, and with legumes. Starchy vegetables should not be combined with nuts, seeds, grains, legumes, or animal proteins. It is common for the starchy vegetables to be combined with meat, fish, eggs, or chicken, but this is likely to complicate protein digestion, due to the different requirements of starchy vegetables and proteins. In most cases, it is best to eat the starchy vegetables first. Starchy vegetables combine fairly well with other cooked vegetables and dairy foods such as milk, cheese, and yogurt.

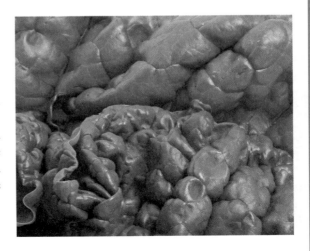

FOOD-COMBINING INFORMATION

FOOD-COMBINING INFORMATION

GRAINS AND PRODUCTS

Whole grains combine very well with vegetables. Rolled oats combine very well with most sub-acid fruits and with milk. Bread combines very well with salads or cheese. Pasta is very suitable when combined with some vegetables. Pizza varieties are numerous; for best digestion, opt for vegetarian with cheese. Meat or vegetable sandwiches or pies are best with spinach, asparagus, cabbage, onion, carrot, leeks, or zucchini.

LEGUMES

The single best combination with legumes is leafy vegetables. Hummus on toast or crackers is a good, cheap, simple combination. Legumes should not be combined with any protein foods as their concentrated starch has digestion requirements that are very different from those required for meat, fish, eggs, poultry, nuts, or seeds. Legumes combine well with dairy foods. The peanut is an ideal snack food when eaten alone or as peanut butter on bread or peanut sauce with rice. Corn chips and beans is a very good combination. Carob powder is ideal with milk drinks. Soy milk combines well with oats or cereals.

NUTS AND SEEDS

The best combination of nuts for a complete protein snack is almonds, Brazil nuts, and cashew nuts (ABC mix). Simple snacks of almonds with an apple or peach are very good. Nuts or seeds combined with leafy vegetables is a very good combination. Do not combine nuts with starch vegetables, legumes, animal proteins, or sweet fruits. Simple combinations of nuts with cookies are all right. A fruit salad with acid fruits and nuts or seeds is very good. Sunflower seeds combine well with oats/milk for breakfast. Ground pumpkin seeds (pepitas) with rice or pasta is very good, especially with leafy vegetables. Tahini is ideal with salads, bread, hummus, or sub-acid fruits.

ANIMAL PROTEINS

Compared to all other food groups, the animal protein foods require the most complex digestion, especially in the stomach. The best combination for animal protein foods is with salads or cooked leafy vegetables, not starch vegetables. A mixed grill is a very complicated meal to digest, especially when starchy vegetables are included. Fish combines very well with cooked leafy or brassica vegetables, or with a garden salad. Eggs should not be combined with other animal proteins. Eggs in cakes, cookies, and vegetable omelets are all right. Avoid combining animal protein foods with one another or with cheese. Fish and chips is a fair combination. Chicken and salads with leafy or brassica vegetables is a good combination.

DAIRY AND OTHER PRODUCTS

Cheese is the most concentrated dairy food. It combines well with salads, bread, or pasta, or with both starch and brassica vegetables. Butter with bread or vegetables is good. Yogurt is best eaten alone or with a simple addition of apple, apricot, or peach. Small portions are fine but best not eaten directly after a large protein meal. Milk chocolate contains concentrated milk fats and should be treated as an occasional snack, not as a meal.

NATURAL FOODS AND INDIVIDUAL FOOD GROUPS

	Group	Foods
	WHOLE GRAINS	barley, bulgur, corn, millet, oats, rice, rye, sorghum, triticale, wheat
	LEGUMES (BEANS/PEAS)	carob, green, kidney, lima, mung, soy, chickpea, lentil, pea, peanut
FRUITS	SUB-ACID FRUITS	apple, apricot, cherry, grape, papaya, peach, pear, mango
FRUITS	SWEET FRUITS	banana, date, fig, prune, raisin, dried fruit
FRUITS	ACID FRUITS	grapefruit, kiwi, lemon, lime, mandarin, tangerine, orange, passionfruit, tomato
FRUITS	MELONS	cantaloupe, casaba, honeydew, watermelon
VEGGIES	STARCHY VEGETABLES	artichoke, beet, carrot, parsnip, potato, pumpkin, winter squash, radish, turnip
VEGGIES	LEAFY VEGETABLES	lettuce, cabbage, celery, chard, spinach, watercress, kale
VEGGIES	FLOWER VEGETABLES	asparagus, broccoli, cauliflower, Brussels sprouts
VEGGIES	OTHER VEGETABLES	bell pepper, cucumber, eggplant, mushroom, okra, onion, summer squash

NOTE: DV refers to the daily value for women 25–50 years, refer to RDI tables on pages 95–96 for adult male and child values.

QUESTION AND ANSWER: NUTRITION AND CARBOHYDRATES

1. What main factors promote good health? (for the answer refer to page 4)

2. Name the five main food groups. (page 4)

3. How do you obtain a balanced diet? (page 4)

4. What are the essential nutrient groups? (page 5)

5. How are carbohydrates made? (page 16)

6. What is a carbohydrate? (page 16)

7. How do you obtain a nutritious diet? (page 5)

8. What is nutrition? (page 4)

9. Define health in one sentence. (page 4)

10. Name five foods in the grains food group. (page 7)

11. Name three foods in the dairy food group. (page 9)

12. List at least three recommendations from the MyPlate program. (page 10)

13. Name the five food groups shown in the MyPlate diagram. (page 11)

14. What food groups are the best sources of carbohydrates? (page 14)

15. Name the food groups that supply no water. (page 14)

16. Describe how the body uses carbohydrates for energy. (page 16)

17. What are the two main types of carbohydrates? (page 16)

18. Name three foods in the carbohydrate food group. (page 7)

19. How do you obtain all the essential nutrients? (page 5)

20. Name two foods to reduce in the daily diet. (page 10)

21. Name two foods to increase. (page 10)

22. List two ways to balance calories. (page 10)

23. Name a one-serving portion in the fruit group. (page 13)

24. Name a one-serving portion in the vegetable group. (page 13)

25. How many servings of grains, per day, are required for teenage boys? (page 12)

26. How many serves of fruit, per day, are required for teenage girls? (page 12)

27. What main food groups supply little or no carbohydrate content? (page 14)

28. Name five foods from the vegetable group. (page 7)

29. How many servings of fruits and vegetables are recommended daily for adult women? (page 12)

QUESTION AND ANSWER: PROTEIN

30. How many amino acids do children need from the diet? (page 90)

31. What is complete protein? (page 85)

32. Name four food groups that supply complete protein. (page 85)

33. How much protein do teenage boys aged 14–18 need daily? (page 86)

34. Name one type of nut that supplies complete protein. (page 92)

35. How many grams of protein does chicken supply, per 100 g? (page 89)

36. Name four essential amino acids. (page 90)

37. Describe what the term NPU means. (page 90)

38. Does excess intake of protein foods lead to weight gain? (page 90)

39. What food group supplies the most protein? (page 89)

40. Name one type of seed that supplies complete protein. (page 92)

41. Do legumes supply complete protein? (page 92)

42. Name one protein food that supplies no cholesterol. (page 88)

43. Name the protein food with the most saturated fat. (page 88)

44. Name the extra amino acid that children need from the diet. (page 90)

45. What essential amino acid is required in the least proportion? (page 90)

46. What is protein made from? (page 85)

47. Name a protein food that contains fiber. (page 88)

48. Name a protein food with over 50% NPU. (page 88)

49. How many amino acids do adults need from the diet? (page 90)

50. Name two amino acids that start with the letter L. (page 90)

51. What protein food has the highest NPU? (page 88)

52. Do all whole grains supply complete protein? (page 90)

53. Name the food with the best supply of the amino acid methionine. (page 92)

54. How many grams of protein does an average roast beef sandwich supply? (page 87)

55. How many grams of protein do fish and chips supply, per 100 g? (page 87)

56. What is the total amount of all amino acids required, in mg? (page 90)

57. How much protein do boys aged 9–13 need daily? (page 86)

58. How much protein do teenage girls aged 14–18 need daily? (page 86)

59. How many grams of protein does milk supply, per 100 g? (page 89)

60. Name one protein food that contains cholesterol. (page 88)

61. Is protein required by the nervous system? (page 87)

62. Name three functions of protein. (page 87)

QUESTION AND ANSWER: LIPIDS (FATS AND OILS)

63. Name the six main food groups that supply lipids (fats and oils). (page 131)

64. What does the term "lipids" refer to? (page 131)

65. Name two common foods that supply lipids. (page 131)

66. Define the term "free radicals." (page 131)

67. Name one oil that is mostly monounsaturated. (page 132)

68. What does the term "cold-pressed" refer to? (page 132)

69. Name the main type of fat in butter. (page 135)

70. Name the main type of fat in margarine. (page 135)

71. Name one nut that contains monounsaturated lipids. (page 135)

72. Name one food that contains saturated fat. (page 135)

73. Is omega-3 an essential fatty acid? (page 132)

74. Describe one function of omega-3. (page 133)

75. Name one function of omega-6. (page 133)

76. What is the main fat in coconut? (page 135)

77. Name the main type of fat in olive oil. (page 135)

78. Describe one step in the process of manufacturing margarine. (page 134)

79. Is omega-6 an essential fatty acid? (page 132)

80. Name one food that contains cholesterol. (page 136)

81. Name one function of cholesterol. (page 135)

82. Describe one problem of excess cholesterol intake. (page 135)

83. Is lecithin part of the human brain? (page 136)

84. Name one function of lecithin. (page 136)

85. What is butter made from? (page 137)

86. How many calories per gram do lipids supply? (page 138)

87. Name one way to reduce excess body weight. (page 138)

88. Does lecithin help to reduce blood cholesterol? (page 136)

89. Can trans fatty acids increase blood cholesterol levels? (page 134)

90. Is omega-3 essential for brain function? (page 133)

91. What are the three main types of lipids? (page 132)

92. Name one vitamin that can protect against free radicals. (page 132)

93. Does margarine contain additives? (page 134)

94. Does an excess intake of soft drinks increase blood cholesterol? (page 135)

95. Name one food that contains mono- and polyunsaturated lipids. (page 135)

96. Does fish supply more omega-3 than omega-6? (page 134)

97. Does meat contain saturated fats? (page 135)

98. Do most dairy foods contain over 50% saturated fats? (page 135)

QUESTION AND ANSWER: MINERALS

99. How many main minerals are required by the human body? (page 147)

100. What is the main mineral in the human body? (page 147)

101. Name one function of the mineral calcium. (page 148)

102. Is calcium required for the functioning of the heart? (page 148)

103. Name one food that is a very good source of calcium. (page 156)

104. Is the mineral chlorine required for proper digestion? (page 149)

105. Does chlorine assist the functions of the liver? (page 149)

106. Is the mineral chlorine affected by heat and cooking? (page 149)

107. Is the mineral copper required for blood development? (page 149)

108. Name one food that contains copper. (page 149)

109. Where is most of the mineral copper stored in the human body? (page 149)

110. Does copper protect the lungs against infection? (page 149)

111. Name one source of organic fluoride. (page 150)

112. Does organic fluoride increase the number of red blood cells? (page 150)

113. Is fluoride essential for the strength and growth of bones? (page 150)

114. Does the mineral iodine help to promote digestion? (page 150)

115. Name the body gland that stores the mineral iodine. (page 150)

116. Name the hormone that the thyroid gland produces. (page 150)

117. Is the mineral iodine required for body growth? (page 150)

118. Is the mineral iron required for the development of red blood cells? (page 151)

119. Does excess cooking deplete the iron content in foods? (page 151)

120. Will the mineral iron protect against colds and infections? (page 151)

121. Does the mineral iron supply oxygen to the muscles? (page 151)

122. Is iron the main blood mineral? (page 151)

123. Name one nut that contains the mineral iron. (page 157)

124. Is vitamin C required for proper iron absorption? (page 151)

125. Does the mineral magnesium protect against muscular cramps? (page 151)

126. Do the heart muscles need the mineral magnesium? (page 151)

127. Name one nut that supplies a very good source of magnesium. (page 157)

128. Can a magnesium deficiency lead to nervous problems? (page 151)

129. Is magnesium essential for the brain? (page 151)

130. Does the mineral manganese assist the process of digestion? (page 152)

131. Is manganese required by the nervous system? (page 152)

132. Does the mineral manganese assist growth and the lengthening of bones? (page 152)

133. Can the mineral manganese improve memory? (page 152)

134. Name one function of the mineral phosphorus. (page 152)

QUESTION AND ANSWER: VITAMINS

135. Does vitamin A increase immunity to disease? (page 162)

136. Is vitamin A important for healthy skin condition? (page 162)

137. Name one function of vitamin A related to the optic system. (page 162)

138. Is vitamin A required for protein digestion? (page 162)

139. Name one very good source of vitamin A. (page 175)

140. What is the name for vitamin A from plant foods? (page 163)

141. Is vitamin A a fat-soluble vitamin? (page 163)

142. Does vitamin C increase the number of white blood cells? (page 164)

143. What part of the eyes needs vitamin C? (page 164)

144. Name one food that is rich in vitamin C. (page 175)

145. Is vitamin C required for healthy blood? (page 164)

146. Does vitamin C assist blood circulation? (page 164)

147. How long does a healthy red blood cell live? (page 165)

148. Is vitamin E a fat-soluble vitamin? (page 165)

149. Does vitamin E increase muscular endurance? (page 165)

150. Is vitamin E required by the reproductive system? (page 165)

151. Does vitamin E protect the skin from ultraviolet radiation? (page 165)

152. What is the best source of vitamin D? (page 166)

153. Name one food source of vitamin D. (page 175)

154. Is vitamin D essential for children's growth? (page 166)

155. Does vitamin D assist the functions of the glandular system? (page 166)

156. What is the main function of vitamin K? (page 166)

157. Name the two main types of vitamin F. (page 167)

158. What is another name for vitamin P? (page 168)

159. Is vitamin BI a water-soluble vitamin and required daily? (page 169)

160. Does vitamin B2 help maintain a healthy skin condition? (page 169)

161. Is vitamin B3 essential for the digestive system and brain? (page 170)

162. Is vitamin B5 required by the glands and nerves? (page 170)

163. What name is vitamin B6 also known by? (page 171)

164. Is vitamin B6 essential for the nervous system? (page 171)

165. Does processing and cooking destroy vitamin B6? (page 171)

166. Is vitamin B12 a water-soluble vitamin? (page 171)

167. Is folate required for healthy red blood cell development? (page 173)

168. Is the vitamin folate destroyed by cooking? (page 173)

169. Is vitamin C required daily? (page 164)

NUTRITION AND DIET SUMMARY

HOW DO I OBTAIN MORE FRUITS IN MY DIET?

			MEAL IDEAS AND SUMMARY OF BENEFITS				
	Fruits	Breakfast (B)	Midmorning Snack (Ms)	Pre Lunch (Pl)	Afternoon Snack (As)	Evening Sweets (Es)	Main Benefits
1	Apples	Juice with pineapple	Fresh with raw almonds	Juice with strawberry	Fresh with cashews	Stewed with yogurt	Promotes a healthy digestive system, provides over 12 nutrients, promotes an alkaline blood balance.
2	Apricots	Juice fresh or canned	Dried or fresh in season	Juice	Dried with fresh apple	Canned with ice cream	Rich in vitamin A, vital for the respiratory system, ideal snack for smokers.
3	Avocado	Ripe on rye toast	Ripe on crackers	Dip with crackers or celery	On bread with cheese	Guacamole with corn chips	Good source of omega-3, helps reduce cholesterol, supplies over 12 nutrients.
4	Banana	Ripe on cereal	Smoothie	With fruit salad	Banana cake	With ice cream	Provides abundant energy, lots of potassium, and numerous nutrients.
5	Berries Cherries Currants Prunes Raisins	Fresh or dried with cereal	Currant or blueberry muffin	Juice with apple	Cookies with slivered almonds	Strawberries with cream	Full of antioxidants, especially blueberries, protects the brain from stress. Rich in vitamin C.
6	Dates Figs	Finely cut served with cereal	Scones or dried or fresh	Dipped in tahini	Date sliced	Dates with custard	Compact energy food, abundant potassium, fiber, and iron. Ideal food to relieve tiredness.
7	Grapes	Juice	Fresh fruit	Juice	Fresh fruit snack	Red wine	Ideal for blood cleansing, supplies antioxidants, manganese, and energy.
8	Grapefruit Lemons	Juice	Lemon meringue slice	Squeezed over fish	Lemon tea	Squeezed over seafood	Cleansing the blood and joint system, good supply of vitamin C and sulfur.
9	Melons Papaya	Juice	Dried papaya slices	Fresh papaya entrée	Watermelon juice	Papaya with fruit salad	Very alkaline foods, ideal for healing, relaxes the skin, nerves, ideal for glands.
10	Olives	Oil on toast	With cheese	Greek salad	On pizza	Salad dressing	Monounsaturated oil
11	Oranges	Juice	Orange teacake	Orange/pineapple juice	Marmalade on crackers	Orange tea	Good source of vitamin C, magnesium, potassium, vitamin A.
12	Peaches Pears	Served on cereal	Fresh fruit snack	Peaches and almonds	Peach/pear/pineapple juice	With ice cream or yogurt	Ideal for the skin, hair, digestion, supplies fiber, antioxidants, vitamin A.
13	Pineapple	Juice with orange	Juice with apple	On pizza or fresh juice	Pineapple fritter	Served with fish	Ideal for the respiratory system, full of sulfur, chlorine, manganese.
14	Tomato	On toast	Juice	In salad	On sandwich	Pasta sauce	Good source of the antioxidant lycopene, which has numerous nutrients.

NUTRITION AND DIET SUMMARY

HOW DO I OBTAIN MORE VEGETABLES IN MY DIET?

	Vegetables	Lunch (L)	Evening Meal (E)	Main Benefits
		MEAL IDEAS AND SUMMARY OF BENEFITS		
15	Asparagus	Asparagus on toast with avocado or grilled cheese. Asparagus with egg mayonnaise and salad.	Asparagus, cottage cheese, and grilled fish with baked squash. Asparagus soup with rye bread.	Cleansing the bladder and kidneys, eyesight, glands, blood vessels, nerves, and brain.
16	Beets	Beet juice with carrot. Grated beet with salad sandwich.	Baked beets, sweet potato with roast chicken and peas. Grated beets in lentil burgers.	Blood building, anticancer, antioxidants, numerous nutrients.
17	Broccoli	Broccoli in stir fry with cashews, bean shoots, onion, rice, and garlic.	Broccoli with melted cheese and baked potatoes, baked fish, and tartar sauce.	Anticancer, antipeptic ulcers, antiviral, chromium, vitamin A, calcium.
18	Brussels sprouts	Brussels sprouts steamed, served with butter, chips, and a salad.	Brussels sprouts sliced in quarters, steamed with mashed potato and chicken fillets, marinated and char-grilled.	Sulfur for cleansing, indoles (phytonutrients that inhibit cancer), folic acid, fiber.
19	Cabbage	Coleslaw salad with kidney bean burgers.	Cabbage rolls, filled with rice, sesame seeds, onion, garlic, parsley, deep fried.	Chlorine, sulfur, vitamin U, cleansing, enzymes.
20	Capsicum (bell peppers)	Add to salad sandwiches, garden salads, pasta.	Baked pepper filled with rice, tomatoes, cabbage, and cheese.	Vitamin C, bioflavonoids for strong blood vessels.
21	Carrots	Carrot juice. Grated carrot with mayonnaise on rye bread.	Steamed carrots with pumpkin seed burgers, rice, chili sauce, and papadam.	Excellent carotene, anticancer, anticolds, liver cleansing, eyes, lungs.
22	Cauliflower	Cauliflower pieces finely chopped into garden salad with pasta and cheese.	Cauliflower lightly steamed, baked in oven with onions, garlic, grilled cheese, served with garlic prawns.	Sulfur, chlorine, cleansing the blood, antiulcers, silicon for hair growth.
23	Celery	Celery juice. Waldorf salad with walnuts, celery, apple, mayonnaise.	Garden salad with finely chopped celery, cottage cheese, red bell pepper, served with fried tofu or zucchini.	Decreases blood pressure, antitumor, eyes, joint system, glands, diabetes.
24	Cucumber	Cucumber juice. Cucumber, cottage cheese dip with crackers.	Cucumber on rye bread with smoked salmon fillets served with grilled tomato and cheese.	Silicon, hair growth, skin condition, diuretic, blood cleansing, digestion.
25	Lettuce	Kebab with lettuce, onion, tomato, tahini sauce, and falafel.	Tacos with sliced lettuce, grated carrot, cheese, tomato, onion, bell pepper, garlic, kidney beans, and sweet chili sauce.	Excellent silicon, hair growth, chlorophyll, iron, folate, vitamin K, sulfur.
26	Leek Onion	Leek soup with whole-grain barley bread. Leeks/onions with burgers.	Add leeks or onions to any baked dish, barbecue meal, vegetable soup, stir-fry, or finely cut in a fresh garden salad.	Antiseptic oils, sulfur, antioxidants, cleansing antibacteria, colds.
27	Potatoes	Potato mashed with tuna in patties; add onion and peas and then pan-fry. Serve with chili sauce and fresh garden salad.	Potato soup with finely cut carrots, onions, parsley, and cabbage, serve with cream or yogurt. Potato bake with grilled zucchini, tomatoes, cheddar cheese, and onions.	Potassium, energy provider but has a very high glycemic index when obtained baked, add oils or cheese to lower GI
28	Pumpkin/ winter squash	Pumpkin soup with toasted rye bread.	Roast pumpkin with veal cutlets, fried mushrooms, garlic, and onions.	Beta-cryptoxanthin, respiratory system, for smokers.
29	Spinach/ chard	Spinach/chard and ricotta cheese baked rolls. Spinach leaves in a fresh garden salad.	Steamed spinach/chard in a quiche or omelet. Spinach or chard with fettuccini pasta and lasagna.	Chlorophyll, lutein, and zeaxanthin, eyes, folate, potassium, vitamin K, iron, anticancer, muscles.

NUTRITION AND DIET SUMMARY

HOW DO I OBTAIN MORE WHOLE GRAINS IN MY DIET?

	Grains	Breakfast (B)	Lunch (L)	Evening Meal (E)	Main Benefits
			MEAL IDEAS AND SUMMARY OF BENEFITS		
30	Barley	Barley toast with honey. Barley beverage.	Barley soup with vegetables and cottage cheese.	Barley and mushroom baked casserole, onions, chives, parsley.	Energy providing, body warmth, low gluten content.
31	Corn	Add lecithin granules and slivered almonds to make the corn flakes a healthy breakfast.	Try corn chips with an avocado dip, or have corn on the cob as a simple lunch.	Corn taco shell with salad, tomato, kidney beans, onion, garlic. Corn tortillas, add minced beef, or kidney beans with salads.	Fresh corn is rich in vitamin A, folate, ideal sweet food for children. Corn bread and chips are low in nutrient value but added foods can make it nutritious.
32	Millet	Use rolled millet with honey, sunflower seed meal, or almond meal as a regular breakfast. In winter, try millet flakes cooked like oats.	Millet salad, with boiled millet, chopped onions, fresh, chopped parsley, basil, bell pepper, Brazil nuts, sprinkle with balsamic vinegar.	Millet pudding, as a sweet, with nutmeg, butter, flour, eggs. Millet pilaf with wine, vegetables, eggplant, and tomato paste.	No gluten content, alkaline food, rich in silicon, iron, folate, and various nutrients, ideal food to add to the diet.
33	Oats	Rolled oats or oat flakes for breakfast with a sprinkle of slivered almonds, a few canned apricots, and a dash of cream and honey. Muesli bar snack.	Oat bread with tahini or peanut butter. Oat salad sandwich with lettuce, cheese, celery, mayonnaise, pepper, and salt.	Oat bread with a fresh garden salad. Original fresh muesli with grated apples, hazelnuts, fruits, milk, or fruit juice and rolled oats.	Promote a steady metabolism, ideal breakfast food, low gluten, rich in silicon and many nutrients, body-building food.
34	Rice	Rice flakes with rice milk, honey, and raisins. Rice pudding with steamed rice, vanilla extract, milk, cream, salt, honey, or sugar.	Rice cakes with tahini. Steamed rice with grilled fish and vegetable fried rice Chinese style with mushrooms, egg, onions, parsley.	Stir-fry rice with prawns, or chicken and vegetables. Rice and kidney beans with grilled tomatoes and cheese.	Alkaline grain, easy to digest, cheap, fair source of nutrients, no gluten content, ideal food for recipes sweet and spicy.
35	Rye	Rye bread toasted with honey and tahini. Rye flakes with milk, apricots or peaches, and honey or raisins. Sourdough rye bread with avocado.	Rye crackers with avocado dip and cheese. Rye bread veggie sandwich with egg or avocado or salmon.	Pumpernickel bread as an entrée with camembert, brie, or other soft cheese and olives. Rye bread with omelet or quiche and salad.	Body-building food, good source of minerals, potassium, excellent fiber, ideal food during menopause.
36	Wheat	Whole-wheat bread with tahini or peanut butter. Whole-wheat breakfast cereal with a sprinkle of wheat germ or almond meal or sunflower meal. Wheat pancakes with honey, maple syrup, tahini, and stewed apples. Homemade rolls with cheese. Cereal with lecithin, hazelnuts, and cream. Croissants with tahini or avocado or honey. Sourdough wheat bread with jam or hazelnut spread.	Whole-wheat bread veggie sandwich with tahini sauce. Pasta with tuna, tomatoes, and garlic. Wheat bread with walnuts and honey. Pizza with olives, mushrooms, bell pepper, onions, and cheese. Wheat crackers with cottage cheese. Hamburger bun with onion and lettuce, beef, tomato. Flat bread with tuna and olive oil.	Wheat pastry for quiche, family size vegetable or chicken pie with onions, mushrooms, peas, zucchini, and spices. Pizza with ham, cheese, and pineapple. Fresh rolls with garlic, veggie, and avocado spread. Pasta with vegetables and cheese. Lasagna with kidney beans and cheese. Spaghetti Bolognese. Macaroni, tuna, and cheese with salad.	Whole wheat is a fair source of many nutrients, iron, B vitamins, vitamin E, good energy food. Processed, refined wheat products are depleted in nutrients, full of gluten, and acid forming. The foods that combine with the wheat can really make it nutritious, such as salads, walnuts, avocado, etc. Try other grains for breakfast; otherwise it's wheat all day long.

NUTRITION AND DIET SUMMARY

HOW DO I OBTAIN MORE LEGUMES IN MY DIET?

	Legumes	Lunch (L)	Evening Meal (E)	Main Benefits
		MEAL IDEAS AND SUMMARY OF BENEFITS		
37	Carob bean	Carob milkshake. Carob smoothie with ice cream.	Carob sprinkled over ice cream. Hot carob soymilk drink.	Alkaline, pectin, removes toxins, rich in calcium, potassium.
38	Chickpeas	Hummus dip with rye bread triangles.	Cooked chickpeas, fried with beef and vegetables.	Complete protein, rich in iron, copper.
39	Green beans	Steamed with butter and spices. Added and served with grilled fish or seafood recipes.	Green beans in quiche, or vegetable soup. As a side serve with chicken or with rice dishes.	Folate, potassium, magnesium, vitamin K, fiber, phosphorus, good diabetic food.
40	Kidney beans	Tacos with lettuce, tomato, kidney beans, chili sauce, garlic, and onions.	Kidney beans with steamed rice, tomatoes, and cheese. Kidney bean burgers.	Complete protein, excellent fiber, (stabilizes blood sugar levels), potassium.
41	Lentils	Lentil patties with fresh salad. Lentils with fried rice and chicken. Lentil sprout soup.	Lentil soup with carrots, celery, bay leaves, vinegar, vegetable stock, onion, olive oil.	Complete protein, very rich in iron, low fat content, helps lower cholesterol.
42	Lima beans	Lima bean soup with onion, carrot, parsley, oil, pepper, basil, thyme, garlic.	Lima bean loaf with sesame seeds, carrot, onions, vege salt (salt mixed with veg. extracts), flour, soy sauce, and garlic.	Excellent iron, complete protein, rich in molybdenum, folate, magnesium.
43	Mung beans	Mung bean sprouts in garden salad with mayonnaise. Mung bean sprout soup with yogurt.	Mung bean dahl with mustard, pepper, turmeric, curry powder, on flat bread with oil. Mung bean patties.	Complete protein, excellent fiber, magnesium, folate, potassium, and copper.
44	Peanuts	Peanut butter on whole-grain rye bread with chopped celery. Peanuts in the shell, roasted.	Peanut sauce over rice dishes with stir-fried vegetables. Roasted peanuts as an appetizer, with beer.	Excellent supply of protein, vitamin B5, B3, copper, folate, vitamin E, manganese, magnesium.
45	Peas	Green peas or snow peas fresh from the pod, served with garden salad.	Pea soup with garlic. Fried rice with peas. Snow peas with fish. Peas with roasted vegetables.	Excellent supply of fiber, potassium, magnesium, folate, vitamin K, copper.
46	Soybeans	Garden salad with fried tofu cubes. Soy milkshake. Soy mayonnaise with vegetable burgers.	Soy sauce with stir-fried vegetables and rice. Soy pastry, apple pie. Soy burgers. Soy vegetable soup.	Excellent complete protein, fiber, lecithin, unique source of genistein, iron, molybdenum, phosphorus, folate.
		MEAL IDEAS AND SUMMARY OF BENEFITS		
47	Sprouts	Wheat or buckwheat sprouts with cinnamon, nutmeg in pancake mix with honey. Wheat sprouts in homemade bread served with a variety of soft cheese.	Sunflower sprouts in garden salad with tahini dressing. Sprouts in soup. Alfalfa sprouts with tahini on rye bread. All sprouts in garden salad with cheese cubes and mayonnaise.	Excellent source of enzymes, good source of trace minerals, B vitamins, antioxidants, pro-vitamin E, K, U, folate rutin, zinc, phytoestrogens.

NUTRITION AND DIET SUMMARY

HOW DO I OBTAIN MORE NUTS IN MY DIET?

	Nuts	Breakfast (B)	Lunch (L)	Evening Meal (E)	Main Benefits
		MEAL IDEAS AND SUMMARY OF BENEFITS			
48	Almonds	Ground almonds sprinkled on breakfast cereal with milk. Ground almonds mixed into pancake mix with stewed apples and cream.	Almonds with crisp apple or peaches. Halva as a lunch sweet. Almonds slivered in fresh garden salad. Cracked almonds in stir-fry with vegetables.	Slivered almonds with grilled fish and fresh salad. Roasted almond pieces with chicken breasts. Almond butter with roasted vegetables. Almonds on rice custard.	Alkaline food, excellent complete protein, magnesium, calcium, phosphorus, iron, zinc, omega-6, vitamin E, fiber, copper, potassium, B vitamins, monounsaturates.
49	Brazil nuts	Ground Brazil nuts in muesli with cream. Cracked Brazil nuts with cereal. Brazil nut butter on toast with honey.	Brazil nuts with almonds and cashews and crisp apple. Cracked Brazil nuts on fresh garden salad or on pasta and cheese.	Ground Brazil nuts sprinkled on seafood entrée. Cracked roasted Brazil nut pieces with boiled rice and honey chicken. Brazil nuts cracked on ice cream.	Excellent source of selenium, antioxidant, essential for diabetics, very good supply of phosphorus, potassium, magnesium, fiber, methionine (amino acid).
50	Cashews	Cashews (raw) cracked and sprinkled on toast with honey or on breakfast cereal, or mixed into peach, apple, apricot fruit salad.	Cashew butter on whole-grain rye bread with garden salad. Cashews raw in fried rice with steamed vegetables and peas. Cashews and apple.	Roasted cashews in crisp garden salad. Cracked raw cashews sprinkled on broccoli and melted cheese. Roasted cashews in curried vegetables. Cashews on ice cream.	Excellent source of copper for the brain, joint system, good source of complete protein, magnesium, phosphorus, omega-6, oleic acid, monoun-saturates.
51	Chestnuts	Roasted chestnuts with morning cereal beverage. Chestnut pieces roasted on muesli.	Roasted chestnut pieces with garden salad and soy mayon-naise. Chestnut pieces with satay sauce and rice.	Roasted chestnut pieces with salmon fillets with egg mayonnaise. Roasted chestnuts by the campfire with a glass of red wine or apple cider.	Low calories, good carbo-hydrate food, potassium, magnesium, folic acid, fiber, vitamin C, low fat content.
52	Hazelnuts	Hazelnut spread on whole-grain toast. Cracked hazelnuts with original fresh muesli recipe. Ground hazel-nuts in pancakes.	Cracked roasted hazelnuts with garden salad. Hazelnuts with crisp apple and peach. Ground hazelnuts with yogurt.	Roasted hazelnut pieces with steamed vegetables and cheese sauce. Cracked hazelnuts with beef steak and mustard. Hazelnuts and ice cream.	Complete protein, very good source of vitamin E, iron, copper, calcium, manganese, B vitamins, zinc, magnesium, fiber.
53	Macadamias	Cracked macadamia nut pieces with breakfast cereal or mixed into pancake. Mac-adamia butter on rye toast or croissants.	Macadamia pieces (raw) with fresh salad. Macadamia oil on salad. Roasted maca-damia with sweet and sour vegetables.	Cracked macadamia with baked fish fillets. Roasted macadamia with rice and beef. Ground macadamia sprin-kled on tofu ice cream and cherries or strawberries.	Excellent source of mono-unsaturated oleic acid and palmitoleic acid, good source of copper, protein, fiber, vitamin E.
54	Pecans	Cracked pecans sprinkled on pancakes with maple syrup. Ground pecans with break-fast cereal or oat muesli.	Pecans with peaches. Roasted pecan pieces with baked greens and tomato with a paprika sauce.	Cracked pecans with baked zucchini, shallots, garlic, and spinach with cheese sauce. Pecan pie with ice cream, or fresh fruits and cream.	Excellent source of copper, good source of phosphorus, magnesium, fiber, complete protein, may help reduce cholesterol.
55	Pine nuts	Pine nuts with grilled tomatoes. Pine nuts with ricotta cheese on whole-grain toast. Pine nuts with grated apple/yogurt.	Pine nuts with garden salad or Greek salad. Pine nuts with grilled fish and tomatoes. Pe-sto or pine nuts with avocado salad.	Roasted pine nuts with fresh smoked salmon and fried mushrooms. Pine nuts with Asian noodles and stir fry vegetables. Pine nuts with chocolate cake.	Excellent supply of phospho-rus, magnesium, complete protein, iron, fiber, manga-nese, good brain food and for the blood system.
56	Pistachios	Pistachio pieces with grilled cheese on rye bread. Pistachio pieces sprinkled on scrambled eggs, with toast.	Pistachio pieces with honey chicken. Pistachios ground with fresh Greek salad or with cottage cheese on rye bread.	Cracked pistachio pieces sprinkled on baked fish with fresh salad. Ground pistachio mixed into sweet pastry. Pistachios on ice cream.	Very good source of phytos-terols, anticancer, anticho-lesterol, very good source of potassium, magnesium, copper, zinc, calcium, and vitamin E.
57	Walnuts	Walnuts on toast with honey. Walnuts with fruit salad or original fresh muesli. Walnuts with tahini on rye toast.	Walnuts in Waldorf salad. Walnuts with grilled cheese on toast. Walnut pieces in car-rot cake or muffins. Walnuts and cream cheese on wheat biscuits.	Walnuts ground and mixed into fish batter with steamed vegetables. Walnuts baked into bread served with soft cheese, such as camem-bert, and wine.	Excellent source of the hard to obtain omega-3, also supplies good amounts of omega-6, folate, iron, phosphorus, manganese, copper.

NUTRITION AND DIET SUMMARY

HOW DO I OBTAIN MORE SEEDS IN MY DIET?

	Seeds	Breakfast (B)	Lunch (L)	Evening Meal (E)	Main Benefits
	MEAL IDEAS AND SUMMARY OF BENEFITS				
58	Pumpkin seeds (Pepitas)	Pepitas ground and served on top of grilled tomatoes with cheddar cheese. Pepitas ground into savory crepes mixed with mushrooms and cream cheese sauce. Cracked pepitas in muesli with fresh grated red apples.	Ground pepitas sprinkled on fresh garden salad served with pasta. Ground pepitas mixed into pasta sauce served over pasta with parmesan cheese. Ground pepitas served on top of pumpkin cream soup.	Roasted pepitas served over grilled zucchini and tomatoes, served with melted cheese or yogurt. Ground pepitas mixed into fish, breadcrumbs, or served over cauliflower cheese sauce. Cracked pepitas sprinkled over omelet with vegetables.	Excellent complete protein, excellent iron content, excellent omega-3 content, zinc, phosphorus, cucurbitacins for prostate gland health, anti-inflammatory power against arthritis and rheumatism.
59	Sesame seeds	Sesame seed paste – tahini – on toasted wholegrain bread with honey. Tahini on pancakes with honey. Tahini on fruit salad.	Fresh garden salad with tahini salad dressing. Tahini cake with tea. Spinach rolls with sesame seeds, sesame seed buns with salad.	Hummus with tahini served with corn chips or rye bread and Greek salad. Tahini in halva as a sweet. Sesame seeds toasted and sprinkled on steamed vegetables with grilled fish.	Excellent complete protein rich in methionine, excellent calcium, copper, iron, zinc, vit. E, lecithin, phytosterols, and special fiber lignans, to lower blood cholesterol.
60	Sunflower seeds	Ground sunflower seeds in pancake mix, served with maple syrup and pears. Sunflower seeds in muesli or sprinkled on commercial breakfast cereal. Sunflower seeds ground in butter mix spread on toast with honey.	Roasted sunflower seeds on French garden salad. Sunflower oil in salad dressing. Ground sunflower seeds in vegetable burger mix with carrot, beet, onions, parsley, spices.	Sunflower seed patties with onion, spinach, and celery, served with soy mayonnaise. Sunflower meal mixed into cream sauce served over grilled fish or fresh smoked salmon. Sunflower seeds sprinkled over ice cream or mixed into a cake, with coffee.	Excellent complete protein, vitamin E, magnesium, phosphorus, silicon, zinc, selenium, full of antioxidant power and fiber plus B-group vitamins plus monounsaturates plus omega-6 and omega-3.

HOW DO I OBTAIN MORE SUPPLEMENTS IN MY DIET?

	Supplements	Breakfast (B)	Lunch (L)	Evening Meal (E)	Main Benefits
	MEAL IDEAS AND SUMMARY OF BENEFITS				
61	Apple cider vinegar	Served as an ingredient in fresh juices, or use as a gargle for sore throats.	Cider vinegar in salad dressing with olive oil or soy oil, or mix cider vinegar with tahini and honey.	Mix a tablespoon of cider vinegar into a commercial salad dressing, or mix with lemon for a seafood cocktail with tartar sauce.	Digestive aid, acid-alkaline blood balance, potassium, healthy skin condition, phosphorus, iron, sodium.
62	Brewer's yeast	Sprinkle a dash into pancake mix or omelet or bread mix.	Sprinkle a dash over salads or into quiche or in patties.	Mix a dash into gravy or breadcrumb mix or in soups or curry.	Excellent source of nearly all B-group vitamins.
63	Dandelion	Use as beverage instead of coffee.	Make dandelion tea or coffee.	Make dandelion coffee.	Vitamin A, iron, potassium, liver tonic, bladder health.
64	Kelp	Add kelp sea salt to scrambled eggs or bread.	Sprinkle kelp over salads, or try kelp crackers.	Use kelp finely sliced in stir-fried vegetables or with noodles.	60 trace elements, excellent source of iodine, 13 vitamins.
65	Lecithin	Add to any egg breakfast or pancake mix.	Sprinkle over garden salads, or add to soups or stews.	Add to gravy, or sprinkle into cheese sauce or pasta sauce.	Excellent to reduce high cholesterol, brain food.
66	Wheat germ	Add to a pancake mix, bread mix, or sprinkle over cereals.	Mix into breadcrumbs with fish meals, or use in cakes.	Sprinkle into stir-fried vegetables or over a fresh garden salad.	Excellent protein, vitamin E, minerals, and vitamins.

INDEX

BIBLIOGRAPHY

Note: When this book was completely revised, the Internet provided many additional resources. It would be difficult to nominate individual sites for mention here, but if you search individual topics on the Internet, always make sure you are getting reliable information.

Altschul, Aaron. M. *Proteins: Their Chemistry and Politics.* New York: Basic Books.

Ballentine, Rudolph. *Diet and Nutrition.* Honesdale, PA: Himalayan Institute Press.

Bethel, May. *The Healing Power of Natural Foods.* Chatsworth, CA: Wilshire Book Company.

Bogert, L. Jean. *Nutrition and Physical Fitness,* 9th ed. Philadelphia, PA: W. B. Saunders Publishing.

Bragg, Paul G. *Healthful Eating Without Confusion.* Health Science Books.

Oxford Dictionaries. *Concise Oxford Dictionary,* 12th ed. New York: Oxford University Press.

Davis, Adelle. *Let's Get Well.* New York: Signet, 1986.

———. *Let's Have Healthy Children.* Mountain View, CA: Ishi Press.

———. *Let's Eat Right to Keep Fit.* Mountain View, CA: Ishi Press.

Dunne, Lavon J. *Nutrition Almanac,* 5th ed. New York: McGraw-Hill Book Company.

Goodhart and M. E. Shils. *Modern Nutrition in Health and Disease.* Philadelphia, PA: Lea and Febiger Publishing.

Heck, Henrietta. *Introduction to Nutrition.* New York: MacMillan Publishing.

Kirshner, H. E. *Book of Nature's Healing Grasses.* Yucaipa, CA: H. C. White Publications.

Macia, Rafael. *The Natural Foods and Nutrition Handbook.* New York: Harper & Row Publishing.

Mateljan, George. *The World's Healthiest Foods.* World's Healthiest Foods.

Null, Gary. *Protein for Vegetarians.* New York: Jove Books.

Walker, N. W. *Become Younger.* Prescott, AZ: Norwalk Press.

Robertson, L., C. Hinders, and B. Godfrey. *Laurel's Kitchen.* Tomales, CA: Nilgiri Press.

Pauling, Linus. *Vitamin C and the Common Cold.* New York: Bantam.

Peterson, Vicki. *The Wholefood Catalogue.* Rigby.

Phillips, David A. *Guidebook to Nutritional Factors in Foods.* Anaheim, CA: Woodbridge Press Publishing Co.

Shelton, H. M. *Food Combining Made Easy,* 3rd ed. Book Pub Company.

Shils, Maurice E., James A. Olson, Moshe Shike, and A. C. Ross, eds. *Modern Nutrition in Health and Disease,* 9th ed. New York: Lippincott Williams & Wilkins.

Sidhwa, Keki. *Fit for Anything.* Health for All Publishing.

Wigmore, Ann. *Naturama Living Textbook.* New York: Avery.

Winter, Ruth. *Beware of the Food You Eat.* New York: Signet Books.

Time-Life Science Library.

The Body (Edey, Maitlland A.)

The Cell (Pfeiffer, John)

Energy (Wilson, Mitchell A.)

Evolution (Moore, Ruth)

Growth (Tanner, J. M.)

Health and Disease (Dubos, Rene, and Maya Pines)

The Mind (Wilson, John Rowan)

Time (Goudsmit, Samuel A., and Robert Claiborne)

Universe (Bergamini, David)

Water (Leopold, Luna B., and Kenneth S. Davis)